Cardiac

Emergency Care

Cardiac

Emergency Care

Edited by EDWARD K. CHUNG, M.D.

Professor of Medicine
Jefferson Medical College of
Thomas Jefferson University
and
Director of the Heart Station
Thomas Jefferson University Hospital
Philadelphia

SECOND EDITION

Lea & Febiger • *Philadelphia* • *1980*

Library of Congress Cataloging in Publication Data

Chung, Edward K
  Cardiac emergency care.

  Includes bibliographical references and index.
  1. Heart—Diseases.   2. Medical emergencies.
3. Coronary care units.   I. Title.
RC682.C55   1980   616.1'2025   79-28235
ISBN 0-8121-0690-3

First Edition, 1975
Spanish Translation, 1978

Published in Great Britain by Henry Kimpton Publishers, London

PRINTED IN THE UNITED STATES OF AMERICA

Print number: 3 2 1

To My Wife, Lisa,
and to My Children,
Linda and Christopher

PREFACE
TO THE FIRST EDITION

It is not the purpose of this book to discuss in depth various subjects in medicine or to describe in detail all possible emergency medical events. The primary intention is to describe common cardiac emergencies which are frequently encountered in our daily practice.

The contents are intended to be clinical, concise, and practical. It is hoped that this book will provide all physicians with up-to-date materials that will assist them directly in the daily care of their patients with cardiac emergency problems.

The book will be particularly valuable to house staff, cardiology fellows, practicing internists, cardiologists, family physicians, and emergency room physicians, as well as coronary care unit nurses. In addition, medical students will derive great benefit from reading this book in learning a general approach to various cardiac emergencies.

I am grateful to all authors for their valuable contributions to *Cardiac Emergency Care*. I also wish to thank my personal secretary, Miss Theresa McAnally, for her devoted and cheerful secretarial assistance. She has been most helpful in handling correspondence with the contributors, as well as in typing several chapters of mine for this book. It has been my pleasure to work with the staff of Lea & Febiger Publishers. In particular, I would like to express my thanks to Mr. R. Kenneth Bussy, Executive Editor, for his indispensable assistance.

Philadelphia   EDWARD K. CHUNG, M.D.

PREFACE

Since 1975, when the first edition of this book was published, there have been significant changes in the therapeutic approach to cardiac emergencies. The best example of those changes is that at present the most common indication for artificial cardiac pacing is the sick sinus syndrome and the brady-tachyarrhythmia syndrome—*not* the Adams-Stokes syndrome due to complete AV block. Thus a new chapter, "The Sick Sinus Syndrome and the Brady-Tachyarrhythmia Syndrome," has been added in this edition.

Another good example of the changes is that the nursing aspects of cardiac emergency care have become extremely important. Thus in-depth knowledge of cardiac emergency care is now an essential part of the training of nurses who deal with cardiac patients, especially in the intensive coronary care and the intermediate coronary care units and in connection with the rehabilitation programs for the various cardiac conditions. Consequently, another chapter, "The Nursing Aspect of Cardiac Emergency Care," has also been added in this edition.

The chapter "Radiologic Diagnosis in Cardiopulmonary Emergencies" has been added because the roentgenographic recognition of various cardiac emergencies is invaluable for cardiac emergency care.

The whole text has been revised considerably, although the basic aims and designs of the book are essentially unchanged. The unique feature of the book is its practical approach, but the book format has been changed somewhat—to a cookbook style—so that busy primary physicians and house officers may be able to use the book as a quick reference source.

Many illustrative ECGs have been replaced, and many new ones have been added. In addition, clinically pertinent tables have been included.

The secretarial and the editorial burdens were borne cheerfully by Miss Theresa McAnally, my secretary and editorial assistant. Her able assistance and effort have been most valuable in the completion of the book. The endless cooperation of the staff of Lea & Febiger—and particularly of Mr. R. Kenneth Bussy, Executive Editor—is greatly appreciated.

Lake Naomi, Mount Pocono, Pa.   EDWARD K. CHUNG, M.D.

CONTRIBUTORS

A.A.J. Adgey, M.D., F.R.C.P., F.A.C.C.
Cardiologist, Department of Cardiology
Royal Victoria Hospital
Belfast, Northern Ireland

Theodore L. Biddle, M.D., F.A.C.P., F.A.C.C.
Associate Professor of Medicine
University of Rochester
School of Medicine and Dentistry
Director, Coronary Care Unit
Strong Memorial Hospital
Rochester, New York

Albert N. Brest, M.D., F.A.C.P., F.A.C.C.
James C. Wilson Professor of Medicine
Director, Division of Cardiology
Thomas Jefferson University
Philadelphia, Pennsylvania

Stanley K. Brockman, M.D., F.A.C.S., F.A.C.C.
Professor of Surgery and
Director, Division of Cardiothoracic Surgery
Thomas Jefferson University
Philadelphia, Pennsylvania

Agustin Castellanos, M.D., F.A.C.C.
  Professor of Medicine
  University of Miami
  School of Medicine
  Miami, Florida

Edward K. Chung, M.D., F.A.C.P., F.A.C.C.
  Professor of Medicine
  Jefferson Medical College of
  Thomas Jefferson University
  Director of the Heart Station
  Thomas Jefferson University Hospital
  Philadelphia, Pennsylvania

Lisa S. Chung, M.D.
  Chief Medical Officer and Medical Director
  U.S. Public Health Service
  Philadelphia, Pennsylvania

Jay N. Cohn, M.D., F.A.C.P., F.A.C.C.
  Professor of Medicine
  Head, Cardiovascular Section
  University of Minnesota School of Medicine
  Minneapolis, Minnesota

Edward Genton, M.D., F.A.C.P., F.A.C.C.
  Professor of Medicine
  Associate Dean for Health Services
  McMaster University
  Faculty of Health Sciences
  Hamilton, Ontario, Canada

* William J. Grace, M.D., F.A.C.P., F.A.C.C.
  Professor of Clinical Medicine
  New York University–Bellevue Medical Center
  Director, Department of Medicine
  St. Vincent's Hospital
  New York, New York

Michael J. Gullotti, M.D.
  Fellow in Cardiology
  Thomas Jefferson University
  Philadelphia, Pennsylvania
* Deceased

George H. Khoury, M.D., F.A.A.P., F.A.C.C.
  Professor of Pediatrics
  Assistant Dean of Continuing Medical Education
  University of Kansas
  School of Medicine
  Wichita, Kansas

Albert S. Klainer, M.D., F.A.C.P.
  Professor of Medicine
  Rutgers Medical School
  Newark, New Jersey
  Chairman, Department of Internal Medicine
  Morristown Memorial Hospital
  Morristown, New Jersey

Louis Lemberg, M.D., F.A.C.P., F.A.C.C.
  Professor of Clinical Cardiology
  University of Miami School of Medicine
  Miami, Florida

J. F. Pantridge, M.D., F.R.C.P., F.A.C.C.
  Professor of Cardiology
  The Queen's University of Belfast
  Belfast, Northern Ireland

Leon Resnekov, M.D., F.R.C.P., F.A.C.C.
  Professor of Medicine
  Joint Director, Section of Cardiology
  University of Chicago School of Medicine
  Chicago, Illinois

Martha I. Spence, R.N., M.N., C.C.R.N.
  Instructor, University of Miami School of Nursing
  Patient Educator Instructor
  Staff Nurse
  Baptist Hospital
  Miami, Florida

David H. Spodick, M.D., F.A.C.P., F.A.C.C.
  Professor of Cardiovascular Medicine
  University of Massachusetts School of Medicine
  Director, Division of Cardiology
  St. Vincent's Hospital
  Worcester, Mass.

Robert M. Steiner, M.D., F.A.C.R.
  Associate Professor of Radiology
  Director, Cardiopulmonary Radiology
  Jefferson Medical College of
  Thomas Jefferson University
  Philadelphia, Pennsylvania

Paul Walinsky, M.D.
  Associate Professor of Medicine
  Co-director, Coronary Care Unit
  Thomas Jefferson University
  Philadelphia, Pennsylvania

Leslie Wiener, M.D., F.A.C.P., F.A.C.C.
  Professor of Medicine
  Thomas Jefferson University
  Philadelphia, Pennsylvania

Paul N. Yu, M.D., F.A.C.P., F.A.C.C.
  Sarah McCort Ward Professor of Medicine
  University of Rochester
  School of Medicine and Dentistry
  Head, Cardiology Unit
  Strong Memorial Hospital
  Rochester, New York

CONTENTS

Chapter *1*

ACUTE PULMONARY EDEMA*

THEODORE L. BIDDLE
PAUL N. YU

GENERAL CONSIDERATIONS

Acute pulmonary edema is a common medical emergency that demands prompt and effective treatment. In this chapter pulmonary edema of both cardiac and noncardiac origin is discussed, with particular emphasis on a practical overview for clinical management.

Four anatomic compartments of the pulmonary circuit have been delineated in an effort to improve our understanding of the pathophysiology of heart failure.[1] The *vascular compartment* consists of the pulmonary arteries, capillaries, and veins that participate in fluid exchange with the interstitital tissue of the lung. The *alveolar compartment* comprises the alveoli, whose walls are made up of epithelial cells with a lipoprotein layer called surfactant. That layer coats the inner alveolar surface and exerts an "anti-atelectasis effect," stabilizing the alveoli and preventing their collapse under conditions of low alveolar volume. The *interstitial space* is interposed between the small pulmonary vessels and the alveoli, and it also contains small lymphatics and conducting airways. The *lymphatic space* is the extensive network of pulmonary lymphatics that

* This work was supported in part by MIRU Contract No. HV 81331, HL 03966 and HL 05500 from the National Heart and Lung Institute, National Institutes of Health, Bethesda, Maryland.

1

drain excess fluid from the alveolar and interstitial compartments. Endothelial cells of the pulmonary capillaries, alveoli, and lymphatics and other cell types have been discussed extensively elsewhere.[1-3] Their specific function, although of great importance, is not described in this review.

Two important cell-mediated responses in pulmonary edema involve the generation of early symptoms and late pathologic changes. The J receptors in the interstitial space act as stretch receptors stimulated by increases in interstitial pressure or fluid resulting in the characteristic tachypnea of acute congestive heart failure.[4] Also, edema fluid promotes the formation of collagen, reticulum, and elastic fibers in the interstitial space. That phenomenon may lead to the interstitial fibrosis common in people with chronic elevation of the pulmonary capillary pressure.

Traditionally, the study of the pathophysiologic aspects of pulmonary edema has been concerned with (1) increased hydrostatic pressure or (2) increased permeability of the alveolar-capillary "membrane." But those factors cannot account for every illness in the wide spectrum of illnesses characterized by pulmonary edema. In general, one or more of four factors are responsible for the production of acute pulmonary edema: (1) elevation of the pulmonary capillary pressure, (2) damage to the pulmonary capillary "membrane," (3) decrease in the plasma osmotic pressure,

Table 1–1.   *Etiology of Acute Pulmonary Edema*

Cardiac causes
Left ventricular failure
Myocardial infarction
Acute decompensation of chronic left ventricular failure—aortic, hypertensive, or cardiomyopathic
Mitral valve disease
Volume overload
Noncardiac causes
Altered permeability of pulmonary capillary membrane
Inhalation of toxic agents
Adult respiratory distress syndrome
Bacteremic sepsis
Uremia
Radiation pneumonitis
Disseminated intravascular coagulation
Decreased plasma oncotic pressure—hypoalbuminemia
Lymphatic obstruction
Uncertain etiology
High-altitude pulmonary edema
Heroin overdose
Pulmonary embolism
Neurogenic causes
Postanesthesia

and (4) impairment of the lymphatic drainage. Our etiologic approach considers both cardiac and noncardiac forms of pulmonary edema (Table 1–1). The cardiac forms are discussed extensively in this chapter. And since a broad knowledge of the many noncardiac forms of pulmonary edema is also necessary for intelligent management, those forms are also considered.

ETIOLOGY OF ACUTE PULMONARY EDEMA

The most common cause of acute pulmonary edema is cardiac disease, whether atherosclerotic, valvular, hypertensive or myopathic in origin. (Pericardial disease is discussed in Chapter 14.) Acute or chronic myocardial "failure" occurs when the left ventricle is unable to eject the normal stroke volume. Thus the diastolic pressure in the left ventricle rises, causing an elevation of the left atrial and pulmonary venous pressures. Normally, the plasma oncotic pressure prevents a substantial diffusion of intravascular fluid across the normal capillary membrane to the interstitial space. With increasing hydrostatic pressure, however, interstitial and intra-alveolar edema may occur. We have measured the amount of lung water in patients with acute myocardial infarction complicated by heart failure.[5,6] The lung water measured by a double isotope technique increased according to the increasing severity of pulmonary congestion as determined by both clinical and radiographic criteria (Figs. 1–1 and 1–2). A significant correlation was found between the pulmonary capillary (wedge) pressure and lung water. In all patients with acute pulmonary edema, the pulmonary wedge pressure was elevated. With clinical improvement, both the pulmonary wedge pressure and the lung water decreased. Increasing arterial hypoxemia has been correlated with more severe pulmonary edema and elevation of lung water.[6]

In patients with left ventricular failure secondary to aortic valve disease, hypertensive cardiovascular disease, or cardiomyopathy, the elevation of the left ventricular end-diastolic pressure eventually leads to an increase in pulmonary capillary pressure and transudation of fluid into the interstitial or alveolar compartments of the lungs. Patients with rheumatic mitral stenosis develop an elevation of the left atrial and then of the pulmonary capillary pressure. The magnitude of mitral valvular obstruction and the increase in hydrostatic force determine in the main the severity of the pulmonary congestion.

Volume overload from excessive intravenous fluid therapy may precipitate acute pulmonary edema but usually only in patients with preexisting myocardial dysfunction or severe valvular disease.

Noncardiac types of pulmonary edema are usually related to alterations

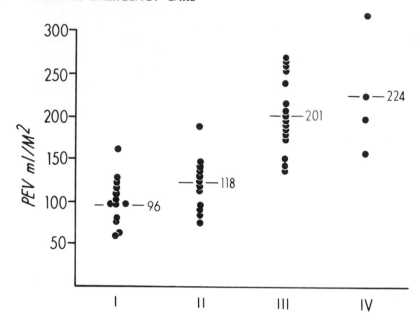

Figure 1-1. Pulmonary extravascular volume (PEV) in patients with acute myocardial infarction. Class I—uncomplicated patients; class II—patients with S_3 gallop and pulmonary rales; class III—patients with frank pulmonary edema; class IV—patients with cardiogenic shock. The mean value in each class of patients is represented by the horizontal line in the designated figure. Note the progressive increase in PEV from class I to class IV patients.

in the permeability of the pulmonary capillary membrane.[2] An offending agent may cause damage to the capillary endothelium or alveolar epithelium without deleterious myocardial effects. Pulmonary congestion therefore could occur in the absence of left ventricular dysfunction. Inhalation of smoke or toxic gases, such as chlorine, phosgene, hydrogen sulfide, metallic oxides, and nitrogen dioxide, may be associated with fulminant pulmonary edema.[7]

The term adult respiratory distress syndrome has been used to denote pulmonary parenchymal damage with interstitial edema of several causes. Pulmonary infection, shock, extracorporeal oxygenation, and mechanical ventilation with a high partial pressure of inspired oxygen have all been associated with the loss of capillary endothelial integrity. The resultant clinical picture of pulmonary edema with progressive respiratory failure is thought to be secondary to altered permeability, yet the exact mechanism of injury has yet to be defined.

Bacterial sepsis with endotoxemia has resulted in pulmonary edema without an elevated pulmonary capillary pressure. Vasoactive peptides (histamine, serotonin, kinins), as well as local endothelial cell damage,

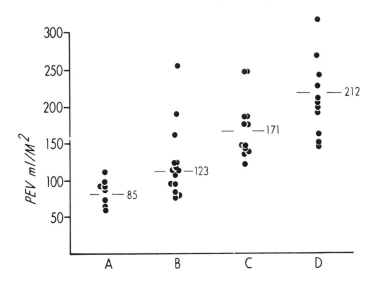

Figure 1–2. Pulmonary extravascular volume (PEV) in patients with acute myocardial infarction classified according to changes in the chest roentgenogram. Class A—normal patients; class B—patients with pulmonary congestion; class C—patients with interstitial edema; class D—patients with frank pulmonary edema. The mean value in each class of patients is represented by the horizontal line in the designated figure. Note the progressive increase in PEV from class A to class D patients.

may be responsible for the pulmonary congestion.[8] Impaired myocardial function in bacteremic sepsis has been demonstrated in experimental animals.[9,10] That direct myocardial depressant effect may be present in some cases of sepsis in man.[12] Uremia, high-dose irradiation, and disseminated intravascular coagulation may also induce pulmonary edema as a result of vascular endothelial injury.

An abrupt fall in plasma protein concentration reducing osmotic pressure may result in pulmonary edema with only moderate volume overload in the absence of left ventricular failure.[2]

Lymphatic obstruction with impaired drainage can experimentally produce pulmonary edema. The clinical counterpart may exist in the pulmonary edema occasionally seen in silicosis and lymphangitic carcinomatosis.[12]

Other syndromes of acute pulmonary edema have been well described clinically, but their precise causes are not known. People without previous cardiopulmonary disease have manifested pulmonary edema on sudden exposure to high altitude. The illness is reversed when those same people descend toward sea level, and other manifestations of heart disease are found to be lacking in them.[13] Similarly, the use of intravenous heroin and overdoses of other narcotics have resulted in florid pulmonary congestion and frequently death in respiratory failure despite normal cardiac function.[14] The pulmonary edema associated with acute pulmonary embolism may occur secondary to changes in vascular permeability or acute pulmonary hypertension.[15] In addition to thromboembolic disease, fluid accumulation has been associated with fat embolism. Injuries to the central nervous system and the use of general anesthesia have also been associated with acute pulmonary edema of unexplained origin.

TREATMENT OF CARDIAC PULMONARY EDEMA

Acute pulmonary edema may be of such rapid onset and life-threatening potential that immediate and intelligent management is mandatory. Severe respiratory distress is often accompanied by frothy, blood-tinged sputum, cold, clammy extremities, and the patient's terror of drowning in his own secretions.

Pulmonary edema is most commonly secondary to disease of the left side of the heart, except for less common noncardiac causes, as mentioned in the previous section. The initial management therefore should involve consideration of the exact cause. The patient may be aware of preexisting cardiac disease, but often acute pulmonary edema is the first manifestation of cardiac disease. Generally, treatment should follow the history taking, physical examination, ECG, and roentgenogram of the chest, but the severity of the illness usually demands some emergency therapy while the results of diagnosic tests are being gathered and evaluated. Information about the drugs commonly used to treat acute pulmonary edema is summarized in Table 1–2.

Improvement in Ventilation

The treatment that is usually applicable to all cases of acute pulmonary edema includes attention to techniques that optimize ventilatory function. For several reasons, the sitting position is usually the most comfortable and effective one for the patient. The sitting position reduces the venous return to the heart, and thus lowers the pulmonary blood volume and congestion. The sitting position also decreases the work of breathing and increases vital capacity.[16] The arterial hypoxemia common to acute pulmonary edema warrants the use of oxygen therapy to increase alveolar oxygenation and prevent the metabolic consequences of sustained tissue hypoxia. Pulmonary congestion from left ventricular dysfunction is thought to produce a ventilation-perfusion imbalance responsible for the hypoxemia. In acute myocardial infarction, the degree of hypoxemia correlates with the severity of the heart failure.[17,18] Oxygen administration

Table 1–2. Drugs Commonly Used in Acute Pulmonary Edema

Drug	Dosage and Administration	Onset of Action	Precautions	Side Effects	Contraindications
Morphine sulfate	4–5 mg IV; dose may be repeated, depending on patient's response	10–15 min	AV block Hypotension Chronic lung disease	Nausea Vomiting Hypotension Respiratory depression	Respiratory acidosis
Furosemide	40 mg IV	Venodilation in 5–10 min Diuresis in 30–60 min	Hypokalemia Hyponatremia	Electrolyte depletion Metabolic alkalosis	Severe hypokalemia
Digoxin	0.5 mg IV initially and 0.25 mg q 2–4 hours for 1 or 2 doses, depending on patient's response	15–30 min	First-degree heart block Ventricular arrhythmia Hypokalemia Acute myocardial infarction	Nausea Vomiting High degree AV block Arrhythmias of digitalis toxicity	Second- or third-degree AV block Severe bradycardia Digitalis intoxication
Nitroprusside	20 μgm/min; starting dose by IV infusion	5 min	Hypotension; Swan-Ganz monitoring mandatory	Hypotension Cyanide intoxication	Shock
Aminophylline	500 mg by slow IV drip over 20–30 min 0.9 mg/kg/hr if sustained therapy required	15–30 min	Arrhythmia Hypertension Acute myocardial infarction	Nausea Vomiting Tachycardia Arrhythmias	Uncontrolled hypertension Severe ventricular arrhythmias (bigeminy or recurrent ventricular tachycardia)

by nasal catheter is usually adequate in mild cases. A Venti mask can be used to measure the exact levels of inspired oxygen if that information is necessary in patients with more severe hypoxemia or associated chronic lung disease. The arterial blood gases should be monitored in patients with advanced pulmonary edema and hypoxemia. The partial pressure of carbon dioxide is usually normal, but a mild respiratory alkalosis is frequently observed, even in lesser degrees of left ventricular dysfunction.[19] If hypercarbia ($pCO_2 > 50$ mm Hg) and severe hypoxemia ($pO_2 < 60$ mm Hg) occur despite oxygen therapy and optimum medical treatment, intubation and mechanical ventilation are usually necessary. Care must be exercised, however, because high levels of inspired oxygen ($>50\%$) and prolonged positive pressure ventilation may result in oxygen toxicity or the adult respiratory distress syndrome.[20-22] Without intubation, the highest actual level of inspired oxygen delivered even with 100% oxygen flow is about 50 to 60%.[21] Thus the risk of oxygen toxicity using the standard disposable face mask is low. If (1) the pCO_2 is between 35 and 40 mm Hg, (2) the pO_2 is maintained above 80 mm Hg, and (3) the pH is normal, adequate ventilatory support has been provided.

Morphine

Morphine provides rapid and reliable improvement in cardiac acute pulmonary edema by several beneficial actions. Venodilatation occurs and reduces the venous return and the pulmonary capillary hydrostatic pressure.[23,24] The work of breathing is decreased by a reduction in hyperventilation through a blunting of the respiratory reflexes as well as through a decrease in pain and anxiety. Small doses (4 to 5 mg) may be given intravenously and be rapidly effective. Use of the subcutaneous or intramuscular routes of injection may result in delayed effectiveness in hypotensive patients with poor peripheral perfusion, but the hazards of drug-induced hypotension or respiratory depression are less likely to occur than when the intravenous route is used. Our practice has been to administer morphine intravenously in severe cases of pulmonary edema if the blood pressure is maintained above 100 mm Hg.

Diuretic Therapy

Diuretics have been used in acute congestive heart failure to promote a reduction in plasma volume and subsequently a decrease in pulmonary capillary pressure. When given intravenously, furosemide and ethacrynic acid can indeed induce a rapid diuresis. It is questionable, however, whether alveolar or interstitial fluid is actually mobilized in the first one or two hours. In any event, a reduction in plasma volume by diuresis would aid in alleviating any further increase in pulmonary capillary pressure. Furosemide has been demonstrated to have additional beneficial effects in patients with left ventricular failure complicating acute myocardial infarction. Since a decrease in pulmonary artery pressure occurs within five to 15 minutes after injection—before any possible diuretic effect could occur—the decrease is probably related to venodilatation.[25] Thus the decrease in venous return and capillary hydrostatic pressure from venodilatation with furosemide, together with furosemide's prompt diuretic effect, provide a valuable form of treatment.

Digitalis

Another major therapeutic approach to the management of acute pulmonary edema involves the use of digitalis to increase myocardial contractility.

Digitalis is recommended in acute congestive heart failure as adjunctive therapy to oxygen, morphine sulfate, and diuretics. Many patients can be successfully treated without digitalis, and in some patients use of the drug may have serious consequences. Patients with acute myocardial infarction, for example, appear to be more sensitive to digitalis, and toxic rhythm disturbances may result.[26,27] In addition, the hemodynamic response to digitalis in acute myocardial infarction is unpredictable.[27,28] With an increase in myocardial contractility, oxygen consumption must also increase, and concern is often expressed that the use of digitalis in acute myocardial infarction may actually extend the area of necrosis. If cardiomegaly exists in congestive heart failure, however, an increase in myocardial oxygen consumption by digitalis increasing contractility is offset by a decrease in oxygen requirement because of the reduction in the size of the left ventricle and in wall tension.[26] The problem is not solved, but it is recommended that digitalis not be used in patients with acute myocardial infarction and mild left ventricular failure that can be managed with diuretics alone. When the severity of acute congestive heart failure warrants the use of digitalis, the more rapid and reliable intravenous route is recommended. Digoxin can be given in an initial dose of 0.50 to 0.75 mg intravenously, with additional 0.25 mg doses in 2 to 4 hours if necessary, depending on the patient's response. Body size, electrolyte imbalance, and the use of other drug therapy must be considered. It is important to remember that a significant inotropic response can be achieved with doses less than those considered to produce full digitalization.

Digitalis can be of benefit in pulmonary edema due to mitral stenosis through control of rapid atrial fibrillation. A decrease in the ventricular rate can allow for improved left ventricular filling and a reduction in the pulmonary venous pressure. In pure mitral stenosis, the inotropic effect of digitalis on the left ventricle probably is of no consequence. Since patients with obstructive cardiomyopathy are made worse by drugs that increase left ventricular contractility, digitalis is contraindicated in patients with that disease, even in the presence of pulmonary edema.

Vasodilator Therapy

Newer techniques of vasodilator therapy for heart failure have been developed. Drugs that reduce either venous or arterial peripheral resistance have been found to be quite beneficial.[29–31] A reduction in arterial resistance decreases the impedance to left ventricular ejection and therefore facilitates ventricular emptying. That phenomenon results in an increased cardiac output and a decreased end-diastolic volume in the left ventricle. Therefore, forward flow (cardiac output) would be increased and pulmonary congestion would be decreased. The initial small decrease in blood pressure the vasodilator drug causes is offset by the increase in cardiac output. Similarly, a reduction in venous resistance has specific benefit. Also, the drugs that produce or cause venodilatation have been found to decrease venous return to the heart and to subsequently reduce the pulmonary artery pressures and pulmonary congestion. Many vasodilator drugs have been investigated, and substantial benefit has been shown to be derived from the use of nitrates, intravenous nitroprusside, phentolamine, trimethaphan, hexamethonium, hydralazine, and prazosin. The nitrates (sublingual and oral and nitroglycerin paste) have a predominant effect on the venous bed, with only slight arterial vasodilatation. Nitroprusside has a more balanced effect, causing a reduction in both venous and arterial resistance. The alpha ganglionic blocker phentolamine, the ganglionic blockers trimethaphan and hexamethonium, and the smooth muscle-relaxant hydralazine promote primarily arteriolar vasodilatation. In acute pulmonary edema of cardiac origin that is not manageable by standard pharmacologic techniques, it would be appropriate to consider vasodilator therapy. The absorption and response to sublingual or oral nitrates is somewhat unpredictable. An infusion of nitroprusside would be beneficial in promoting a decrease in venous return and pulmonary congestion by venodilatation as well as an increase in cardiac output by arteriolar vasodilatation.

The intravenous administration of nitroprusside by infusion pump starting at 20 μg per minute can be carried out cautiously, with constant monitoring of the blood pressure. The infusion rate can be increased every 10 minutes until symptomatic improvement occurs; the blood pressure is maintained at no lower than 100 to 120 mm Hg.

The alpha ganglionic blockers that reduce only arteriolar resistance are of less benefit in acute pulmonary edema. While sympathomimetic effects often accompany the use of phentolamine, undesirable side effects make alpha ganglionic blockers a second choice. Hydralazine and prazosin are primarily of benefit in the management of refractory chronic left ventricular failure.

Nitroprusside should not be considered as a first-line drug in the management of acute pulmonary edema. Its use may be hazardous if not closely monitored by experienced physicians who can readily perform right heart catheterization and take precise measurements of the pulmonary wedge pressure and the cardiac output. Structural defects, such as acute papillary muscle dysfunction and ventricular septal rupture complicating acute myocardial infarction, are uniquely amenable to treatment with nitroprusside. In acute papillary muscle dysfunction, a reduction in systemic peripheral resistance with nitroprusside facilitates left ventricular emptying and decreases regurgitant flow through the incompetent mitral valve. Rupture of the ventricular septum complicating acute myocardial infarction considerably increases the pulmonary blood flow and congestion because of the left-to-right shunt. In our laboratory we have demonstrated a reduction in both left-to-right shunt flow and pulmonary congestion in acute septal rupture treated with intravenous nitroprusside. The initial studies with those new drugs are promising, and the drugs warrant further investigation.

Aminophylline

Aminophylline is known to have cardiovascular, renal, and pulmonary effects, and it can have a specific beneficial effect in acute pulmonary edema. Bronchodilatation results from smooth muscle relaxation and provides a specific use for aminophylline in acute pulmonary edema complicated by bronchospasm. If wheezing suggestive of bronchospasm is resistant to the standard treatment, 500 mg of aminophylline may be given by slow intravenous drip over a period of 20 to 30 minutes. Should prolonged administration be necessary, 0.9 mg/kg/hr is a recommended dosage. The drug also increases the heart rate and myocardial contractility, yet it decreases peripheral vascular resistance by smooth muscle relaxation. The net result is usually an increase in blood pressure because of increased cardiac output despite the peripheral vasodilatation. The diuretic effect of aminophylline is due to a direct effect on the renal tubule independent of the increase in renal blood flow that results from the rise in cardiac output. Caution must be exercised because the rapid administration of aminophylline may precipitate cardiac arrhythmias. It would be wise to avoid the drug in acute myocardial infarction because of the risk of ventricular arrhythmias. Aminophylline should not be given for its cardiac or diuretic effects alone since safer and more effective drugs that have those effects are available.

Phlebotomy

In severe cases of acute congestive heart failure, phlebotomy may be helpful when other measures are ineffective. Cautious venesection of 300 to 500 ml of blood can be effective in decreasing venous return and therefore pulmonary capillary pressure. Plasmapheresis separates red cells from plasma and makes the red cells available for retransfusion. Patients who have a severe volume overload can be bled 500 ml initially; and after plasmapheresis their packed cells can be retransfused during subsequent phlebotomies. That technique provides a continued reduction in plasma volume without a significant loss of red cells.

If pharmacologic therapy is not immediately available, the application of venous occlusive tourniquets can be of help. Tourniquets applied in a rotating fashion on three of four extremities for brief periods are an effective way of reducing venous return. Care must be taken not to occlude arterial flow; and prolonged venous occlusion could result in thrombosis and embolic phenomena. The application of rotating tourniquets is a temporizing measure; it should be used only if the more standard therapy is unavailable or ineffective.

Mechanical Ventilation

On occasion, acute pulmonary edema is so severe that respiratory failure occurs despite optimum management. Profound hypoxemia ($PO_2 < 50$ mm Hg) with increasing hypercarbia ($PCO_2 > 50$ mm Hg) despite optimum ventilatory therapy usually indicates that intubation and mechanical ventilation are necessary. It is important to remember that carbon dioxide retention is uncommon with acute pulmonary edema alone, and a PCO_2 of 50 mm Hg or greater implies the presence of pulmonary disease as well as heart failure. Heavy sedation may be required to totally control respiration, but better ventilation and gas exchange should result. Positive end-expiratory pressure (PEEP) of 5 to 20 cm applied with the respirator has additional advantages in refractory hypoxemia. PEEP increases the functional residual capacity of the lungs, which serves to increase the airway and alveolar diameters. Thus alveolar collapse is reduced, and an improvement in the distribution of ventilation decreases physiologic shunting and hypoxemia. The increase in end-expiratory pressure may also decrease the venous return. To a degree, that decrease would be beneficial in reducing hydrostatic pressure and pulmonary congestion. On the other hand, the use of mechanical ventilation may be harmful if the reduction in venous return is so great that left ventricular filling is impaired and cardiac output decreases. However, the judicious use of PEEP is usually beneficial in improving ventilation-perfusion abnormalities, and it is recommended.[32]

TREATMENT OF NONCARDIAC PULMONARY EDEMA

Pulmonary edema of noncardiac origin is so often confusingly similar to congestive heart failure that a description of it is in order. As stated, an alteration in the pulmonary-capillary membrane permeability is probably the most common cause of noncardiac pulmonary edema. The three basic features of the management of the condition, regardless of its cause, are (1) removal of the offending agent, (2) ventilatory support, and (3) consideration of therapy with anti-inflammatory drugs. Generally, pulmonary edema is a secondary feature of the illness and it is treated differently from the pulmonary congestion of cardiac decompensation. Industrial exposure to caustic chemicals may produce alveolar or capillary damage sufficient to induce a chemical pneumonia, edema, and hypoxemia.[7] Although oxygen therapy is of the utmost importance, digitalis, morphine, and diuretics are usually of little benefit. In some cases, corticosteroids are recommended to reduce the intense inflammatory reaction. The prognosis is good if the extent of hypoxemia and the need for mechanical ventilatory support are not great. The term adult respiratory distress syndrome refers to severe respiratory dysfunction and hemorrhagic pulmonary edema that are end results of many respiratory and cardiovascular insults. Again, pulmonary edema occurs from extensive pulmonary vascular or parenchymal damage; it is not secondary to left ventricular dysfunction with pulmonary venous congestion. Appropriate therapy involves treatment of the primary illness and ventilatory support with oxygen, mechanical ventilation, positive end-expiratory pressure, and tracheostomy if necessary. The condition has been the subject of extensive review elsewhere, and it is not discussed further here.[20–22,32]

Increased membrane permeability and myocardial depression of uncertain cause contribute to the pulmonary edema that is occasionally present in bacteremic sepsis. Adequate ventilation, corticosteroids, and often inotropic drugs to improve myocardial contractility are important in managing the cardiovascular manifestations of sepsis.[7,11] Disseminated intravascular coagulation, uremia, and irradiation therapy may all induce alveolar and capillary damage sufficient to increase "membrane" permeability. The clinical manifestations of acute pulmonary edema must not be interpreted as those of cardiac decompensation, because therapy should not include the techniques for reducing pulmonary capillary pressure or increasing myocardial contractility previously discussed.

Hypoalbuminemia and lymphatic obstruction are potential sources of pulmonary congestion, but clinically they are quite rare.

Other syndromes of acute pulmonary congestion are of uncertain or mixed origin. High-altitude pulmonary edema usually occurs when the person rapidly ascends to extreme heights. The syndrome is most common in the young, with its onset frequently occurring at night, after a strenuous day. Oxygen therapy is of supportive value, and morphine or diuretics are of some benefit, but the best treatment—return toward sea level—should not be delayed.[13]

Acute pulmonary edema secondary to the use of intravenous heroin has, unfortunately, become a frequent illness in major cities. Other narcotics, including oral preparations, have less commonly resulted in the syndrome. Heroin coma with miotic pupils is followed in 12 to 24 hours by tachypnea, severe pulmonary congestion, and profound hypoxia. Treatment of the overdose itself should include the use of a narcotic antagonist. Oxygen therapy, tracheal suction, and, frequently, mechanical ventilation are necessary for treatment of the pulmonary edema.[14]

Acute pulmonary embolism may result in severe pulmonary edema despite preexisting normal cardiac function. It has been postulated that acute pulmonary hypertension is responsible for the transudation of fluid, but an exact explanation for the pulmonary edema is lacking.[15] Mechanical obstruction from the thromboembolism and reflex pulmonary vasoconstriction from hypoxia or vasoactive drugs (serotonin, histamine) have been suggested. Generally treatment should include oxygen and anticoagulation therapy; mechanical ventilatory support, angiography, and embolectomy should be considered only in cases of shock or severe respiratory failure.

Injuries to the central nervous system and general anesthesia have also been associated with unexplained pulmonary edema.[2] As in other cases of uncertain origin, the therapy should be supportive.

BEDSIDE CARDIAC CATHETERIZATION IN ACUTE PULMONARY EDEMA

The development of a flow-directed balloon-tipped cardiac catheter that can be safely floated into the pulmonary artery of a critically ill patient has significantly improved patient care. Specific diagnostic and therapeutic help can be derived from bedside cardiac catheterization in regard to (1) the measurement of ventricular function, (2) the use of fluid therapy for the hypotensive patient, and (3) the diagnosis of mechanical defects complicating acute myocardial infarction.

On inflation of the catheter balloon, the catheter tip is guided in the direction of the blood flow until the balloon lodges in a vessel of equal diameter. The tip of the catheter no longer records pulmonary artery pressure since that wave is totally damped through the air-filled balloon. The catheter tip records the downstream pressure—the pulmonary capillary, or wedge, pressure. Use of the wedge pressure as an indirect but relatively reliable indication of left ventricular diastolic pressure is a helpful way to measure intracardiac pressure and left ventricular function. A second lumen within the catheter has an orifice 30 cm from the catheter tip that corresponds anatomically to the right atrium when the tip is in the pulmonary artery. Thus right atrial pressure can also be measured. That port also adds an injection site for the measurement of cardiac output by the thermodilution technique, with the use of a thermistor at the catheter tip.

Bedside cardiac catheterization is also an important guide to the use of fluid therapy for the hypotensive patient. Often, pulmonary disease clouds the picture in hypotension, and occasionally pulmonary edema is not only pressure dependent. Swan-Ganz pressure monitoring is helpful when the cause of the hypotension is unclear and intravenous fluid therapy is a potential risk, such as in a patient with cardiac disease. When the wedge pressure is in the 18 to 20 mm Hg range, further administration of fluid will probably not increase the blood pressure.

When a patient with acute myocardial infarction develops a loud systolic murmur, bedside cardiac catheterization can often distinguish between acute mitral regurgitation and ventricular septal rupture. In the latter, there is a step-up in oxygenation between the right atrium and the right ventricle because of the left-to-right shunt at the ventricular level. The patient with acute mitral regurgitation often exhibits a large, regurgitant "V" wave on the pulmonary wedge pressure tracing.

Although a single measurement of pulmonary wedge pressure and cardiac output is helpful, it is obvious that more relevant data about the patient's response to therapy can be achieved by a number of measurements.

SUMMARY

1. The most common cause of acute pulmonary edema is cardiac disease, whether atherosclerotic, valvular, hypertensive, or myopathic in origin. Noncardiac types of pulmonary edema are not secondary to true left ventricular failure but are usually related to an alteration in the permeability of the pulmonary capillary "membrane."

2. Acute pulmonary edema may be of such rapid onset and life-threatening potential that immediate and intelligent management is mandatory. Consideration of the exact cause is important, but usually the severity of the illness demands some emergency therapy while the results of diagnostic tests are being gathered and interpreted.

3. The treatment that is usually applicable to all cases of acute pulmonary edema includes techniques to optimize ventilatory function. The sitting position is usually the most comfortable and effective one for the patient; and oxygen administration by nasal catheter is recommended

as a start. If chronic lung disease or severe pulmonary edema with hypoxemia are present, it may be necessary to monitor arterial blood gases and more accurately administer oxygen therapy by Venti mask with accurate measurements of inspired oxygen.

4. Morphine can provide rapid and reliable improvement in cardiac acute pulmonary edema when it is given intravenously in small doses (4 to 5 mg). The drug promotes venodilatation, reducing the venous return and therefore the pulmonary capillary hydrostatic pressure. Morphine also reduces the work of breathing by decreasing pain and anxiety and by reducing hyperventilation through a blunting of the respiratory reflexes.

5. The rapid action of intravenous diuretics has a twofold benefit in acute pulmonary edema. The administration of furosemide is accompanied by a reduction in pulmonary artery pressure in 5 to 15 minutes following injection, the reduction is probably related to venodilatation. Furosemide can also induce a rapid diuresis that by reducing intravascular volume can further decrease pulmonary hydrostatic pressure.

6. Digitalis is recommended in acute congestive heart failure as adjunctive therapy to oxygen, morphine sulfate, and diuretics. Many patients with mild pulmonary congestion can be successfully treated without digitalis, and in some patients the drug may have serious consequences. Patients with acute myocardial infarction appear to be more sensitive to digitalis, and drug-induced rhythm disturbances may result. In addition, the hemodynamic response to digitalis in acute myocardial infarction is unpredictable. In severe cases of acute pulmonary edema, it is recommended that 0.50 to 0.75 mg of digoxin be given intravenously as the initial dose and an additional 0.25 mg be given in 2 to 4 hours if necessary.

7. Vasodilator therapy has been found to be effective in patients with heart failure refractory to standard management. Drugs that produce or cause venodilatation decrease the venous return and subsequently reduce the pulmonary capillary pressure and pulmonary congestion. A drug that reduces arterial resistance decreases the impedance to left ventricular ejection, resulting in an increased cardiac output and a decreased end-diastolic volume of the left ventricle. In acute pulmonary edema of cardiac origin that is not manageable by standard pharmacologic techniques, the intravenous administration of nitroprusside by infusion pump, with constant monitoring of the blood pressure and, if possible, of the pulmonary wedge pressure has been found to be quite effective.

8. Aminophylline can be of benefit when acute pulmonary edema is complicated by bronchospasm. Bronchodilatation results from smooth muscle relaxation, and if necessary aminophylline may be given by slow intravenous drip of 500 mg over a period of 20 to 30 minutes. A sustained infusion of the drug is also possible; caution must be exercised because rapid administration of the drug may precipitate cardiac arrhythmias.

9. In severe cases of acute congestive heart failure, phlebotomy may be helpful when other measures are ineffective. Cautious venesection of 300 to 500 ml of blood can be effective in decreasing venous return and pulmonary capillary pressure. Plasmapheresis of the withdrawn blood permits retransfusion of packed cells if phlebotomy must be repeated.

10. The application of venous occlusive tourniquets can be of benefit if drug therapy is not immediately available. Tourniquets applied in a rotating fashion on three of the four extremities for 15 to 20 minutes provides a way of temporarily reducing the venous return and pulmonary congestion.

11. Occasionally, acute pulmonary edema is so severe that respiratory failure occurs despite the best management. Profound hypoxemia with increasing hypercarbia despite optimum ventilatory therapy usually indicates that intubation and mechanical ventilation are necessary. Positive end-expiratory pressure (PEEP) has additional advantages in refractory hypoxemia. PEEP increases the functional residual capacity of the lungs and the airway and alveolar diameters. Thus alveolar collapse is reduced, and an improvement in the distribution of ventilation decreases physiologic shunting and hypoxemia.

12. The most common cause of noncardiac pulmonary edema is an alteration in pulmonary capillary permeability. In general, the basic features of management include removal of the offending agent, ventilatory support, and consideration of therapy with anti-inflammatory drugs. The term adult respiratory distress syndrome denotes a heterogeneous group of clinical disorders characterized by severe respiratory dysfunction and pulmonary edema. The hypoxemia may be severe, and, in addition to ventilatory support, treatment of the underlying disease process must be considered.

13. Bedside cardiac catheterization can help to separate noncardiac causes of acute pulmonary edema from cardiac ones. It can also serve as an important guide to therapy. Measurements of intracardiac pressure and cardiac output can be readily made with small risk to the patients. It is recommended that patients undergo bedside cardiac catheterization whenever heart failure or hypotension is refractory to standard management.

REFERENCES

1. Robin, E.D., Cross, C.E., and Zelis, R.: Pulmonary edema. Part I. N. Engl. J. Med. 288:239, 1973.
2. Robin, E.D., Cross, C.E., and Zelis, R.: Pulmonary edema. Part II. N. Engl. J. Med. 288:292, 1973.
3. Szidon, J.P., Pietra, G.G., and Fishman, A.P.: The alveolar capillary membrane and pulmonary edema. N. Engl. J. Med. 286:1200, 1972.

4. Fishman, A.P.: Pulmonary edema, the water-exchanging function of the lung. Circulation 46:390, 1972.
5. Biddle, T.L., Khanna, P.K., Yu, P.N., Hodges, M., and Shah, P.M.: Lung water in patients with acute myocardial infarction. Circulation 49:115, 1974.
6. Biddle, T.L., Hodges, M., Yu, P.N., Chance, J.R., Kronenberg, M.W., and Roberts, D.L.: Hypoxemia and lung water in acute myocardial infarction. Am. Heart J. 92:692, 1976.
7. Cordasco, E.M., and Stone, F.D.: Pulmonary edema of environmental origin. Chest 64:182, 1973.
8. Christy, J.H.: Pathophysiology of gram-negative shock. Am. Heart J. 81:694, 1971.
9. Siegal, H.H.: Modifying myocardial response to endotoxin. Clin. Research 13:220, 1965.
10. Solis, R.J., and Downing, S.E.: Effects of E. coli endotoxin on ventricular performance. Am. J. Physiol. 211:307, 1966.
11. Winslow, E.J., Loeb, H.S., Rahimtoola, S.H., Kamath, S., and Gunnar, R.M.: Hemodynamic studies and results of therapy in 50 patients with bacteremic shock. Am. J. Med. 54:421, 1973.
12. Rusznyak, I., Foldi, M., and Szabo., G.: Physiology and pathology. In L. Youlten (ed.), Lymphatics and Lymph Circulation, 2nd ed. Oxford, Pergamon Press, 1967.
13. Wilson, R.: Acute high-altitude illness in mountaineers and problems of rescue. Ann. Intern. Med. 78:421, 1973.
14. Addington, W.W., Cugell, D.W., Bazley, E.S., Westerhoff, T.R., Shapiro, B., and Smith, R.T.: The pulmonary edema of heroin toxicity: An example of the stiff lung syndrome. Chest 62:199, 1972.
15. Sasahara, A.A.: Pulmonary vascular responses to thromboembolism. Mod. Concepts Cardiovasc. Dis. 36:55, 1967.
16. Ramirez, A., and Abelmann, W.H.: Cardiac decompensation. N. Engl. J. Med. 290:499, 1974.
17. Valencia, A., and Burgess, J.H.: Arterial hypoxemia following acute myocardial infarction. Circulation 40:641, 1969.
18. Fillmore, S.J., Shapiro, M., and Killip, T.: Arterial oxygen tension in acute myocardial infarction. Serial analysis of clinical state and blood gas changes. Am. Heart J. 79:620, 1970.
19. Ramo, B.W., Myers, N., Wallace, A.G., Starmer, F., Clarke, D.O., and Whalen, R.E.: Hemodynamic findings in 123 patients with acute myocardial infarction on admission. Circulation 42:567, 1970.
20. Pontoppidan, H., Geffin, B., and Lowenstein, E.: Acute respiratory failure in the adult. Part I. N. Engl. J. Med. 287:690, 1972.
21. Pontoppidan, H., Geffin, B., and Lowenstein, E.: Acute respiratory failure in the adult. Part II. N. Engl. J. Med. 287:743, 1972.
22. Pontoppidan, H. Geffin, B., and Lowenstein, E.: Acute respiratory failure in the adult. Part III. N. Engl. J. Med. 287:799, 1972.
23. Goodman, L.S., and Gilman, A. (eds.): The Pharmacological Basis of Therapeutics, 4th ed. New York. Macmillan, 1970.
24. Zelis, R.F., Mason, D.T., Spann, J.F., and Amsterdam, E.A.: The effects of morphine on the venous bed in man. Demonstration of a biphasic response. Am. J. Cardiol. 25:136, 1970.
25. Dikshit, K., Vyden, J.K., Forrester, J.S., Chatterjee, K., Prakash, R., and Swan, H.J.C.: Hemodynamic effects of furosemide in cardiac failure. N. Engl. J. Med. 288:1087, 1973.
26. Smith, T.W.: Digitalis glycosides. Part I. N. Engl. J. Med. 288:719, 1973.
27. Smith, T.W.: Digitalis glycosides. Part II. N. Engl. J. Med. 288:942, 1973.
28. Hodges, M., Friesinger, G.C., Riggins, R.C.K., and Dagenais, G.R.: Effects of intravenously administered digoxin on mild left ventricular failure in acute myocardial infarction in man. Am. J. Cardiol. 29:749, 1972.
29. Gold, H.K., Leinbach, R.C., and Sanders, C.A.: Use of sublingual nitroglycerin in congestive failure following acute myocardial infarction. Circulation 46:839, 1972.

30. Chatterjee, K., Parmley, W.W., Ganz, W., Forrester, J., Walinsky, P., Crexells, C., and Swan, H.J.C.: Hemodynamic and metabolic responses to vasodilator therapy in acute myocardial infarction. Circulation 48:1183, 1973.
31. Franciosa, J.A., Limas, C.J., Guiha, N.H., Rodriguera, E., and Cohn, J.N.: Improved left ventricular function during nitroprusside infusion in acute myocardial infarction. Lancet I:650, 1972.
32. Leftwich, E.I., Witorsch, R.J., and Witorsch, P.: Positive end-expiratory pressure in refractory hypoxemia. A critical evaluation. Ann. Intern. Med. 79:187, 1973.

Chapter 2

PULMONARY EMBOLISM AND INFARCTION

EDWARD GENTON

GENERAL CONSIDERATIONS

The anatomy of the lung assures that particulate matter entering the venous blood will lodge somewhere in the pulmonary arterial tree. Numerous substances may enter the venous blood and become pulmonary emboli, including amniotic fluid, fat globules, tumor fragments, foreign materials (such as ballistic missiles or plastics from catheters), or thrombotic materials detached from their sites of formation. Of those, by far the most important ones in regard to incidence and significance are the thromboemboli.

Thromboemboli may arise from a number of locations, including the veins of the lower extremities, pelvic plexus, and upper extremities and the right heart chambers. The lower extremities are the source in the majority of patients, and fewer than 15% of all emboli arises from all the other sites combined. Pelvic vein thrombosis occurs in the presence of pelvic inflammation, especially in infection or malignant disease. Veins in the upper extremities are an unusual source of symptomatic emboli, because thrombosis in deep veins is uncommon and because emboli that do form there are usually small. Thrombi form in the right heart in association with obvious heart disease. Embolism from the right atrium may occur in patients with atrial fibrillation, embolism from the tricuspid valves may occur in patients with either bacterial or marantic endocarditis, and embolism from the right ventricle may occur in patients with myocardiopathy or with myocardial infarction that has involved the ventricular septum or the right ventricular muscle.

Thrombosis in veins of the lower extremities occurs with great frequency, especially in hospitalized or otherwise immobilized patients. The factors that contribute to the formation of thrombi in veins include (1) damage to the blood vessel wall, such as occurs in soft tissue trauma, (2) fractures, (3) thermal or chemical substances or microorganisms that trigger the coagulation mechanism, (4) hypercoagulability, which includes increased platelet reactivity, activation of clotting factors, and circulation of thromboplastic materials released from some malignant tissue, from placenta, or perhaps from other necrotic tissue, and (5) stasis of venous blood, which probably contributes to and magnifies the effect of vessel wall damage and hypercoagulability by leading to further damage or by preventing the removal of activated clotting factors and thereby allowing their concentration to increase locally. A number of clinical situations are identifiable in which the thrombogenic factors are particularly likely to exist alone or in combination (Table 2–1). When found alone, each of those factors marks the patient as being at risk for venous thrombosis, and when they exist in combination, the risk is greatly magnified.

In most of the high-risk situations, the venous thrombosis begins in the veins of the calf, and usually it remains there; or, if emboli form, they are small and seldom constitute a life-threatening or even major risk. However, in approximately 20% of patients there is extension of the venous thrombi into the "proximal" veins, which includes the popliteal, femoral, and iliac veins. In some patients, such as those who have trauma or who have had surgery of the hip, thrombi often begin in proximal femoral vessels. When the thrombi involve proximal vessels, the likelihood of

Table 2–1.   *Factors Predisposing to Venous Thromboembolism*

Increasing age
Immobilization
Trauma
Major surgery
Malignant disease
Congestive heart failure
Hematologic disorders (associated with polycythemia, thrombocytosis, or hemolysis)
Prior venous thromboembolism
Hyperestrogenemia (associated with pregnancy, the use of oral contraceptives, or estrogen replacement therapy)
Miscellaneous factors (e.g., obesity and dehydration)

embolism increases to probably more than 30 or 40%, the size of the emboli is greater, and the clinical consequences are more serious.

In many, perhaps most instances, thrombosis involving the deep veins of the lower extremities remains clinically silent. Clinicians cannot rely on the presence of "typical" evidence of venous thrombosis (e.g., pain, redness, or swelling) to alert them to the diagnosis. They must have a high level of suspicion, and they must use surveillance techniques to recognize incipient venous thrombi in patients considered at high risk. Ideally, effective methods of prophylaxis should be used to prevent the development of venous thrombi.

Pulmonary embolism is extremely common, but it is virtually impossible to make a reliable estimate of its frequency since the majority of cases are probably silent and self limiting. Some studies indicate that as many as 20% of surgical patients develop emboli postoperatively, which represents nearly 50% of the patients who develop venous thrombosis in their lower extremities. The overall incidence of pulmonary embolism in general autopsy series is about 10%, and it rises to 50% or more in patients who die from decompensated cardiac or respiratory problems or malignant disease. Many emboli are considered incidental (i.e., as not having contributed to the patient's death), although major pulmonary embolism causes more than 5% of hospital deaths and contributes significantly to another 5% of deaths. Many patients with fatal pulmonary embolism have associated debilitating disease, but in about 50% of those patients, had pulmonary embolism been prevented, survival could have been expected. In the majority of cases of fatal pulmonary embolism, there is autopsy evidence that suggests prior embolism, indicating that it is the recurrent rather than the initial embolus that proves fatal.

When death occurs from pulmonary embolism, it is rapid; more than 50% of the deaths occur within the first hour of the onset of symptoms and 75% of the deaths occur within two hours. Another 20 to 25% of deaths occur over the next 48 hours, and the remaining small percentage of deaths occur after several days. Thus salvaging the majority of patients requires the use of preventive measures, ideally before the initial episode; and if not prevention, then early diagnosis and prevention of recurrence.

PATHOPHYSIOLOGY

The consequences of embolism to the pulmonary circulation are a reduction or cessation of the blood flow to the pulmonary tissue distal to the site of the embolism and a resultant alteration in respiratory and hemodynamic function. The magnitude of the changes produced varies. It is largely dependent on the cross-sectional area of the pulmonary circulation affected, which is the amount of embolic material and the preexisting condition of the pulmonary circulation. In a normal pulmonary bed, a compromise of more than 50% is needed for a significant hemodynamic alteration to be produced. However, when the lung has been previously affected by disease, such as congestive heart failure or chronic obstructive pulmonary disease, an embolism of lesser magnitude may produce a significant functional change.

The major alteration in respiratory function from embolism is an increase in alveolar dead space due to the continued ventilation of nonperfused or underperfused segments of lung, which creates an alteration in gas exchange. The magnitude of that phenomenon is somewhat modified by constriction of terminal airways, brought about probably by a reduction in carbon dioxide tension and hypoxemia in the embolized area of lung and possibly by vasoactive humoral drugs, such as histamine and serotonin. There is often alveolar collapse of the involved lung that is thought to be related to a decrease of surfactant, which leads to congestive atelectasis.

Usually associated with pulmonary emboli is arterial hypoxemia, with resultant widened alveolar-arterial oxygen tension difference and reduced arterial PO_2. The degree of the hypoxemia is usually related to the magnitude of the pulmonary embolization, but that correlation is not constant; occasionally massive embolism is associated with a normal PO_2 and instances of submassive embolism are associated with marked hypoxemia. The mechanism of hypoxemia has not been definitely elucidated, but it is probably multifactorial and related to ventilation-perfusion abnormalities from intrapulmonary shunts and possibly to the consequence of hyperperfusion of non-embolized lung zone.

The hemodynamic consequence of pulmonary embolism is an immediate increase in resistance to blood flow through the pulmonary circulation, which is reflected in an elevation of the right ventricular pressure. In the extreme, this can produce acute cor pulmonale. It is not certain whether other factors besides the mechanical ones are involved in the increase in pulmonary resistance. It has been speculated that diffuse reflex or humorally stimulated vasoconstriction may occur. It is possible that vasoconstriction may occur rapidly with embolism and subside to a large extent or completely within minutes or several hours in most patients. The hemodynamic effect of embolism is relative to the magnitude of obstruction of existing circulation. Thus in patients whose pulmonary vascular bed was substantially compromised before embolism, a profound alteration in hemodynamics may be produced with even small numbers of emboli.

In most organs, the interruption of blood flow is associated with rapid tissue necrosis or infarction. In the lung, necrosis is the exception rather than the rule, probably because oxygen to lung tissue derives from several sources, including the pulmonary arterial blood, the bronchial arterial blood, and probably the airways. Loss of one of those sources, such as occurs with pulmonary embolism does not reduce the oxygen supply critically, and tissue necrosis usually does not occur. However, because of the insult to the pulmonary tissue, products of inflammation may enter the alveoli and produce congestive atelectasis. In most instances, that phenomenon proceeds not to necrosis and healing through organization but to resorption of the materials over a period of days, with restoration of normal histology and of normal function if the obstructing embolus resolves. Thus pulmonary consolidation usually reflects congestive atelectasis, and it occurs in approximately 10% of people with pulmonary emboli, usually in association with occlusion of medium-sized pulmonary vessels (less than 1 ml), especially in the presence of prior cardiopulmonary abnormalities.

THE COURSE OF PULMONARY EMBOLISM

In most instances the fate of an individual embolus is spontaneous resolution, either completely or to a major extent. The resolution is thought to occur principally from physiologic fibrinolysis, which, through the action of plasmin, digests the fibrin from the embolus. Some emboli fragment and produce showers of smaller emboli, which move downstream, thus relieving the more proximal obstruction. The remaining emboli undergo organization and attachment to the vessel wall, which leads in time to a fatty streak or web or band at the site of the initial embolus. The rate of resolution of emboli varies considerably, probably in relationship to not only the size of the embolus but also to whether it is firmly lodged in a vessel or allows laminar flow around the lesion, to whether it is intact or has fragmented during embolism, and, most important, to the age of the thrombus at the time of embolism. Emboli that are more than three to five days old probably resolve slower than fresher ones—and there also may be variations from patient to patient. In any case, the resolution is slight for the first 24 to 48 hours but substantial within five to seven days. Although in rare instances complete resolution may occur rapidly, it is seldom complete in less than two weeks, but often complete within eight weeks. Generally, the larger the initial embolic insult, the more slowly resolution occurs. It is likely that resolution may proceed for several months. In 10 to 15% of patients, some obstruction remains permanently, especially in patients with preexisting cardiopulmonary disease and in patients with massive embolism. Rarely, there is no significant resolution of massive embolism, and persistent obstruction of flow to a segment or lobe of the lung or, occasionally, to the entire lung may be seen. Chronic persistent pulmonary hypertension is a theoretical consequence of pulmonary embolism, especially when there have been multiple recurrences, but fortunately the condition is rarely seen. Obliterative pulmonary hypertension is most often the result of many small to medium sized emboli.

In most patients the return of the hemodynamic measurements to normal or near normal parallels the rate of resolution of the embolism.

CLINICAL MANIFESTATIONS

Understanding the pathophysiologic consequences of pulmonary embolism permits the physician to take a rational approach to predicting and interpreting the clinical manifestations. The most useful means of classifying emboli is based on their size and the degree of obstruction they bring to the pulmonary circulation. On that basis, pulmonary embolism may be divided into massive and submassive. Massive embolism implies the obstruction of 50% or more of the cross-sectional area of the pulmonary arterial circulation. The obstruction would involve the occlusion of the main pulmonary artery, or the right or left pulmonary artery or two or more lobar branches. Submassive embolism produces occlusion of a lesser degree. It is important to emphasize that the clinical consequences of embolism do not entirely parallel the absolute obstruction produced but depend to a considerable extent upon the preexisting condition of the pulmonary circulation and on the suddenness with which obstruction occurs.

SYMPTOMS AND SIGNS OF MASSIVE PULMONARY EMBOLISM

The clinical picture in massive embolism varies widely, and, not unusually, symptoms may be fleeting and minimal. The characteristic feature of massive embolism is sudden and severe dyspnea, which may be associated with apprehension, stupor, or syncope. There is tachypnea or gasping respiration, the blood pressure may be low, or shock may exist, and usually diaphoresis and cyanosis are present. There may be crushing substernal chest pain, often indistinguishable from that of myocardial infarction. The arterial pulse is rapid and of small volume; the jugular venous pulse may reveal elevated venous pressure and, often, prominent A and V waves. Rarely is the right ventricular activity palpable, but occasionally a shock of pulmonary closure is felt. A scratchy systolic murmur, which may be mistaken for a pericardial friction rub, is sometimes audible in the pulmonary area. The second heart sound may be widely split and the pulmonary closing sound accentuated. Rarely, a murmur of pulmonary incompetence is heard, or a systolic ejection murmur at the left base may be present due to partial occlusion of the pulmonary outflow tract. Occasionally, a pansystolic murmur of functional tricuspid incompetence and a right venticular gallop may be heard along the lower left sternal border.

PHYSICAL FINDINGS IN SUBMASSIVE PULMONARY EMBOLISM

In submassive embolism, the clinical manifestations are often minimal or absent, or they may be quite transient, lasting only a few minutes. Again, tachypnea with or without dyspnea and tachycardia are the major and often the only clinical manifestations. The patient may have a fever of varying severity. It is always useful to look for evidence of venous thrombosis in the lower extremities. When embolism of a medium-sized pulmonary artery has occurred, pulmonary infarction may develop. When pulmonary infarction is present, pleuritic chest pain, cough, and hemoptysis develop from several hours to as long as 72 hours after the embolism. Examination reveals a pleural friction rub and, often, signs of consolidation of pulmonary tissue. Pleural effusion may develop over a period of hours or days (Table 2–2).

A number of subtle clinical findings associated with pulmonary embolism have been identified in the literature. Although they do not occur frequently, their appearance should alert the clinician to the possible presence of pulmonary embolism. The findings are (1) worsening of congestive heart failure or respiratory failure, (2) the development of digitalis intoxication without explanation, or (3) atrial fibrillation in cardiac patients. It has also been suggested that hospitalized patients who develop sudden tachycardia that lasts for only a few minutes or several hours or who experience a spike in temperature should be suspected of having pulmonary emboli.

LABORATORY FINDINGS

A number of routine laboratory tests may have abnormal results in the presence of pulmonary embolism, but no test is sufficiently sensitive or

Table 2–2. *Symptoms of Pulmonary Embolism*

Symptom	Minor Embolism	Major Embolism	Massive Embolism
Dyspnea	+	+ +	+ + – + + + +
Cough	+	+ +	±
Pleurisy	±	±	0
Fever	+	+	+
Hemoptysis	±	+	±
Collapse	0	±	+ +

0 = absent; + = present and severity.

specific to establish or exclude the diagnosis. The white blood count is usually normal, but it may be elevated to 15,000 to 20,000. The serum fibrinogen-fibrin antigen level is usually elevated, which may be helpful in excluding pulmonary embolism if the level is normal, but the test lacks specificity. The lactic dehydrogenase level is often elevated, and, less often, the SGOT and serum bilirubin levels are elevated. In most patients, the arterial blood gases show some derangement. Typically, the arterial PCO_2 is reduced, and there is arterial hypoxemia, with the arterial PO_2 reduced below 90 mm Hg in more than 85% of patients. On the other hand, 10 to 15% of patients with established pulmonary embolism have PO_2 values within the normal limits, and even more important, many conditions may be associated with a reduced PO_2, making it necessary to interpret the results cautiously; the diagnosis should never be decided by the PO_2 value alone.

The ECG is altered in about 50% of patients with major pulmonary embolism, but those changes may be fleeting, disappearing within minutes or hours. In the presence of right heart strain, there is usually sinus tachycardia and occasionally supraventricular tachyarrhythmia. The initial QRS vector may rotate leftward and produce Q waves in lead III, II (occasionally), and aVF. The terminal QRS forces may move rightward and produce a terminal S wave in lead I and a prominent R wave in lead III. T wave changes are due to a leftward axis, which produces inversion of T waves in leads III, II (at times), and aVF. Occasionally, a right bundle branch block may occur, and in the presence of right atrial enlargement, there may be P pulmonale, manifested by peaking of P waves in leads II, III, and aVF. Those changes, singly or in combination, produce the characteristic pattern changes of pulmonary embolism, including the S_1, Q_3, T_3 pattern and acute right axis deviation, but in most patients the ECG changes, if present, are limited to nonspecific S-T or T waves changes.

Although there are no findings in the routine chest roentgenogram specific for pulmonary embolism, a chest film is useful for each person in whom the condition is considered. A number of conditions that mimic pulmonary embolism (such as pulmonary edema and pneumothorax) may be thus identified. In pulmonary embolism, the most common finding is a normal chest roentgenogram. A number of changes may occur to suggest the diagnosis or to provide another bit of evidence to support it. The occlusion of a proximal pulmonary artery results in the reduction of blood flow to the distal lung, which may be suggested on the chest roentgenogram by oligemia of a lobe or entire lung. If seen in association with plethora or hyperperfusion of other areas of the lung, the oligemia is a useful radiologic sign. More subtle are the differences in size of comparable vessels and dilatation of the main pulmonary arteries. In the presence of loss of lung volume from pneumoconstriction, the diaphragm on the affected side may be elevated and there may be areas of platelike atelectasis in the involved area of the lung. In congestive atelectasis, parenchymal infiltrations, presenting as infiltrates of varying sizes and shapes (they may be round, linear, or, occasionally, wedge shaped) are observed. Pleural effusions of small to moderate size that cannot be explained by other conditions are a useful clue.

RADIOISOTOPE LUNG SCAN

An alteration in lung perfusion, as measured by isotopic scanning techniques, is regularly present in pulmonary thromboembolism. When particulate material labeled with a gamma-emitting isotope of particle size 10 to 50μ in diameter is injected intravenously, it is distributed throughout the lung in a manner corresponding to the blood flow through the pulmonary circulation. Scanning readily identifies underperfused areas and produces a visual display of blood flow distribution. If four views—anterior, posterior, and two lateral views—are obtained using scintillation cameras, as is currently done, the test may be completed rapidly, even in very sick patients. A technically adequate lung scan is a sensitive indicator of pulmonary embolism. A normal lung scan virtually excludes the diagnosis of pulmonary embolism, and in the presence of pulmonary embolism, it reliably quantifies the perfusion abnormality present. Thus the technique is useful in establishing the initial diagnosis, for detecting recurrent embolism, and for studying the rate of resolution of embolic obstruction. Therefore virtually all persons suspected of having a pulmonary embolism should have a lung scan. Unfortunately, the technique has poor specificity since many other conditions also produce perfusion abnormalities, and false-positive scans occur in many conditions, including chronic pulmonary or cardiac disease, pneumonia, and asthma. Theoretically, an embolus involving only the main pulmonary artery may be missed by lung scan, but in practice that has rarely occurred.

The specificity of lung scanning may be increased by performing a combined perfusion-ventilation scan. Ventilation scanning is accomplished by the use of inhaled isotopes such as Xenon 133, which is distributed to the parts of the lungs that are being ventilated. The distribution of the gas and, especially, the washout of radioactivity from the lungs are recorded. The sequential lung images, compared to those observed in a perfusion study, allow identification of areas that are being ventilated but not perfused, as would occur in pulmonary embolism, from areas that are neither ventilated or perfused, which would suggest numerous other causes. If a major defect of segmental size is shown by the perfusion scan and if there is a mismatch with ventilation, the probability of pulmonary embolism is high. But when a ventilation defect is present in an area of underperfusion, parenchymal or airway disease (but not pulmonary embolism) is likely.

PULMONARY ANGIOGRAPHY

Injection of adequate quantities of radiocontrast medium into the pulmonary artery is the most sensitive and definitive way to identify the presence and location of pulmonary emboli. Caution must be used in regard to the position of the catheter, the rate of injection, and the volume of contrast material to assure that good filling of the entire pulmonary circulation is accomplished. A number of angiographic changes are consistent with pulmonary emboli. The most specific is a filling defect within a pulmonary artery, which outlines a partially occluding embolus. Abrupt cutoff of a major vessel from an impacted embolus is reasonably definitive. Angiographic changes that are less specific but consistent with pulmonary emboli are delayed filling of an area of lung and abnormal tapering of a vessel. Delayed emptying from a pulmonary artery or from the venous system is an unreliable sign of embolism. A complete study may require selective angiographic study of areas of the lung suspected of having an embolus but not adequately delineated by injection from a catheter located in the main pulmonary artery.

APPROACH TO THE DIAGNOSIS OF PULMONARY EMBOLISM

Even when the presence of pulmonary embolism is strongly suspected on clinical grounds, it is always desirable to obtain ''objective'' evidence of the condition to avoid misdiagnosis and to justify the risks and ramifications of antithrombotic therapy. A reasonable approach to the diagnosis of pulmonary embolism includes taking a careful history, a physical examination, the performance of a routine chest roentgenogram, ECG, measurement of the arterial blood pH and gas tension, and a four-view perfusion lung scan accompanied, when possible or necessary, by a ventilation scan. In cases in which the diagnosis remains uncertain, venography of the deep veins of the lower extremities or other tests to detect occlusion of proximal veins in the lower extremities, such as impedance plethysmography, often are helpful in deciding on the treatment (Table 2–3). Finally, pulmonary arteriography should be considered if the diagnosis remains in doubt after the studies just listed have been done or at times as an initial procedure if the patient is in shock or otherwise unstable and is being considered for thrombolytic therapy or embolectomy. If the lung scan is normal or shows only minor abnormalities, treatment should be withheld. If a major segmental defect is

Table 2–3. *Diagnostic Approach to Pulmonary Embolism*

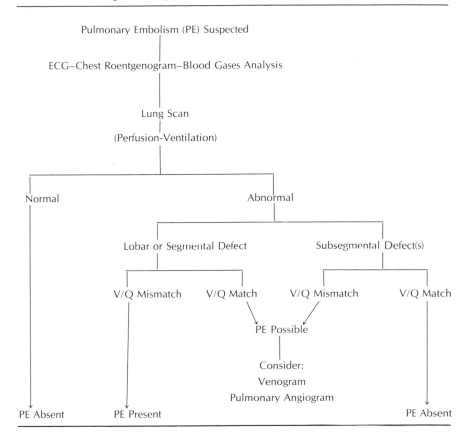

shown by a perfusion lung scan and an associated mismatch is shown by a ventilation scan, it is reasonable in most instances to proceed with treatment. If the clinical picture is equivocal, or if the results of the ventilation perfusion scan are indeterminate, angiography should be carried out. An advantage of angiography, in addition to locating emboli, is that the hemodynamic consequences of the embolus can be quantified. The angiogram is not usually done on an emergency basis, except when surgery is anticipated. Considering the usual rate of resolution of emboli, it is generally possible to delay the performance of an angiogram for one to three days without affecting the success of the study. During that time, the patient can be treated as though he had an embolus. That approach reduces the complication rate of angiography and increases the likelihood of a successful study. It is not unusual that after all available techniques have been performed, the diagnosis remains uncertain. In such cases, clinical judgment must be applied, taking into consideration how the decision will affect the risk-benefit ratio for the patient in question.

DIFFERENTIAL DIAGNOSIS

Pulmonary embolism may mimic many other conditions, and, conversely, a variety of disorders may mimic pulmonary embolism. The type of lesions to be considered in the differential diagnosis depend on whether they simulate massive or submassive embolism. With massive embolism, the differential diagnosis includes the disorders that produce a rapid onset of cardiopulmonary embarrassment. Those disorders include myocardial infarction, dissecting aneurysm of the aorta, pneumothorax, and cardiovascular collapse from hypovolemic shock, such as follows hemorrhage or septicemia. Submassive embolism may be simulated by disorders that produce pleural pain, hemoptysis, fever, or any other abnormality in the roentgenogram or perfusion lung scan. Included in that group of disorders are atelectasis of the lung, pneumonitis, and pleural effusion of any cause.

THERAPY

The major objective in the management of pulmonary embolism is prevention of its occurrence, using effective prophylaxis. Once pulmonary embolism has developed, the primary objective is prevention of further embolism, the secondary objective is relief of the symptoms produced by the embolism, and the third objective (in selected cases) is either acceleration of the rate of resolution of the embolism or removal of the embolism.

PRIMARY PROPHYLAXIS IN PULMONARY THROMBOEMBOLISM

Since the majority of emboli derive from the lower extremities, their prevention would best be accomplished by preventing the development of venous thrombosis or arresting the extension of thrombi into proximal veins and thereby reducing the likelihood of embolism. Since patients at high risk for venous thrombosis are identifiable, it is desirable that such patients receive prophylaxis before the thrombogenic stimulus or as soon after it as possible. (Some examples of thrombogenic stimuli are trauma, elective surgery, and bedrest). The prophylaxis should be continued for as long as the patient remains at high risk. A number of approaches to prophylaxis may be used; the selection should be geared to the needs of the particular patient. The approaches include:

1. The use of oral anticoagulants, which are probably the most effective drugs for primary prophylaxis. Their onset of action is delayed for several days from the initiation of treatment. They should be administered in doses to achieve and sustain a prolongation of the prothrombin time that is two to two and one-half times the control values.

2. The use of low doses of heparin, 5000 units administered subcutaneously every 8 to 12 hours to achieve and sustain low plasma levels of the drug. The onset of action is immediate. The drug is effective in patients at moderate but not extremely high risk, such as patients who have just had hip surgery or who have a malignant disease.

3. The use of dextran, molecular weight 40–70,000, 500 ml a day for two or three days, then every other day for the period of risk. The drug is immediately effective, but its overall effectiveness is probably somewhat less than that of the oral anticoagulants.

4. The use of mechanical methods, especially those that prevent stasis of the lower extremities by pneumatic compression of the lower extremities.

5. The use of platelet-suppressant drugs. A number of drugs (e.g., aspirin) alter platelet reactivity. It has been suggested that aspirin in a dose of 600 to 1200 mg a day reduces the incidence of venous thromboembolism. However, the effectiveness of aspirin has not been conclusively established, and it should not be considered a first-line prophylactic drug.

TREATMENT OF ACTIVE VENOUS THROMBOSIS

The greatest need of the patient with acute pulmonary embolism who survives to receive medical attention, is the prevention of recurrent embolism. Heparin therapy is remarkably effective in achieving that objective, and it should be begun when the presence of pulmonary embolism is suspected, in most cases even before the objective studies have been completed. Heparin therapy should be initiated by an intravenous bolus of the drug in an amount to achieve anticoagulation. Administration of 7500 to 10,000 units achieves anticoagulation in the vast majority of patients; and many think it is useful to administer initially a larger than necessary bolus to achieve anticoagulation for the first 12 to 24 hours of treatment. It is advisable to document the anticoagulation by performance of an appropriate coagulation test 15 to 30 minutes after the initial dose. Heparin anticoagulation should be maintained by continuous heparin infusion, 1000 to 1500 units an hour, or by bolus injections of 5000 to 7500 units at 4-to-6 hour intervals. Both approaches are probably equally effective in preventing recurrence; the continuous infusion approach may be associated with a lower incidence of bleeding because it obviates the peaks of anticoagulant activity associated with intermittent injections. Therefore patients considered at high risk for bleeding, such as patients in the postoperative stage or those with multiple trauma, would be the best candidates for continuous infusion. The dosage should be adjusted to maintain the Lee-White clotting time at 25 to 30 minutes or the partial thromboplastin time at 60 to 80 seconds during a continuous infusion or just before an intermittent dose. Heparin should be continued for five to 10 days to allow attachment and organization of the thrombus in the lower extremities. After that, a period of secondary prophylaxis is desirable for practically all patients. The prophylaxis is best accomplished with oral anticoagulant therapy, which should be begun three to five days before the heparin therapy is terminated to assure the full antithrombotic effect. Oral anticoagulant therapy should be continued for a period of at least six weeks or until the provocation to thrombosis has been eliminated. Patients who resume full activity, who have no residual evidence of venous thrombosis in the lower extremities, and who no longer have an underlying predisposition, can usually have treatment withdrawn after six to eight weeks. Other patients should continue treatment for three to six months, and patients who have had recurrent embolism when anticoagulant therapy was withdrawn should continue with the therapy indefinitely.

Procedures that compromise the vena cava are available; they include surgical ligation, plication using various types of clips, and the insertion, in a jugular-vein approach, of a plastic "umbrella" into the inferior cava below the renal arteries. Those procedures are seldom indicated for patients with pulmonary embolism since heparin therapy is so effective. Caval procedures should be reserved for patients for whom anticoagulation therapy is absolutely contraindicated or for patients who have had a recurrent large embolus, as documented by an objective test, such as a perfusion lung scan or angiogram, during optimal heparin therapy. Caval ligation is probably indicated in patients with obliterative pulmonary hypertension, which has been shown by serial cardiac catheterization studies to progress in spite of long-term anticoagulation.

ACCELERATING THE REMOVAL OF EMBOLIC OBSTRUCTION

For patients who have massive embolism, and circulatory failure and whose condition has not stabilized or has further deteriorated after a trial of several hours of supportive therapy and heparinization, removal of the obstruction may be desirable (and for some patients it may be lifesaving). Emboli may be removed by:

1. Embolectomy, which is indicated in patients with massive embolism who have suffered cardiac arrest or shock and who do not stabilize with supportive treatment. In such patients, the diagnosis should be documented by angiography; and the patient is often best temporarily supported with partial cardiopulmonary bypass.

2. Thrombolytic therapy. Both streptokinase and urokinase administered according to standard regimens have been shown to accelerate the resolution rate of pulmonary embolism. Results are best if treatment is begun early, and certainly within three to five days after the embolic episode. The treatment should be continued for 12 to 24 hours in most patients. The drugs are administered intravenously, usually into a distal vein, but they may be given through an indwelling catheter in the pulmonary artery. To minimize bleeding complications, vascular invasion and other trauma to the patient should be carefully avoided. Following thrombolytic therapy, anticoagulation with heparin, followed by oral anticoagulants, is necessary.

RESUSCITATIVE MEASURES IN COLLAPSE FROM PULMONARY EMBOLISM

A patient who has suffered cardiovascular collapse from pulmonary embolism or who is in cardiac arrest when seen should have vigorous external cardiac massage, which, it has been suggested, may fragment the emboli in proximal vessels and allow them to move more distally, where their hemodynamic effects may be lessened.

SYMPTOMATIC THERAPY IN PULMONARY EMBOLISM

The symptoms of an embolic episode can usually be effectively treated with routine measures. Those measures include the alleviation (1) of pleuritic pain with analgesics (often narcotics), (2) of ischemic angina-like pain with oxygen, which also reduces arterial hypoxemia, (3) of acidemia with bicarbonate and with improved tissue perfusion and oxygenation, and (4) of cardiovascular decompensation by treating the acidemia and hypoxemia—and in some instances by the use of inotropic drugs. The inotropic drugs include digitalis, used cautiously, isoproterenol, which serves as a bronchodilator and a pulmonary artery vasodilator, and dopamine. Bronchoconstriction may be alleviated by heparin, as well as by intravenous aminophylline.

PROGNOSIS

The mortality in untreated pulmonary embolism is difficult to determine because it seems certain that the majority of episodes go undetected and because, fortunately, the process is self limited. However, in symptomatic cases of pulmonary embolism, it appears that withholding heparin treatment is associated with a recurrence rate in excess of 50%, which may prove to be fatal in 20 to 30% of cases. In patients in whom the diagnosis is made and heparin treatment given, the recurrence rate in most series is less than 5%, and fatal recurrence is less than 1%. The outlook for survival is excellent. The mortality in patients with submassive embolism is essentially that of the underlying condition rather than of the pulmonary embolism; and even with massive embolism, the mortality is usually around 10% and it is lower than 20% even in patients who were in shock at the beginning of the episode. Over the weeks or months following treatment, most or all of the pulmonary obstruction is resolved in more than 80% of patients, and only a small percentage have significant residual obstruction to pulmonary flow. During the period of secondary prophylaxis, 5 to 10% of patients have recurrent episodes of venous thromboembolism. Any suspected episodes should be carefully documented by objective measures since they often are not actual recurrences, and misdiagnosis has unfortunate implications and consequences. The long-term outlook for patients after completion of secondary prophylaxis again is excellent; fewer than 10% have subsequent embolic episodes. Any person who has had a venous thromboembolism should have appropriate prophylaxis when he enters a high-risk situation, such as elective surgery, prolonged bedrest, or immobilization for any cause, such as an acute medical illness, a fracture or trauma.

SUMMARY

1. Pulmonary thromboembolism arising from thrombi in the deep veins of the lower extremities is a frequent occurrence in immobilized patients, regardless of their primary disease.

2. Embolism left untreated is often recurrent, leading to high mortality and significant morbidity.

3. The diagnosis of embolism is difficult to make because of the subtleness of the clinical manifestations, which are either absent or nonspecific.

4. Often the first clinical manifestation of embolism is collapse of the patient from recurrent embolism.

5. Suspected pulmonary embolism should be confirmed by objective diagnostic methods, of which the lung scan is the most useful because it is highly sensitive. A normal scan excludes the diagnosis; and although it is nonspecific, an abnormal scan indicates the magnitude of the perfusion abnormality.

6. Pulmonary angiography is the most definitive test; it is indicated when the lung scan results leave the diagnosis in doubt.

7. The ECG, chest roentgenogram, and blood gases measurements are useful adjuncts to diagnosis.

8. Ideally, embolism should be prevented by the use of prophylactic measures in patients at high risk for venous thrombosis.

9. Once embolism has occurred, heparin treatment to arrest the thrombosis and to prevent recurrent embolism is indicated in all patients since the outlook for survival and full recovery is excellent, even in patients with massive embolism, if recurrence is prevented.

10. In selected cases, removal of the emboli by thrombolytic therapy or embolectomy is indicated.

SUGGESTED READINGS

Frantantoni, J., and Wessler, S. (eds.): Prophylactic therapy of deep vein thrombosis and pulmonary embolism. U.S. Department of Health, Education, and Welfare Publication No. (NIH) 76–866, 1975.

Sasahara, A.A., Sonnenblick, E.H., and Lesch, M. (eds.): Pulmonary Emboli. New York, Grune & Stratton, 1975.

A National Cooperative Study: The urokinase/pulmonary embolism trial. Circulation 47 (Suppl. II), 1973.

Gallus, A.S., and Hirsh, J.: Venous thromboembolism. Semin. Thrombosis Hemostasis. II:203, 1976.

Chapter 3

CARDIOGENIC SHOCK

JAY N. COHN

Shock is best defined as a state of abnormal circulatory function in which impairment of tissue blood flow has resulted in a disturbance in organ function and has initiated a series of feedback mechanisms that may lead to progressively more severe perfusion abnormality.[1] The diagnosis of shock, therefore, can be made only in the presence of a disturbance in organ function, and once the diagnosis is established, it may be assumed that the syndrome is progressive. In its broader sense, the term cardiogenic, when applied to shock, implies that an abnormality in cardiac function is an important factor in the development and progression of the shock state. However, it is likely that cardiac function is impaired to a varying degree in all patients with shock, regardless of cause. Therefore, all shock may be considered at least in part cardiogenic shock. In more restrictive usage, however, the term cardiogenic is taken to indicate that form of shock precipitated by an acute myocardial infarction. In the following review, I shall consider in general the physiology of shock and then discuss in particular the syndrome of shock associated with acute myocardial infarction.

THE DIAGNOSIS OF SHOCK

The diagnosis of shock must be based on the demonstration of inadequacy of tissue blood flow. The normal cardiac output in the adult of between 5 and 6 liters per minute is distributed to the regional vascular beds on the basis of flow requirements. If cardiac output falls below normal levels, or if peripheral requirements increase out of proportion to the increase in cardiac output, then certain regional beds become less adequately perfused. Mild degrees of inadequate perfusion may be well tolerated without symptoms, and even considerable depressions of cardiac output on a more chronic basis may be surprisingly well tolerated by readjustment of peripheral requirements. Acute reductions in cardiac output are less well tolerated, but even in acute illnesses the degree of reduction in cardiac output that precipitates the syndrome of shock may be variable.[2] Such variability probably relates to the distribution of the reduced cardiac output, the person's neurohumoral response to that reduction, and the unique requirements of the person's peripheral tissues. Obviously, the flow deficiency that precipitates shock usually begins some time before the full syndrome is detectable. It is during the early preshock phase, when tissue blood flow may not yet be critically reduced, that therapy may be most effective in reversing the disorder. Possible therapeutic intervention before the diagnosis of shock is established is discussed later in the chapter. Nonetheless, the diagnosis of shock must be based on clear clinical or laboratory evidence of reduced blood flow.

When renal blood flow decreases, renal conservation of sodium and oliguria develop. An hourly urine output of less than 20 ml with a urinary sodium concentration of less than 20 mEq per liter is evidence of a critical reduction in renal blood flow. The careful timed measurement of urine output is therefore critical to the early diagnosis of shock, especially because the renal vascular bed may be constricted early in shock and reduction of renal blood flow may therefore occur before any change in arterial pressure is detected. The splanchnic, cutaneous, and skeletal muscle circulations also are under the influence of the sympathetic nervous system. Flow in those beds also may be critically reduced, even though arterial pressure is still at normotensive levels. Reduction in cutaneous blood flow can be detected from the color and temperature of the skin. Skeletal muscle and splanchnic flow are vital in the maintenance of normal lactate metabolism. A reduction in those flows leads to a rise in blood lactate levels and the development of metabolic acidosis, which may be detected from arterial blood gases.[3] Early in the course of shock, the arterial blood may reveal an isolated reduction in PCO_2 that is indicative of hyperventilation, but the pH subsequently begins to fall and the patient enters a more rapid downhill phase of tissue underperfusion. The skin and muscle flow in the upper extremities is also critical in the maintenance of arterial pulses in the upper extremities and of an auscultatory blood pressure. The thready radial and brachial pulses and unobtainable auscultatory blood pressure associated with shock are due more often to intense upper extremity vasoconstriction than to hypotension.[4]

Table 3–1.   *Manifestations of Regional Flow Deficiency in Shock*

Renal manifestations
    Oliguria (<20 ml/hr)
    Sodium conservation (<20 mEq/liter urine)

Cutaneous manifestations
    Cool extremities
    Diaphoresis
    Peripheral cyanosis

Skeletal muscle manifestations
    Reduced peripheral pulse volume
    Reduced auscultatory blood pressure
    Lactic acidosis

Splanchnic manifestations
    Lactic acidosis
    Ileus
    Mesenteric infarction

Cerebral manifestations
    Agitation, confusion
    Coma
    Hypoventilation

Coronary manifestations
    Myocardial ischemia
    Arrhythmias

The cerebral and coronary beds are less affected by sympathetic nervous system activity and are more under the influence of aortic perfusion pressure. The confusion, restlessness, and somnolence associated with shock is usually due to arterial hypotension, but sometimes inadequate cerebral blood flow may be detected even before the blood pressure falls; thus the sensorium of the patient is another critical guide to the diagnosis of shock. Coronary arterial flow decreases as the blood pressure falls, and in the later stages of shock that arterial hypotension is an important factor in progressive deterioration of cardiac function.[5] Indeed, most of the peripheral vascular reactions that contribute to the regional flow deficiencies in shock represent the body's attempt to prevent hypotension, for once hypotension develops, a rapid deterioration of the cardiovascular system can be expected and survival may be very short. The manifestations of regional flow deficiency in shock are summarized in Table 3–1.

THE HEART IN SHOCK

Regardless of the cause of shock, the heart plays a pivotal role in its progression. In pure hemorrhagic shock, for instance, the reduction in the venous return precipitates a fall in the cardiac output, which induces the peripheral vascular reactions that are clinically detected as the shock syndrome. If the circulating blood volume is quickly restored to normal levels, no change in cardiac function may be detected. However, if there is some delay in the correction of the inadequate blood volume and if the hypotension persists for any length of time, cardiac function begins to deteriorate.[6] Because of the sympathetic discharge that accompanies the low cardiac output, the contractility of the myocardium is increased. If the increase in contractility cannot be reflected in an increase in arterial pressure because of a low circulating blood volume, the coronary blood flow may be inadequate to provide the oxygen required to maintain enhanced cardiac contractility.[7] Therefore, the myocardial function may begin to deteriorate, and the left ventricular end-diastolic pressure may begin to rise. That increase in the left ventricular diastolic pressure is a further impediment to the coronary blood flow since the effective coronary perfusion pressure is the aortic diastolic pressure minus the left ventricular diastolic pressure.[8] Progressive subendocardial ischemia may develop, because it is the subendocardium that is most vulnerable to reductions in effective perfusion pressure. The resultant failure of the left ventricle may then contribute to the peripheral flow deficiency, and a cardiogenic factor comes to play a role in what was initially pure hypovolemic shock. That same chain of events may affect the performance of the heart in all kinds of shock, even those that are initiated by acute myocardial infarction. The balance between myocardial oxygen supply and oxygen delivery is thus a critical factor in the progression of shock,[9] and that balance takes on even more significance in the patient with coronary disease, as will be discussed later. The factors that impair cardiac function in shock are summarized in Table 3–2.

The simplest bedside way to evaluate cardiac function is to relate the cardiac output or the stroke volume to the ventricular filling pressure (Fig. 3–1).[10] Information about the bedside evaluation of cardiac function is summarized in Table 3–3. In the right ventricle, the filling pressure represents the central venous pressure or the mean right atrial pressure. In the left ventricle the filling pressure can be assessed either from a measurement of the left ventricular end-diastolic pressure or the pulmonary wedge pressure. With the increasing popularity of invasive methods

Table 3–2.   *Factors That Impair Cardiac Function in Shock*

Low aortic perfusion pressure
High left ventricular diastolic pressure
Hypoxemia
Acidosis
Arrhythmias (tachyarrhythmias or bradyarrhythmias)
The use of depressant drugs

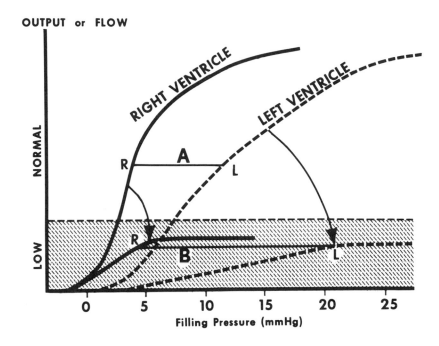

Figure 3–1.   The effect of acute myocardial infarction on right and left ventricular function curves. Both curves are depressed downward and to the right (arrows), but the depression of the left ventricle curve usually is greater than that of the right so that the difference between the left and right ventricular filling pressures (line B) is greater after myocardial infarction than in the normal heart (line A). In true "pump failure," output remains in the low (shaded) zone even at very high filling pressures.

Table 3–3.   *Bedside Evaluation of Cardiac Function*

Evaluation of Filling Pressure	Evaluation of Output
Right	Skin temperature
Central venous pressure	Pulse volume
Jugular venous pressure	Urine output
Hepatojugular reflux	State of consciousness
	Arterial blood gases analysis
Left	
Pulmonary artery diastolic	
or wedge pressure	
Left ventricular diastolic pressure	
Rales	
Pulmonary congestion	
(as shown on the roentgenogram)	
Delayed mitral valve closure	
(as shown on the echocardiogram)	

for bedside evaluation of cardiac function, it is now relatively simple to assess both right and left ventricular function in patients with shock. The cardiac output need not be measured directly but can be assessed qualitatively from an evaluation of the adequacy of regional perfusion. Thus thready pulses, cool skin, low urine output, and metabolic acidosis all may be used as signs of a low cardiac output. Right and/or left ventricular filling pressure must be measured directly with catheters advanced blindly at the bedside by well-established techniques. The right ventricular filling pressure often can be assessed by a careful evaluation of the deep jugular venous pulse as the patient is carefully positioned in bed. Nonetheless, direct measurement of that pressure is usually more satisfactory. In patients with cardiac dysfunction developing as a result of sepsis or of prolonged shock regardless of cause, the right and left ventricular functions appear to be relatively equally impaired. Therefore, both the right and left ventricular function curves are shifted to the right, and the central venous pressure and the left ventricular filling pressure bear a normal relationship to each other, with the pulmonary wedge pressure averaging between 5 and 10 mm Hg higher than the right atrial pressure.[11] In patients with acute cor pulmonale, right ventricular filling pressure is inordinately elevated, and it often rises to levels higher than the left ventricular filling pressure. In contrast, patients with acute myocardial infarction usually manifest a left ventricular filling pressure that is considerably higher than the right ventricular filling pressure. Therefore the central venous pressure is not a reliable guide to the adequacy of myocardial function in the patient with acute myocardial infarction (Fig. 3–1).

VOLUME CHALLENGE

The relative importance of cardiac dysfunction and inadequate venous return in the genesis of the low cardiac output of shock is difficult to evaluate when the ventricular filling pressure is not greatly elevated. The degree of cardiac impairment can best be assessed by sharply augmenting venous return while the ventricular filling pressures and the signs of peripheral blood flow adequacy are monitored.[12] That acute challenge of plasma volume expansion serves two vital purposes in the patient with shock: (1) it provides therapy for the patient whose low cardiac output is due at least in part to inadequate venous return, and (2) it helps to distinguish hypovolemic shock from that due to right or left ventricular dysfunction. A favorable clinical response without much rise in ventricular filling pressure indicates hypovolemia. In contrast, a rise in filling pressure without improvement in the blood flow deficiency indicates cardiac dysfunction, and the ventricle whose filling pressure rises more rapidly is the one that is predominately involved.

Table 3–4.   *Rules for Volume Challenge in Shock*

Monitor the cardiac filling pressure.
Monitor the cardiac output or a bedside sign of output (Table 3–3).
Use a colloid.
Infuse rapidly (25–50 ml/min).
Stop the infusion if the central venous pressure (CVP) rises >3 mm/50 ml.
Stop the infusion if the CVP >20 mm Hg.
Stop the infusion if the pulmonary wedge pressure >20 mm Hg.
Stop the infusion if there is an adverse response: rales, falling blood pressure.
Monitor the blood gases frequently.

In general, patients with a left ventricular filling pressure over 25 mm Hg should not be subjected to volume expansion, because little rise in cardiac output would be expected and there is danger of inducing pulmonary edema.[13] If the left ventricular filling pressure is less than 20 mm Hg, or if the central venous pressure is less than 10 mm Hg and the patient exhibits no signs of left ventricular failure, a cautious trial of volume expansion is indicated. That should be accomplished by administering albumin, dextran, or some other colloidal solution in 50-ml boluses and measuring the ventricular filling pressure after each bolus. As long as the left-side pressure remains below 20 mm Hg, or the central venous pressure rises by less than 3 mm Hg per bolus, the challenge should be continued until the flow deficiency has been corrected. Cessation of the infusion before one of those events has occurred represents an inadequate therapeutic trial.

It is vital that the challenge be carried out rapidly. Thus a 500-ml expansion should take no longer than 20 minutes to complete. Only by such rapid infusion can one be certain that the vascular compartment is expanded and that the venous return is acutely augmented. Since volume-responsive shock is the only form of shock that can be treated with complete success, it is imperative not to miss a case by circumventing an indicated volume challenge. The rules for volume challenge in shock are summarized in Table 3–4.

THE HEMODYNAMICS OF ACUTE MYOCARDIAL INFARCTION

Myocardial infarction is characterized by a rise in left ventricular end-diastolic pressure and a fall in stroke volume.[14] The left ventricular failure is an almost invariable accompaniment of myocardial infarction involving the left ventricle, even when symptoms of heart failure are not detectable at the bedside. More rarely, myocardial infarction involves the right ventricle and leads to predominant right ventricular dysfunction.

Although myocardial infarction has traditionally been viewed as a finite process in which the insult has occurred prior to the patient's hospitalization, recent evidence suggests that the area of ischemia and infarction may enlarge significantly during the first few days of hospitalization.[15] The balance between myocardial oxygen consumption and oxygen supply must therefore be viewed as a dynamic process that may be affected by hemodynamic events that characterize the early phase of convalescence. Thus the elevated end-diastolic pressure, which seems to bear a direct relationship to the severity of the myocardial infarction, may impede subendocardial blood flow and enlarge the area of infarction. Similarly, a reduction in aortic diastolic pressure as a result of a falling cardiac output may also lead to a critical reduction in the coronary blood flow. Structural changes also may affect the hemodynamics. Changes in stiffness of the infarcted area may determine whether the area resists stretch, whether it bulges during ejection, and whether it can dilate adequately during diastole. Changes in function of the mitral valve apparatus because of ischemic insult to the papillary muscle may lead to valvular regurgitation.

MECHANISMS OF SHOCK AFTER ACUTE MYOCARDIAL INFARCTION

When the peripheral blood flow becomes critically reduced after acute myocardial infarction, the prognosis is grave. A mortality of between 80 and 95% despite intensive medical therapy has been reported from a number of institutions. Autopsy studies of patients dying of myocardial infarction shock usually have revealed extensive damage to the left ventricle, with more than 40% of its mass infarcted.[16] Those findings have suggested to some that the appearance of shock indicates that the infarction is so extensive that medical therapy is doomed to failure. Nonetheless, the fact that most shock after myocardial infarction develops in the hospital some hours after the onset of clinical signs suggests that the initial insult is indeed compatible with life and that some subsequent changes in the heart or in the peripheral circulation contribute to the further reduction of the peripheral blood flow. That concept allows one to postulate that the large infarcts observed at the time of autopsy are made up of an original central zone of infarction and a surrounding infarcted area that may have become progressively larger during the course of hospitalization. If that thesis is correct, a strong plea could be made for instituting aggressive therapy early in the course of myocardial infarction before progressive myocardial damage reduces ventricular function so much that survival is impossible. Such an approach would, of course, depend on the availability of an effective form of therapy.

The syndrome of shock after acute myocardial infarction must be viewed as a multifactorial event. Some events are preventable, some are treatable, and some may be beyond help with current therapy.

The Initial Central Zone of Infarction

The initial central zone of infarction usually represents the pathologic equivalent of the episode for which the patient sought medical advice. Since the muscle in the central infarcted zone probably is destroyed within minutes after the initial episode, no therapy to preserve that myocardium is likely to be successful. Depending on the area of the central infarction, varying degrees of left ventricular dysfunction ensue. If the central infarction represents more than 40% of the mass of the left ventricle, or if old and new infarctions render more than 50% of the left ventricle noncontractile, it is unlikely that the patient will survive the acute episode. Indeed, under those circumstances it is probably unlikely that the patient will even survive long enough to reach the hospital. Therefore a patient who has reached the hospital some minutes or hours after his acute episode should be viewed as having a central infarcted zone not large enough to be incompatible with survival.

Peri-infarction Ischemic Zone

Around the central zone of necrosis is an ischemic area in which the balance between the myocardial oxygen consumption and the oxygen supply is tenuous but in which infarction has not yet occurred. Contraction in that ischemic zone may be severely depressed or absent. Thus the ventricle may function as if the infarction were larger than it really is. If events occur that increase the oxygen consumption of this ischemic zone or reduce the delivery of oxygen to this ischemic zone, the area may progress from reversible to irreversible infarction.

Hypovolemia

The circulating plasma volume may be reduced after acute myocardial infarction because of the release of catecholamines, sweating, the reduced fluid intake, or the administration of diuretics.[17] When myocardial function is impaired, the left ventricle requires a higher-than-normal end-diastolic volume or end-diastolic pressure in order to maintain an adequate cardiac output. If the venous return is impaired because of that hypovolemia, the left ventricular filling may fall below its optimal level, and the cardiac output may be correspondingly reduced. Hypovolemia is rarely the major factor in the development of shock after acute myocardial infarction, but it may be a significant factor often enough that it must be kept in mind and evaluated by the use of a measurement of the left ventricular filling pressure.

Peripheral Vasoconstriction

When the cardiac output falls, reflex activation of the sympathetic nervous system ensues. The myocardium is thus stimulated by adrenergic mechanisms to increase its contractility, and the peripheral vascular bed is constricted in order to maintain the arterial pressure despite the reduction in cardiac output. Such a mechanism to maintain arterial pressure is critical to the maintenance of life, because severe hypotension is incompatible with survival. However, the sympathetic nervous system reaction often is inappropriately intense, and the arterial pressure may rise to a level above that required to maintain tissue perfusion. Pressure work and oxygen consumption of the left ventricle is thus inordinately increased, and an imbalance between oxygen consumption and oxygen delivery may lead to a further deterioration of the left ventricular function.

Inadequate Vasoconstriction

Some people, particularly those who are elderly or have a chronic debilitating disease, such as diabetes, may exhibit impairment of the peripheral vasoconstrictor response to a falling cardiac output.[2] In those people, the blood pressure falls with the cardiac output, and the reduced aortic pressure may lead to further impairment of the myocardial oxygen delivery and a progressive enlargement of the area of infarction. Thus while too much vasoconstriction may be deleterious, so also may too little vasoconstriction.

Arrhythmias

Disturbances in cardiac rhythm may play an important role in the falling cardiac output of shock. Bradyarrhythmias, tachyarrhythmias, and frequent ventricular premature beats may all contribute to the inadequacy of a heart that might otherwise be functioning at a level sufficient to maintain peripheral perfusion. Heart rates below 70 beats per minute may be deleterious when the stroke volume is limited, and even isolated ventricular premature beats may be dangerous in patients with severe ischemia, because the premature beat may consume oxygen without doing any useful work. Rapid heart rates greatly increase the myocardial oxygen consumption and may set up a vicious cycle of progressive ischemia and progressive deterioration of the cardiac function.

Drugs

The administration of drugs that depress myocardial contractility may play an important role in the development of the shock syndrome. Drugs that may be given safely to patients with a more normal myocardial function may be hazardous to the patient whose function is at a critical level. The antiarrhythmic drugs, such as lidocaine, quinidine, procainamide, and, particularly, propranolol, may all be culprits. Great caution, therefore, should be exercised in the use of those drugs in patients with mild arrhythmias, particularly when the arrhythmias are a manifestation of left ventricular failure. It is also important to recognize that the cardiac dysfunction that may result from the pharmacologic action of those drugs may long outlast the biologic life of the drug since positive feedback mechanisms initiated during the period of cardiac dysfunction may continue and progress even though the direct myocardial action of the drug is no longer operating.

Hypoxemia and Acidosis

A reduction in the oxygen saturation of arterial blood and lactic acidosis, both of which phenomena commonly complicate the course of myocardial infarction shock, may further depress myocardial function and thus may play a role in the progression of the shock syndrome.[18]

PUMP FAILURE AFTER ACUTE MYOCARDIAL INFARCTION

The term pump failure is diagnostically less restrictive than the term shock because the former term does not necessarily require the documentation of hypotension and organ perfusion failure. Indeed, no clear-cut diagnostic criteria for pump failure exist. The term is reserved for the patient with acute myocardial infarction who has severe left ventricular dysfunction but not necessarily shock. A left ventricular filling pressure over 25 mm Hg with a depressed stroke volume would, in some investigators' view, fulfill the criteria.

What is most critical in the diagnostic category pump failure is that the mortality is very high. Although it does not reach the 85% level reported in shock, the 21-day mortality does range from about 30 to 60%. The high risk may well justify aggressive intervention to attempt to restore peripheral perfusion and, if possible, to reduce the myocardial ischemia. Although data on the response of the "pump-failure" group to therapy are not available, it is likely that the prognosis would be more easily improved by therapy in that group than it would be in the group of patients who develop the full-blown shock syndrome. The following sections, therefore, discuss therapy to combat left ventricular failure and flow deficiency after myocardial infarction, regardless of whether the stringent criteria for shock are met.

MONITORING THE PATIENT WITH PUMP FAILURE

The patient with pump failure complicating acute myocardial infarction cannot be treated adequately without knowledge of the bedside measurements discussed in the following paragraphs.

Arterial Pressure

The cuff pressure is an unreliable guide to the arterial pressure in the patient with pump failure. An indwelling cannula in the brachial, radial, or femoral artery attached to a strain-gauge transducer and a display oscilloscope or recorder is a necessity.

Left Ventricular Filling Pressure

The central venous pressure is a crude and unreliable guide to the left ventricular function in acute myocardial infarction. A balloon-tipped catheter in the pulmonary artery or an arterial catheter advanced retrogradely from the femoral artery into the left ventricle provides a measurement of the left ventricular filling pressure that is vital in selecting therapy and following the patient's course.[19,20]

Urine Output

An indwelling bladder catheter is needed to assess the adequacy of renal perfusion, which serves as a guide to the course of shock.

Blood Gases

Determinations of the arterial blood gases should be obtained at frequent intervals to assure that oxygenation is adequate and acidosis has been corrected.

MANAGEMENT OF PUMP FAILURE

General Considerations

Information about the treatment of myocardial infarction shock is summarized in Table 3–5.

Table 3–5. *Rules for the Treatment of Myocardial Infarction Shock*

Maintain adequate oxygenation (monitor the arterial blood gases).

Correct tachyarrhythmia (>140 beats per min) or bradyarrhythmia (<60 beats per min).

Measure the arterial pressure directly and keep the systolic pressure above 90 mm Hg.

Measure the pulmonary wedge pressure and keep it between 15 and 20 mm Hg.

Correct acidosis (monitor the arterial blood gases).

Use albumin if necessary to adjust the pulmonary wedge pressure.

Use sodium nitroprusside (20–200 μg/min) if the systolic arterial pressure >100 mm Hg.

Use dopamine or dobutamine (10–15 μg/kg/min) if the systolic pressure <100 mm Hg. Add sodium nitroprusside if necessary.

Use norepinephrine if the arterial pressure cannot be maintained.

Consider mechanical support or emergency surgery.

Table 3–6. *Drugs Commonly Used to Treat Shock*

Drug	Dosage
Vasodilator drugs	
Sodium nitroprusside (Nipride)	20–200 μg/min IV
Hydralazine (Apresoline)	10–50 mg IM
Phentolamine (Regitine)	0.5–2 mg/min
Inotropic drugs	
Dopamine (Intropin)	10–30 μg/kg/min
Dobutamine (Dobutrex)	5–15 μg/kg/min
Inotropic-vasodilator drug	
Isoproterenol (Isuprel)	1–5 μg/min
Inotropic-vasoconstrictor drugs	
Norepinephrine (Levophed)	5–30 μg/min
Metaraminol (Aramine)	100–1000 μg/min
Diuretic drugs	
Furosemide (Lasix)	20–200 mg IV

The most important early goal of the physician is correction of those contributory factors that may yield to relatively simple therapy. Rhythm and rate must be controlled at most effective levels. Acidosis and hypoxia must be treated. Antiarrhythmic drugs (Chapter 7) that may depress myocardial function should be stopped, or at least the dosage should be reduced to minimally effective therapeutic levels. An attempt should be made to adjust ventricular filling pressure to optimal levels by the use of plasma volume expanders if the pressure is low or by the application of tourniquets or phlebotomy if the pressure is very high.

Corticosteroids have been recommended as appropriate therapy for all kinds of shock and low-flow states. Their use in cardiogenic shock is not based on controlled observations, but evidence does exist that pharmacologic doses of steroids (methylprednisolone, 30 mg/kg in a single dose) may prolong the "reversibility" of shock by stabilizing lysosomal membranes. Therefore, steroids might well be administered along with other more specific therapy in the patient with severe shock that is not likely to yield promptly to conventional treatment. Information about the drugs commonly used to treat shock is summarized in Table 3–6.

Vasodilator Drugs

When peripheral blood flow is reduced and arterial pressure still is supported at normotensive levels (pump failure, "preshock"), vasodilator drugs have proved to be an effective pharmacologic approach to therapy.[21] Most experience has been gained with the use of sodium nitroprusside (Nipride) given in a continuous intravenous infusion of from 20 to 200 μg/min. Similar responses to nitroglycerin and the long-acting nitrates have been observed, but dosage titration with those latter drugs is more difficult. Phentolamine (Regitine) and trimethaphan (Arfonad) have also been used for their vasodilating properties.

The vasodilator drugs improve left ventricular performance by lowering the impedance against which the left ventricle must eject blood. Since arterial pressure is reduced and cardiac contractility is little altered, the oxygen consumption of the heart is lowered at the same time that its output is increased. The goal of therapy with vasodilators is to reduce the left ventricular filling pressure and to increase the cardiac output without inordinately reducing the arterial pressure. The drug dose should be adjusted to attain that goal, and great care must be exercised to avoid hypotension, which can be hazardous in the patient with acute myocardial infarction.

Isoproterenol is also used as a vasodilator drug, but because of its prominent inotropic and chronotropic properties, it is more appropriate to discuss it in the next section.

Inotropic Drugs

The use of inotropic drugs to treat pump failure would appear to be rational, but recent evidence has suggested that such therapy may be harmful in patients with acute myocardial infarction.[15] All inotropic drugs augment myocardial oxygen consumption by virtue of their effect on contractility, and further oxygen wasting may result from induced increases in heart rate and arterial pressure.[7] Thus inotropic drugs may aggravate the intramyocardial imbalance between myocardial oxygen consumption and oxygen delivery. Enlargement of the area of infarction or ischemia could result.

Digitalis. The cardiac glycosides increase cardiac contractility but do not produce much increase in the cardiac output in patients with cardiogenic shock.[22] They possess peripheral vasoconstrictor properties that may be deleterious, and they may precipitate arrhythmias, especially in hypotensive patients. The cardiac glycosides therefore have little place in the acute management of the pump failure of myocardial infarction although they may still be useful in the treatment of supraventricular arrhythmias (Chapter 7).

Isoproterenol. Isoproterenol, a potent inotropic drug, dilates the peripheral vascular bed, especially skeletal muscle, but it also increases the heart rate and automaticity. Although it has proved to be a very effective drug in treating low-output states not due to ischemic heart disease, its use in myocardial infarction is hazardous because of the marked rise in myocardial oxygen consumption it induces. Its only rational use is in the patient with normal intra-arterial pressure and marked peripheral vasoconstriction in whom low doses may be effective in restoring blood flow without much increase in heart rate.

Norepinephrine and Metaraminol. Norepinephrine and metaraminol produce both inotropism and peripheral vasoconstriction. When they are administered to a hypotensive patient, the induced increase in myocardial oxygen consumption usually is counterbalanced by a rise in coronary blood flow because of the restoration of the aortic diastolic pressure. Thus those drugs may be tolerated by the ischemic ventricle for short periods.[23] However, the regional blood flow often is reduced and the shock state usually is not reversed.

Dopamine and Dobutamine. Dopamine (Intropin) and dobutamine (Dobutrex) are sympathomimetic amines that have a more selective inotropic effect than either norepinephrine or isoproterenol. Dopamine exerts peripheral vasoconstriction at higher doses, but it has a renal vasodilator effect at lower doses.[24] Dobutamine has only a modest peripheral vasodilator effect at higher doses.[25] Both drugs increase cardiac output, but the increase is more linearly related to dose with dobutamine; dobutamine also produces less increase in heart rate and a greater fall in left ventricular filling pressure than dopamine. On the other hand, dopamine is more effective in raising arterial pressure in hypotensive patients because of its vasoconstrictor effect. Therefore, dobutamine may be the sympathomimetic drug of choice when an increase in cardiac output is desired, whereas dopamine may be the drug of choice when hypotension accompanies severe left ventricular failure.

Glucagon. Glucagon produces an unreliable inotropic effect, but since it is well tolerated and easily administered, a 5-mg intravenous dose as a test for responsiveness may be worthwhile. If a beneficial effect is observed, a continuous infusion of the drug may be administered; however, there has been little experience with prolonged infusions of the drug. Nausea is a frequent side effect.

Vasoconstrictor Drugs

The only indication for administering a vasoconstrictor drug to the patient with pump failure after acute myocardial infarction is hypotension. Rapid restoration of arterial pressure is critical to the patient's survival in that condition, and a vasoconstrictor drug counteracts hypotension most rapidly. However, peripheral vasoconstriction increases the work load on the left ventricle and may both increase myocardial oxygen consumption and reduce cardiac output. Norepinephrine, which also possesses inotropic properties, is the drug of choice. It should not be administered, however, unless hypotension is documented by intra-arterial pressure measurement or unless signs of cerebral underperfusion exist. Angiotensin and methoxamine, which are relatively devoid of direct cardiac effects, probably have no place in the management of pump failure complicating myocardial infarction.

Mechanical Cardiac Assistance

When pump failure persists after correction of those factors that can be specifically treated, after adjustment of the left ventricular filling pressure to above 20 mm Hg and after a short trial of pharmacologic therapy with vasodilator, inotropic, or vasoconstrictor drugs, then consideration should be given to mechanical cardiac assistance.

Intra-aortic balloon pumping has proved to be an effective means of improving the circulatory status of patients with cardiogenic shock.[26] However, long-term survival has been less common, probably because of the extensiveness of the cardiac damage at the time balloon pumping has been instituted. Many experts feel that early intervention with a mechanical assistance device is preferable to waiting until the patient's condition has deteriorated during ineffective medical therapy.

At present, it is probably advisable for mechanical assistance to be used only in institutions with well-trained medical and cardiac surgical teams. Patients probably should not be subjected to mechanical assistance if they have a history of chronic heart failure with considerable cardiomegaly.

Cardiac Surgery

Emergency surgery for the patient with pump failure has been advocated in some institutions. Revascularization of an ischemic zone and excision of dyskinetic areas of the left ventricle have in some cases led to survival that otherwise seemed unlikely. Cardiac surgery is the only hope for patients who respond initially to intra-aortic balloon pumping but cannot sustain their circulation when the pump is turned off. The surgical therapeutic approach is discussed in detail in Chapter 18.

SUMMARY

1. Shock represents a syndrome of inadequate peripheral blood flow in which insufficient cardiac output is precipitated by inadequate venous return or impairment of cardiac function or by a combination of the two.

2. The diagnosis of shock can be made only when a deficiency of perfusion results in demonstrable abnormalities in organ function, but subtle reductions in perfusion usually precede the appearance of clinical shock, and therapy introduced in the preshock phase may be most effective.

3. In acute myocardial infarction, an impairment of left ventricular function is an important factor in the genesis of shock, but reduction in venous return, abnormalities in peripheral vascular regulation, disturbances in rhythm, adverse effects of antiarrhythmic drugs, and abnormalities in oxygenation and acid-base balance all may contribute to the circulatory failure. When a state of low peripheral blood flow persists after those nonmyocardial factors have been corrected, the diagnosis of pump failure can be made.

4. Managing the patient with pump failure requires the monitoring of directly measured arterial pressure, left ventricular filling pressure (pulmonary wedge pressure), hourly urine output, and blood gases.

5. Pharmacologic management includes the use of vasodilator drugs if intra-arterial pressure is adequate and the cautious use of inotropic or inotropic-vasoconstrictor drugs if arterial pressure is low. New inotropic drugs provide some choice in the selection of therapy, but the risks of an increase in myocardial oxygen consumption always must be considered when those drugs are employed.

6. Mechanical cardiac assistance and emergency cardiac surgery have been the only rational approaches to the patient whose circulation continues to deteriorate despite appropriate pharmacologic therapy.

7. Intra-aortic balloon pumping has been widely employed, but no controlled studies are available to document the long-term benefit of the procedure.

8. Earlier intervention with aggressive invasive management may eventually prove to be effective, but careful prospective studies must be carried out.

REFERENCES

1. Thal, A.P., and Kinney, J.M.: On the definition and classification of shock. Prog. Cardiovasc. Dis. 9:527, 1967.
2. Cohn, J.N., and Luria, M.: Studies in clinical shock and hypotension. IV. Variations in reflex vasoconstriction and cardiac stimulation. Circulation 34:823, 1966.
3. Shubin, H., Afifi, A., Rand, W., and Weil, M.: Objective index of hemodynamic status for quantitation of severity and prognosis of shock complicating myocardial infarction. Cardiovasc. Res. 2:329, 1968.
4. Cohn, J.N.: Blood pressure measurement in shock. Mechanisms of inaccuracy in auscultatory and palpatory methods. J.A.M.A. 199:972, 1967.
5. Berne, R.M.: Regulation of coronary blood flow. Physiol. Rev. 44:1, 1964.
6. Guyton, A.C., and Crowell, J.W.: Cardiac deterioration in shock. I. Its progressive nature. Int. Anesthesiol. Clin. 2:159, 1964.
7. Sonnenblick, E.H., and Skelton, C.L.: Myocardial energetics: Basic principles and clinical implications. N. Engl. J. Med. 285:668, 1971.
8. Salisbury, P.F., Cross, C.E., and Rieben, P.A.: Acute ischemia of inner layers of ventricular wall. Am. Heart J. 66:650, 1963.
9. Haddy, F.J.: Physiology and pharmacology of the coronary circulation and myocardium, particularly in relation to coronary artery disease. Am. J. Med. 47:274, 1969.
10. Sarnoff, S.J., and Berglund, E.: Ventricular function. I. Starling's law of the heart studied by means of simultaneous right and left ventricular function curves in the dog. Circulation 9:706, 1954.
11. Cohn, J.N., and Tristani, F.E.: Studies in clinical shock and hypotension. VI. Relationship between left and right ventricular function. J. Clin. Invest. 48:2008, 1969.
12. Cohn, J.N., Luria, M.H., Daddario, R.C., and Tristani, F.: Studies in clinical shock and hypotension. V. Hemodynamic effects of dextran. Circulation 35:316, 1967.
13. Russell, R.O., Jr., Rackley, C.E., Pombo, J., Hunt, D., Potanin, C., and Dodge, H.T.: Effects of increasing left ventricular filling pressure in patients with acute myocardial infarction. J. Clin. Invest. 49:1539, 1970.
14. Hamosh, P., and Cohn, J.N.: Left ventricular function in acute myocardial infarction. J. Clin. Invest. 50:523, 1971.
15. Maroko, P.R., Kjekshus, J.K., Sobel, B.E., Watanabe, T., Covell, J.W., Ross, J., Jr., and Braunwald, E.: Factors influencing infarct size following experimental coronary artery occlusion. Circulation 43:67, 1971.
16. Page, D.L., Caulfield, J.B., Kastor, J.A., DeSanctis, R.W., and Saunders, C.A.: Myocardial changes associated with cardiogenic shock. N. Engl. J. Med. 285:133, 1971.
17. Agress, C.M., Rosenburg, M., Binder, M.J., Schneiderman, M., and Clark, W.: Blood volume changes in protracted shock resulting from experimental myocardial infarction. Am. J. Physiol. 166:603, 1951.
18. Wildenthal, K., Mierzwiak, D.S., Myers, R.W., and Mitchell, J.H.: Effects of acute lactic acidosis on left ventricular performance. Am. J. Physiol. 214:1352, 1968.
19. Swan, H., Ganz, W., Forrester, J., et al.: Catheterization of the heart in man with the use of a flow-directed balloon tipped catheter. N. Engl. J. Med. 283:447, 1970.
20. Cohn, J.N., Khatri, I.M., and Hamosh, P.: Bedside catheterization of the left ventricle. Am. J. Cardiol. 25:66, 1970.
21. Cohn, J.N.: Vasodilator therapy for heart failure: The influence of impedance on left ventricular performance. Circulation 48:5, 1973.
22. Cohn, J.N., Tristani, F.E., and Khatri, I.M.: Cardiac and peripheral vascular effects of digitalis in cardiogenic shock. Am. Heart J. 78:318, 1969.
23. Mueller, H., Ayers, S.M., Giannelli, S., Conklin, E.F., Mazzara, J.T., and Grace, W.J.: Effect of isoproterenol, 1-norepinephrine, and intraaortic counterpulsation on hemodynamics and myocardial metabolism in shock following acute myocardial infarction. Circulation 45:335, 1972.
24. Goldberg, L.I.: Cardiovascular and renal actions of dopamine: Potential clinical applications. Pharmacol. Rev. 24:1, 1972.

25. Akhtar, N., Chaudhry, M.H., and Cohn, J.N.: Dobutamine: Selective inotropic action in patients with heart failure. Circulation 48(Suppl. IV): 538, 1973.
26. Kuhn L.A.: Current status of diastolic augmentation for circulatory support. Am. Heart J. 81:281, 1971.

Chapter 4

A RATIONAL APPROACH TO THE PREHOSPITAL MANAGEMENT OF THE CORONARY ATTACK

J. F. PANTRIDGE
A. A. J. ADGEY

GENERAL CONSIDERATIONS

More than two-thirds of the premature deaths from acute myocardial infarction occur before the patient reaches the hospital. Sixty-three per cent of the deaths among men 50 years old or less occur within one hour of the onset of symptoms,[2] and among people of both sexes under 65 years old, with an initial coronary attack 61% of the deaths occur within the hour.[16] Hospital coronary care units cannot affect significantly the community mortality from acute myocardial infarction, which is around 40%,[14] since the median time between the onset of the illness and hospital admission may be more than eight hours.[29,30]

Asystolic arrest usually related to acute AV block is responsible for a few sudden deaths, but more than 90% of the early deaths from coronary artery disease are due to ventricular fibrillation.[1] Clinical and experimental evidence indicates that after coronary occlusion the size of the infarction is likely to be determined within the first few hours and that early therapeutic intervention may have a salutary effect on the size.[27,34]

The objectives of prehospital coronary care are therefore to attack the problem of sudden death outside the hospital and to provide treatment for the patient with acute myocardial infarction at the earliest possible moment after the onset of symptoms.

SUDDEN DEATH

Sudden death from ventricular fibrillation outside the hospital will continue to be a major problem since there is no ideal long-term antiarrhythmic drug for the patient with known coronary artery disease. Furthermore, ventricular fibrillation may be the first manifestation of ischemic heart disease.

In 1966 it was shown for the first time that the correction of ventricular fibrillation outside the hospital is possible.[32,33] That demonstration led to a proliferation of mobile coronary care units, particularly in the United States. Static units also appeared outside the hospital in football stadiums and in other places where large crowds gather.[47]

Paramedical personnel who operate prehospital coronary care units concentrate on the resuscitation of patients with cardiac arrest. Remarkable success has been achieved with such units. Each year in Seattle, which has a population of about 500,000, more than 100 patients with ventricular fibrillation that occurred outside the hospital are resuscitated. Involvement of lay people in cardiopulmonary resuscitation is part of most prehospital coronary care schemes.[45]

The limitations of cardiopulmonary resuscitation have not been sufficiently recognized. External cardiac massage and ventilation will maintain the viability of the cerebrum for 20 minutes or longer.[22] The arterial pressure during chest compression is about 80 mm Hg, and between compressions it is 10 to 20 mm Hg.[22] Even a highly sophisticated mechanical device with a duration of compression 50% of cycle time will not produce a mean arterial pressure of 70 mm Hg.[44] A mean coronary perfusion pressure less than 70 mm Hg is unlikely to give adequate perfusion of the ischemic myocardium. Progression of myocardial injury during cardiopulmonary resuscitation may explain the inverse relationship between the duration of cardiopulmonary resuscitation and the long-term survival rate.

Aware of the limitations of cardiopulmonary resuscitation and aiming at the immediate correction of ventricular fibrillation, one of us (JFP) has concentrated on the development of small and inexpensive (and therefore readily available) defibrillators. The first defibrillator that was used outside the hospital is shown in Figure 4–1. It operated on two 12-volt car batteries and a static inverter. It weighed 64 kg. Continued development of portable defibrillators in our laboratories has resulted in an instrument

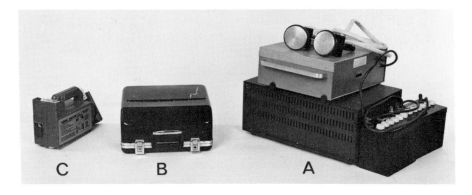

Figure 4–1.   Defibrillators developed in the cardiac department of the Royal Victoria Hospital in Belfast. A. The first "portable" defibrillator, weight 64 kg. B. Defibrillator weighing 25 kg. C. Belfast defibrillator Mark II, weighing 3.2 kg.

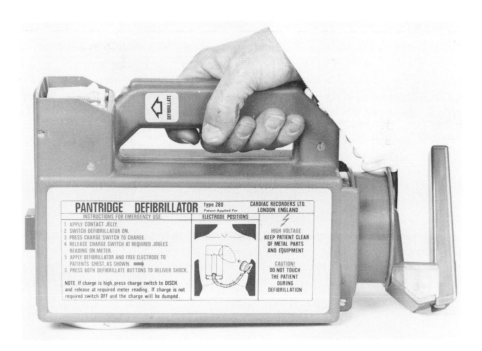

Figure 4–2.   Belfast defibrillator Mark II, weight 3.2 kg.

that weighs 3.2 kg (Figs. 4–1 and 4–2). It stores 400 Wsec, and it delivers 330 Wsec through a resistance of 50 ohms.

In the investigation of the miniaturization of defibrillators and in the quest for a pocket defibrillator, one of us (JFP) considered it imperative to determine whether the 400 Wsec stored energy currently advocated was necessary. Thus in 1974 a prospective study of the efficacy of low-energy shocks was initiated. Preliminary data indicated that 98% of episodes of ventricular fibrillation might be removed by a delivered energy not greater than 165 Wsec.[37]

Animated controversy now exists regarding the energy requirements for successful defibrillation. The majority of workers advocate the use of the maximum stored energy of the defibrillator, usually 400 Wsec.[3,11,12,18,42] The maximum energy delivered through a resistance of 50 ohms by commercially available defibrillators ranges from 270 Wsec (American Optical) to 330 Wsec (Pantridge Portable).[4] Workers at Purdue claim that one-third of patients cannot be defibrillated by the conventional devices.[43] They state that the maximum energy delivered from the usually available defibrillators is inadequate to defibrillate 35% or more of patients weighing over 50 kg and ineffective in 60% of patients weighing 90 to 100 kg. They therefore recommend that defibrillators be capable of delivering 500 to 1000 Wsec and presumably storing 600 to 1200 Wsec.[13] Such devices would therefore be much larger, less portable, more expensive, and less readily available.

The recommendations of Ewy and Tacker[13] are not supported by the data of other workers.[4,5,6,9,21,36,37] The complete Belfast study, which involved 394 episodes of ventricular fibrillation among 214 patients, showed that shocks of 100 Wsec stored energy were successful in 81% of episodes of ventricular fibrillation.[4] A single shock of 100 Wsec stored succeeded in 67% of episodes. Shocks of 200 Wsec stored energy succeeded in 95% of episodes, and a single shock of 200 Wsec succeeded in 85% of episodes. Body weight was not related to the success of defibrillation with 200 Wsec stored energy. Among the few patients in the Belfast study who failed to be defibrillated by low energy shocks, there was not a single example of failure with 400 Wsec stored. The maximum delivered energy was 330 Wsec. The lack of a relationship between the energy required for defibrillation and the body weight is apparent in other reports. There are records of successful defibrillation by conventional defibrillators in patients who weigh 108 to 225 kg.[7,8,9,23]

The controversy regarding energy levels for ventricular defibrillation is of considerable importance. Apart from the disadvantages of reduced portability and availability, larger defibrillators carry the risk of cardiac damage. In the experimental situation, increasing the energy of direct current shock was associated with an increasing frequency of arrhythmias.[15,25] The higher the energy level, the greater the amount of myocardial damage.[10] In the clinical situation, there was a direct relationship between the energy used for synchronized direct current conversion and the incidence of postcardioversion arrhythmias and S–T segment displacement.[26,40]

It has been contended that when the initial shock is of low energy it may need to be repeated and that two low-energy shocks cause more damage than does a single shock of identical total energy. But animal experiments do not support the contention. When a given amount of energy is delivered by high-energy shocks, the resultant myocardial damage is greater than when the same total energy is delivered by twice the number of low-energy shocks.[38]

The Belfast data do not support the proposition that defibrillators should store more than 400 Wsec. Indeed, the data suggest that that energy level is excessive for the majority of patients with ventricular fibrillation.

The widespread availability of small inexpensive defibrillators is therefore to be encouraged. Indeed, in certain factories and offices it might be appropriate to have a defibrillator mounted beside the fire extinguisher (Fig. 4–3).

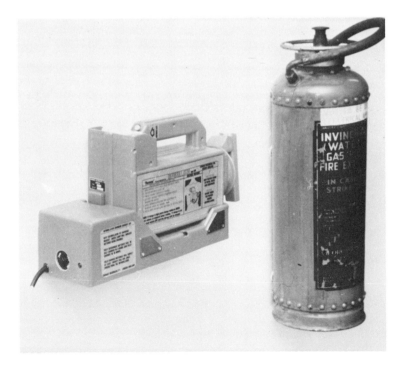

Figure 4–3.   Defibrillator on charging unit mounted beside a fire extinguisher.

MANAGEMENT OF ACUTE MYOCARDIAL INFARCTION

The therapeutic measures in acute myocardial infarction aim at the relief of pain, correction of the autonomic disturbance, and control of the arrhythmias.

Pain

The immediate relief of pain is particularly important in the management of acute myocardial infarction. Pain may accentuate or initiate autonomic disturbances, and the autonomic disturbances so frequent at the onset may respond to relief of pain alone. The catecholamine release may be diminished by the immediate control of pain. Analgesics should also be used to relieve distress and fear. The ideal analgesic has a rapid effect without causing nausea, vomiting, or hemodynamic disturbance. Morphine is the analgesic most frequently used, but adverse effects with its use have been documented. Profound hypotension and bradycardia may follow the administration of morphine, particularly if the patient is moved. Adverse hemodynamic effects may also occur following the administration of pethidine to patients with acute myocardial infarction. Diamorphine is the most satisfactory of the narcotic drugs, particularly for the control of severe pain. Given in a standard intravenous dose of 5 mg it has little adverse effect on the cardiovascular system. It has a more rapid action and less emetic effect than morphine does. Nausea and vomiting are relatively common at the onset of acute myocardial infarction. Since vomiting is associated with adverse circulatory effects, its immediate control is important. An analgesic is, therefore, given in combination with an antiemetic. Cyclizine has been used, but it has a sympathomimetic effect that is undesirable in patients with normal or already increased heart rates. Metoclopramide monohydrochloride (Maxolon) is a suitable alternative to cyclizine.

Narcotic drugs cannot be given by paramedical personnel. However, in some countries paramedical personnel are permitted to administer nitrous oxide.

Autonomic Disturbance

Among patients with acute myocardial infarction seen within 30 minutes of the onset of symptoms, only 17% have a normal heart rate and normal blood pressure. Nearly 50% show evidence of parasympathetic overactivity with bradycardia, or hypotension, or both, and 22% have a systolic blood pressure not over 80 mm Hg. More than one-third of patients seen within 30 minutes of the onset of symptoms show sympathetic overactivity with tachycardia or transient hypertension or both.[35]

Sinus bradycardia does not require therapy unless the patient also has hypotension or ventricular irritability. However, uncomplicated bradyarrhythmia is uncommon in the early minutes of the acute heart attack. Sinus bradycardia may be corrected by atropine given in aliquots of 0.3 mg to 0.6 mg intravenously. Atropine is often indicated in AV junctional bradycardia since the loss of atrial transport function usually accentuates hypotension. During the administration of atropine, monitoring of the heart rate is imperative to ensure that an appropriately high rate is avoided. Early complete AV block frequently responds to atropine, but the dosage required is significantly greater than that required to correct either sinus or AV junctional bradycardia. The majority of patients with an acute diaphragmatic infarction complicated by complete AV block who are seen soon after the onset of symptoms and who respond to atropine do not require the insertion of prophylactic transvenous pacemakers.

Bradyarrhythmia at the onset of the acute coronary attack may be associated with a lowering of the ventricular fibrillation threshold.[19] Tachycardia resulting from sympathetic overactivity has also an adverse effect on the ventricular fibrillation threshold.[20] A rapid heart rate, either occurring spontaneously or following the administration of an excess of atropine, may precipitate ventricular fibrillation. Tachycardia is likely to affect adversely the magnitude of the infarct. During movement, sinus tachycardia has been shown to occur in more than one-third of patients with acute infarction.[31] Pain relief prior to movement does not reduce significantly the incidence of the rapid heart rate produced by movement. Tachycardia due to sympathetic overactivity, including that occurring on movement, may be controlled by an appropriate beta-blocking drug.

Ventricular Arrhythmias

Ventricular ectopic beats in patients with heart rates less than 60 beats per minute may be abolished by raising the heart rate. An inappropriate rise in the rate may be avoided if the drug is given in aliquots of 0.3 to 0.6 mg intravenously.

Ventricular ectopic beats that occur immediately after the onset of acute infarction in patients with sympathetic overactivity and heart rates greater than 100 beats per minute are frequently abolished when the heart rate is reduced by the careful administration of a beta-blocking drug.

Lidocaine is used for the control of ventricular ectopic beats occurring in the presence of a normal heart rate. The usual dosage is a bolus of 100 mg intravenously, followed by an infusion of 2 mg/min. However, refractory ventricular ectopic beats may require additional boli or an increase in the rate of infusion. Lie and his co-workers[24] gave a bolus of 100 mg intravenously followed by an infusion of 3 mg/min for 48 hours. They claim that that regimen prevents primary ventricular fibrillation in the coronary care unit. However, primary ventricular fibrillation immediately after the onset of symptoms of acute infarction may be more difficult to prevent.

Ventricular tachycardia is relatively uncommon immediately after the onset of acute myocardial infarction. However, when it occurs at that time, it is likely to be complicated by profound hypotension. The administration of antiarrhythmic drugs in that situation or other situations associated with metabolic acidosis may be hazardous. Ventricular tachycardia in the acute phase of infarction is best managed by direct current cardioversion and correction of the metabolic acidosis. Outside the hospital, unsynchronized direct current shock is frequently used.

LIMITATION OF THE SIZE OF THE INFARCT

Appropriate early pharmacological intervention with the relief of pain, the correction of autonomic disturbances, and the prevention or abolition of arrhythmias may limit the area of myocardial damage and thus diminish the incidence of cardiogenic shock.[34] The usual recorded incidence of cardiogenic shock in hospitalized patients with myocardial infarction is 10 to 15%.[41] Yu[47] found that among patients who reported to a life-support station within two hours of the onset of infarction, the incidence of shock was 7% and the hospital mortality was 9.3%. Those seen two hours or more after the onset of symptoms had an incidence of shock of 12.2% and a hospital mortality of 19.2%. Grace and Chadbourn[17] found that among patients with acute infarction managed by a mobile coronary care unit, those seen within the first hour had a hospital mortality of 6%, whereas those seen more than one hour after the onset of symptoms had a hospital mortality of 20%.

A Belfast study showed that among 271 patients under 70 years old with acute myocardial infarction who were managed by a mobile coronary care unit and seen within one hour of the onset of symptoms, the incidence of cardiogenic shock was 3.3% and the hospital mortality was less than 10%.[35] The Belfast findings contrast with the data from the Bristol study, in which a mortality of 25.6% was recorded among comparable patients who sought medical advice within one hour but who did not obtain intensive care within that time.[28]

SUMMARY

1. In the consideration of coronary artery disease, most emphasis is placed on preventive measures. The logic of primary prevention is irrefutable. However, since the etiology of coronary artery disease is multifactorial, it is unlikely that much progress will be made in its prevention in the immediate future.

2. The hospital coronary care unit was an important advance, but it must be supported by some form of prehospital coronary care scheme to enable the patient to get intensive care quickly and at the time when the risk of death is greatest.

3. The logistics of prehospital coronary care will depend on the local situation. In many areas, it may be difficult to staff mobile coronary care units with medical personnel. But it has been shown, particularly in the United States, that paramedical personnel are capable of resuscitating patients who have succumbed to ventricular fibrillation. Prehospital units manned by paramedical personnel have the most impact when a significant proportion of laymen have been instructed in the technique of cardiopulmonary resuscitation.

4. However, the limitations of cardiopulmonary resuscitation, the importance of defibrillation at the earliest possible moment, and thus the necessity for the widespread availability of defibrillators need to be emphasized.

5. Whether paramedical personnel are able to manage the arrhythmias and the autonomic disturbance so frequently present in acute myocardial infarction remains in doubt. There is at present no standardized approach to the correction of those difficulties. Careful titration of the dose of the drugs used is required.

6. Since the arrhythmias and the autonomic disturbance affect the magnitude of the infarct and therefore the incidence of shock and pump failure and the long-term prognosis, there will continue to be a place for mobile coronary care units staffed by physicians. That will be particularly true if the physicians are oriented toward further elucidating the problems of acute myocardial infarction and developing a simplified therapeutic regimen for stabilizing the rhythm and the hemodynamic state and correcting the autonomic disturbance. If such a regimen should evolve, it might be initiated not only by paramedical personnel but also in some situations by the patient himself. Highly efficient automatic spring injectors exist, but what drugs should be carried in the syringes and what their dosages should be are problems to be solved.

7. Any consideration of prehospital coronary care is incomplete without reference to public education directed at reducing the delay between the onset of symptoms and the request for medical help. The American Heart Association has publicity programs for that purpose.

8. The advice frequently given to a stricken person to proceed immediately to the emergency room of the nearest hospital[39] is far from prudent since 22% of patients seen within 30 minutes of the onset of chest pain have a systolic blood pressure of not over 80 mm Hg.[35] It seems more appropriate to advise the victim to lie down immediately and to ask someone else to summon medical help immediately

9. The involvement of the family doctor in coronary care is also

important. If paramedical personnel are able to deal with ventricular fibrillation, the family doctor should also be able to do so. In rural areas, family doctors could be trained to staff mobile coronary care units.

10. Early initiation of coronary care will not only enable more patients to survive to reach a hospital but also limit the size of the infarction in many patients, allowing them to be discharged from the hospital sooner.[46]

REFERENCES

1. Adgey, A.A.J., Nelson, P.G., Scott, M.E., Geddes, J.S., Allen, J.D., Zaidi, S.A., and Pantridge, J.F.: Management of ventricular fibrillation outside hospital. Lancet i:1169, 1969.
2. Bainton, C.R., and Peterson, D.R.: Deaths from coronary heart disease in persons fifty years of age and younger. N. Engl. J. Med. 268:569, 1963.
3. Benson, D.M., Halloran, M., and Miklos, B.: Evaluation of training volunteer ambulance attendants in advanced life support. *In* Proceedings of the National Conference on Standards for Cardiopulmonary Resuscitation (CPR) and Emergency Cardiac Care (ECC). Dallas, American Heart Association, 1975, p. 31.
4. Campbell, N.P.S., Webb, S.W., Adgey, A.A.J., and Pantridge, J.F.: Transthoracic ventricular defibrillation in adults. Br. Med. J. ii:1379, 1977.
5. Crampton, R.S., and Hunter, F.P., Jr.: Low-energy ventricular defibrillation and miniature defibrillators. J.A.M.A. 235:2284, 1976.
6. Crampton, R.S., Barada, F.A., Jr., and Hunter, F.P., Jr.: The coronary care unit: Current trends. *In* H. Just and H.P. Schuster (eds.), Intensiv Medizin in der Inneren Medizin. Stuttgart, Thieme, 1977. p. 12.
7. Crampton, R.S.: Personal communication, 1978.
8. Curry, J.J., and Quintana, F.J.: Myocardial infarction with ventricular fibrillation during pregnancy treated by direct current defibrillation with fetal survival. Chest 58:82, 1970.
9. DeSilva, R.A., and Lown, B.: Energy requirement for defibrillation of a markedly overweight patient. Circulation 57:827, 1978.
10. DiCola, V.C., Freedman, G.S., Downing, S.E., and Zaret, B.L.: Myocardial uptake of technetium-99M stannous pyrophosphate following direct current transthoracic countershock. Circulation 54:980, 1976.
11. Duggan, J.J., and Barrett, M.C.: A community approach to coronary care. *In* Proceedings of the National Conference on Standards for Cardiopulmonary Resuscitation (CPR) and Emergency Cardiac Care (ECC). Dallas, American Heart Association, 1975, p. 189.
12. Dunning, A.J.: The treatment of ventricular fibrillation. *In* L.E. Meltzer and A.J. Dunning (eds.), Textbook of Coronary Care. Amsterdam, Excerpta Medica, 1972. p. 376.
13. Ewy, G.A., and Tacker, W.A., Jr.: Transchest electrical ventricular defibrillation. Am. Heart J. 91:403, 1976.
14. Fulton, M., Julian, D.G., and Oliver, M.F.: Sudden death and myocardial infarction. Circulation 40 (Suppl. IV):182, 1969.
15. Gold, J.H., Schuder, J.C., Stoeckle, H., Granberg, T.A., Hamdani, S.Z., and Rychlewski, J.M.: Transthoracic ventricular defibrillation in the 100 kg calf with unidirectional rectangular pulses. Circulation 56:745, 1977.
16. Gordon, T., and Kannel, W.B.: Premature mortality from coronary heart disease. The Framingham study. J.A.M.A. 215:1617, 1971.
17. Grace, W.J., and Chadbourn, J.A.: The first hour in acute myocardial infarction (AMI): Observations on 50 patients. Circulation 42 (Suppl. III):160, 1970.
18. Green, H.L., Hieb, G.E., and Schatz, I.J.: Electronic equipment in critical care areas: Status of devices currently in use. Circulation 43:A101, 1971.
19. Han, J., Millet, D., Chizzonitti, B., and Moe, G.K.: Temporal dispersion of recovery of excitability in atrium and ventricle as a function of heart rate. Am. Heart J. 71:481, 1966.

20. Kent, K.M., Smith, E.R., Redwood, D.R., and Epstein, S.E.: Electrical stability of acutely ischemic myocardium: Influences of heart rate and vagal stimulation. Circulation 47:291, 1973.
21. Kerber, R.E., and Sarnat, W.: Clinical studies on defibrillation dose: Effects of body weight and heart weight (Abstr.). *In* Proceedings Second Purdue Cardiac Defibrillation Conference, Purdue, Indiana, 1977. p. 10.
22. Kouwenhoven, W.B., Jude, J.R., and Knickerbocker, G.G.: Closed-chest cardiac massage. J.A.M.A. 173:1064, 1960.
23. Lappin, H.A.: Ventricular defibrillators in heavy patients. N. Engl. J. Med. 291:153, 1974.
24. Lie, K.I., Wellens, H.J., Van Capelle, F.J., and Durrer, D.: Lidocaine in the prevention of primary ventricular fibrillation: A double-blind randomized study of 212 consecutive patients. N. Engl. J. Med. 291:1324, 1974.
25. Lown, B., Neuman, J., Amarasingham, R., and Berkovits, B.V.: Comparison of alternating current with direct current electroshock across the closed chest. Am. J. Cardiol. 10:223, 1962.
26. Lown, B.: Cardiac Devices Panel of the Food and Drug Administration, Washington, D.C., F.D.A., 1978.
27. Maroko, P.R., Kjekshus, J.K., Sobel, B.E., Watanabe, T., Covell, J.W., Ross, J., Jr., and Braunwald, E.: Factors influencing infarct size following experimental coronary artery occlusions. Circulation 43:67, 1971.
28. Mather, H.G., Pearson, N.G., Read, K.L.Q., Shaw, D.B., Steed, G.R., Thorne, M.G., Jones, S., Guerrier, C.J., Eraut, C.D., McHugh, P.M., Chowdhury, N.R., Jafary, M.H., and Wallace, T.J.: Acute myocardial infarction: Home and hospital treatment. Br. Med. J. iii:334, 1971.
29. McDonald, E.L.: The London Hospital. *In* D.G. Julian and M.F. Oliver (eds.), Acute Myocardial Infarction: Proceedings of a Symposium. Edinburgh, Livingstone, 1968. p. 29.
30. McNeilly, R.H., and Pemberton, J.: Duration of last attack in 998 fatal cases of coronary artery disease and its relation to possible cardiac resuscitation. Br. Med. J. iii:139, 1968.
31. Mulholland, H.C., and Pantridge, J.F.: Heart-rate changes during movement of patients with acute myocardial infarction. Lancet i:1244, 1974.
32. Pantridge, J.F., and Geddes, J.S.: Cardiac arrest after myocardial infarction. Lancet i:807, 1966.
33. Pantridge, J.F., and Geddes, J.S.: A mobile intensive-care unit in the management of myocardial infarction. Lancet ii:271, 1967.
34. Pantridge, J.F.: The effect of early therapy on the hospital mortality from acute myocardial infarction. Q. J. Med. 39:621, 1970.
35. Pantridge, J.F., Webb, S.W., Adgey, A.A.J., and Geddes, J.S.: The first hour after the onset of acute myocardial infarction. *In* P.N. Yu and J.F. Goodwin (eds.), Progress in Cardiology, vol. 3. Philadephia, Lea & Febiger, 1974. p. 173.
36. Pantridge, J.F., Adgey, A.A.J., Geddes, J.S., and Webb, S.W.: Management of acute infarction. *In* The Acute Coronary Attack. Bath, England, Pitman Medical, 1975. p. 66.
37. Pantridge, J.F., Adgey, A.A.J., Webb, S.W., and Anderson, J.: Electrical requirements for ventricular defibrillation. Br. Med. J. ii:313, 1975.
38. Pantridge, J.F.: Cardiac Devices Panel of the Food and Drug Administration, Washington, D.C., F.D.A., 1978.
39. Paul, O.: Prehospital management of acute myocardial infarction. Med. Clin. North Am. 57:119, 1973.
40. Resnekov, L., and McDonald, L.: Complications in 220 patients with cardiac dysrhythmias treated by phased direct current shock, and indications for electroconversion. Br. Heart J. 29:926, 1967.
41. Scheidt, S., Alonso, D.R., Wilner, G., and Killip, T.: New concepts of cardiogenic shock: Preservation of ischemic myocardium. Bull. New York Acad. Med. 50:247, 1974.
42. Standards for Cardiopulmonary Resuscitation (CPR) and Emergency Cardiac Care (ECC): Advanced life support. J.A.M.A. 227 (Suppl. 7):857, 1974.

43. Tacker, W.A., Jr., Galioto, F.M., Jr., Giuliani, E., Geddes, L.A., and McNamara, D.G.: Energy dosage for human trans-chest electrical ventricular defibrillation. N. Engl. J. Med. 290:214, 1974.
44. Taylor, G.J., Tucker, W.M., Greene, H.L., Rudikoff, M.T., and Weisfeldt, M.L.: Importance of prolonged compression during cardiopulmonary resuscitation in man. N. Engl. J. Med. 296:1515, 1977.
45. Thompson, R.G., Hallstrom, A.P., and Cobb, L.A.: Beneficial effect of bystander-initiated CPR in out-of-hospital ventricular fibrillation (Abstr.). Circulation 56 (Suppl. III):114, 1977.
46. Wilson, C., and Pantridge, J.F.: ST segment displacement and early hospital discharge in acute myocardial infarction. Lancet ii:1284, 1973.
47. Yu, P.N.: Life support stations. Arch. Intern. Med. 134:234, 1974.

Chapter 5

THE CORONARY CARE UNIT

LESLIE WIENER

With few exceptions,[1-3] intensive coronary care has been accepted as an integral part of customary hospital practice. It has been more than a decade since the opening of the first coronary care unit (CCU). Since then, the CCU has changed from a place where high-risk patients were grouped to insure prompt cardiopulmonary resuscitation to an intricate treatment center where various cardiac arrhythmias (see Chapters 7 to 9) that may lead to cardiac arrest and early pump failure are treated more effectively.

This chapter reviews many aspects of the development of the CCU. It describes the operations of the unit, classifies the various cardiac arrhythmias that are commonly associated with acute myocardial infarction, and discusses some of the current methods of treatment of those arrhythmias. Information about drugs commonly used in the CCU is summarized in Table 5–1. Emphasis is also placed on new methods for managing the still unsolved problem of pump failure. Consideration is given to the iatrogenic hazards of the CCU technique, including errors in interpreting the oscilloscope and electrical leakage. Finally, the present and future value of the CCU is examined.

PERSONNEL

At present, there are wide differences in the implementation of the concept of intensive coronary care. The differences are not only in the

71

Table 5–1. *Drugs Commonly Used in the Coronary Care Unit*

	Loading Dose (Intravenous)	Maintenance Dose (Intravenous)	Loading Dose (Oral)	Maintenance Dose (Oral)
Antiarrhythmia Drug Regimens				
Lidocaine	50–100 mg (bolus)	1–4 mg/min		
Quinidine			300 mg q̄ 3 hr for three doses	300–400 mg q̄ 6 hr
Procainamide (Pronestyl)	100 mg/5 min (limit 1000 mg)	2–4 mg/min	1000 mg	250–500 mg q̄ 3 hr
Diphenyl-hydantoin (Dilantin)	100 mg q̄ 5 min for 5 doses (limit 1000 mg)	400 mg/day	500 mg	400 mg/day (divided dose)
Propranolol (Inderal)	0.5 mg/0.5 min for 4 min or less			40–320 mg/day (divided dose)
Digoxin	0.5–1 mg in 3 doses over 8 hr		1 mg in 3 doses over 8 hr	0.25 mg/day
Disopyramide (Norpace)			300 mg	100–200 mg q̄ 6 hr
Inotropic Drug Regimens				
Norepinephrine		4–16 µg/min		
Metaraminol		Dosage varies		
Isoproterenol		1–6 µg/min		
Epinephrine		17–21 µg/min		
Dopamine		15–35 µg/min (initial dose and B effects) 35–70 µg/min (moderate dose and B effects) 140–350 µg/min (high dose and α effects)		
Vasodilator Drugs				
Nitroprusside		20–200 µg/min		
Phentolamine		5 mg q̄ 4 hr		
Nitrates				2.5–20 mg (PO) q̄ 3 hr 2.5–5 mg (SL) q̄ 2 hr
Drugs Useful in Congestive Heart Failure				
Furosemide (Lasix)	20–40 mg/2 min 40 mg 2 hr later if necessary			20–80 mg/day
Ethacrynic acid (Edecin)	50–100 mg/2 min			50–200 mg/day
Aminophylline	250–500 mg/ 10–20 min			500-mg suppositories

physical design of the facilities or in the type of hospital but also in the methods of operation. The success of the coronary care unit has, to a large extent, been dependent on a team approach. Lack of a plan that allocates to each member specific functions and responsibilities results in increased morbidity and mortality. The ideal CCU team consists of a director, specially-trained nursing personnel, paramedical assistants, attending physicians, and house staff. The duties of the various members of the CCU team are discussed in the following paragraphs.

The CCU Director

The director of the CCU is a physician with special interest in and medical knowledge of emergency cardiology. His responsibilities are to:

1. Develop administrative policies of the CCU, determining (a) the purposes and objectives of the CCU, (b) the admitting privileges of physicians, and (c) the priorities for the admission of patients according to special diagnostic categories

2. Review the utilization of all CCU services

3. Establish protocols for treatment and assign specific duties to various members of the team

4. Organize and participate in training programs for the safe and effective use of diagnostic and therapeutic equipment

5. Supervise the collection and analysis of clinical data needed for the retrospective evaluation of care provided in the CCU

6. Recommend what monitoring and supportive equipment is to be used in the unit

7. Act as a consultant in the implementation of specialized monitoring and therapeutic techniques

8. Introduce and use new methods for coronary care

The CCU Nursing Supervisor and Specially Trained Nursing Personnel

The duties of the CCU nurses are to:

1. Recognize premonitory, potentially lethal, cardiac arrhythmias as well as the early signs and symptoms of circulatory failure

2. Initiate prophylactic emergency medical treatment

3. Initiate cardiopulmonary resuscitation when necessary, including direct current shock defibrillation (Chapter 10)

4. Evaluate the effectiveness of the therapies used

5. Decide when a physician is to be notified

Paramedical Assistants: Specially Trained Cardiac Technicians, Electronic Technicians, and Biomedical Engineers

The duties of the specially trained cardiac technicians are to:

1. Contribute to the team effort by setting up and maintaining the more elaborate items of monitoring equipment

2. Chart the course of patients who require invasive cardiac catheterization monitoring

3. Assist in the actual catheterization procedure by preparing sterile set-ups of special trays and by balancing and calibrating equipment for pressure recordings and cardiac output

4. Insure the steady and continuous operation of the monitoring devices by checking them at regular intervals.

The duties of the biomedical engineers are to:

1. Plan and supervise the construction, maintenance, inspection, and repair of equipment

2. Provide supplemental education for staff members who work with life-support equipment

3. Help the CCU director in instructing the CCU personnel about electrical safety

4. Help the CCU director in observing staff members periodically in the performance of their duties when using electrical instruments

5. Develop and test new items of electronic equipment

6. Act as consultants when the purchase of medical equipment is considered

7. Establish a program of regular periodic inspections and testing of equipment for safety and performance

8. Keep a permanent record or log that indicates date, the condition of the apparatus, and the tests made

9. Tag all devices that have been approved for use and repair or modify electronic equipment when necessary

10. Supervise the electronics technicians

The Attending Physicians

The duties of the attending physician are to:

1. Provide general and specific recommendations pertinent to the care of their patients

2. Delegate some of their usual responsibilities to a central medical authority (e.g., the director of the CCU, who in turn directs the members of the team who in emergencies have the power to initiate the established protocols for treatment)

3. Participate as needed in the CCU committee meetings and conferences in order to strengthen the team approach

House Officers: Cardiology Fellows, Medical Residents, and Interns

The duty of the house officers is to implement the care directives established by the CCU treatment protocols, the CCU director, and the attending physician.

ADMISSION AND DISCHARGE POLICIES

It has been clearly demonstrated that death following acute myocardial infarction occurs early in the clinical course. Approximately 70% of the deaths occur in the first five days after the patient's admission to the hospital, or earlier.[4] The remaining deaths occur during the subsequent weeks of hospitalization, and those late deaths are due to circulatory failure and concomitant secondary arrhythmias.[5] Accordingly, aggressive prophylactic management of cardiac arrhythmias cannot be expected to significantly affect the outcome in the group of patients who develop those conditions. Because the period immediately following the onset of symptoms is so important clinically, it is crucial that the unit policy encourage the earliest possible admission of persons suspected of having myocardial infarction.[6] Since there is a striking decrease in mortality after the first two days of myocardial infarction, it appears less crucial to admit a patient whose myocardial infarction is estimated to be more than two days old.[7]

Because of the considerable pressure for admitting persons with suspected or proved myocardial infarction, the discharge policy of the unit is also important—because it determines how many patients can be accommodated. In general, patients with proved transmural myocardial infarction should be monitored for at least 72 hours or until two days have passed since the successful suppression of a life-threatening arrhythmia.

DIAGNOSIS OF ACUTE MYOCARDIAL INFARCTION

In a significant percentage of cases (38%) it is difficult to diagnose acute myocardial infarction. Killip and Kimball[8] have established criteria for placing acute myocardial infarction in one of three separate categories:

1. Acute transmural infarction. Chest pain, abnormal Q waves, changing ECG, and enzyme elevation.

2. Acute myocardial infarction (probably subendocardial). Chest pain, S–T segment and T wave abnormalities, changing ECG, and enzyme elevation.

3. Possible myocardial infarction. Chest pain, abnormal ECG, and nonspecific enzyme changes.

In groups 1 and 2, the hospital mortality was 30%, whereas in group 3 the mortality was only 3%. Thus the mortality statistics by which the efficacy of CCU may be judged depend on the accuracy of a diagnosis of myocardial infarction.

CARDIAC ARRHYTHMIAS (See also Chapters 7 to 9)

The principal contribution of the CCU to the successful management of acute myocardial infarction is that it permits the early recognition and prompt control of cardiac arrhythmias leading to cardiac arrest.

Typically, cardiac arrhythmias can be described according to their site of origin, for example, atrial, AV junctional, and ventricular arrhythmias. Conduction disturbances can be described according to the site and the degree of block manifested; for example, first-, second-, and third-degree AV block, AV nodal or infranodal block, bundle branch block, and bifascicular or trifascicular block.

Tachyarrhythmias (See also Chapter 7)

Tachyarrhythmic disturbances are common during acute myocardial infarction. They include:

1. Paroxysmal ventricular tachycardia (six or more consecutive ventricular premature beats at a rate of more than 160 beats per minute) or ventricular fibrillation should be terminated immediately.

2. Premalignant ventricular premature beats include ventricular ectopic beats that occur with a frequency of more than six per minute, ventricular group beats, multifocal ventricular premature beats, and ventricular beats with R–on–T phenomenon.

3. Ventricular premature beats are observed in about 80% of patients with acute myocardial infarction.[9]

4. Nonparoxysmal ventricular tachycardia (accelerated ventricular rhythm or idioventricular tachycardia) and parasystolic ventricular tachycardia usually produce a relatively slow rate (usually 70 to 130 beats per minute), and they are self limited in most cases. Therefore active treatment is usually not necessary.

5. Persisting sinus tachycardia and atrial tachyarrhythmias (fibrillation or flutter) are often present in conjunction with developing left ventricular failure, but atrial tachyarrhythmias are often transient and self limited.

Treatment of Tachyarrhythmias. Aggressive management of tachyarrythmias requires early, on-line arrhythmia detection followed by prompt therapeutic intervention as follows:

1. Lidocaine (Xylocaine), 50 to 100 mg in up to three successive doses are given for paroxysmal ventricular tachycardia or premalignant ventricular premature beats. Thereafter, an intravenous drip of lidocaine

(diluted in 5% dextrose in water solution, 1 to 4 mg/min) is recommended as a preventive measure.

2. For life-threatening ventricular arrhythmias (e.g., ventricular fibrillation or flutter, and paroxysmal ventricular tachycardia with extremely rapid ventricular rate), immediate application of direct current shock is often life saving (Chapters 7 and 10).

3. When the arrhythmia persists following attempts at weaning the patient from lidocaine, procainamide or quinidine should be added, or they should replace lidocaine.[10]

4. If there are side effects from procainamide and/or quinidine, disopyramide may be substituted.

5. Ventricular tachyarrhythmias refractory to antiarrhythmic drugs and/or direct current shock, may occasionally be successfully treated with an artificial pacemaker with an overdriving pacing rate (Chapter 11).

6. Digitalization is required for persisting supraventricular tachyarrhythmias, particularly atrial fibrillation with rapid ventricular response. Quinidine or procainamide may be necessary for pharmacologic conversion and suppression of atrial tachyarrhythmias in some cases. If the atrial tachyarrhythmia persists, cardioversion with direct current shock may be needed in some cases.

7. In most cases, no active treatment is necessary for nonparoxysmal or parasystolic ventricular tachycardia. Similarly, nonparoxysmal AV junctional tachycardia requires no treatment.

8. In rare cases of refractory ventricular tachyarrhythmias, various surgical approaches (e.g., ventricular aneurysmectomy) may be considered.

Bradyarrhythmias (See also Chapter 8)

The prognosis of bradyarrhythmias developing during myocardial infarction varies primarily as a function of the location and extent of infarction.

1. During myocardial infarction, sinus bradycardia and AV junctional escape rhythm may evolve as a consequence of increased vagal tone.

2. First-degree AV block, Wenckebach (Mobitz type I) AV block, and nonparoxysmal AV junctional tachycardia are frequently observed in patients with acute diaphragmatic (inferior wall) myocardial infarction.

3. Mobitz type II AV block results from extensive anterior myocardial infarction and it often accompanies severe circulatory failure.

4. In complete AV block, diaphragmatic myocardial infarction produces AV nodal block, whereas anterior myocardial infarction produces infranodal block. Complete AV block in anterior myocardial infarction is

frequently preceded by various intraventricular blocks (bundle branch block, bifascicular block, and incomplete trifascicular block).

5. The sick sinus syndrome may be produced by myocardial infarction, and it is more common in diaphragmatic myocardial infarction (Chapter 9).

Treatment of Bradyarrhythmias

1. Sinus bradycardia and AV junctional escape rhythm are initially best treated with intravenous atropine.[11] If the bradycardia persists because of a fall in cardiac output, intravenous isoproterenol is preferable to atropine.

2. An artificial pacemaker is indicated when:[12]

   a. A Mobitz type II AV block is evident
   b. A Wenckebach (Mobitz type I) AV block or complete AV block in diaphragmatic myocardial infarction becomes symptomatic and drug therapy fails to maintain the ventricular rate above 60 beats per minute
   c. Drug therapy increases coronary insufficiency and/or myocardial irritability
   d. Complete AV block in acute anterior myocardial infarction is present
   e. The sick sinus syndrome and the brady-tachyarrhythmia syndrome are present
   f. Refractory tachyarrhythmias (usually ventricular) are present

The Brady-Tachyarrhythmia Syndrome

The term brady-tachyarrhythmia syndrome is used when the arrhythmia consists of a tachyarrhythmia component and a bradyarrhythmia component on the same ECG tracing. The brady-tachyarrhythmia syndrome is commonly a late manifestation of the sick sinus syndrome (Chapter 9).

HEMODYNAMIC MONITORING FOR CIRCULATORY FAILURE

Pulmonary Artery Pressure and Pulmonary Artery Wedge Pressure

The development of a flow-directed, balloon-tipped catheter that can easily be introduced at the bedside into the pulmonary artery without fluoroscopic monitoring may achieve for hemodynamic monitoring what the ECG has achieved for the bedside detection of cardiac arrhythmias. In acute myocardial infarction, knowledge of the left ventricular filling pressure is essential for the reliable measuring of the myocardial performance. On-line measurement of that pressure provides a quantitative means of anticipating pulmonary edema. Monitoring of the pulmonary artery pressure also allows optimum volume support in low-flow, low-pressure states as well as continuous assessment of the hemodynamic effects of complex therapeutic interventions (pharmacologic, electrical, and surgical).

Before the advent of a simple means of bedside monitoring of pulmonary artery pressure, the central venous pressure had been widely used as a guide to fluid therapy. In particular, it was assumed that pulmonary edema could be recognized from elevations in the right heart filling pressure. However, the use of central venous pressure monitoring for that purpose assumes that the right ventricular function reflects changes in the left ventricular function. Forrester and his co-workers[13] presented clear evidence that the central venous pressure correlates poorly with the pulmonary artery wedge pressure after acute myocardial infarction. Furthermore, not infrequently even directional changes in central venous pressure are misleading.

Although the balloon-tipped, flow-directed catheter may be advanced simply into the pulmonary artery with reasonable safety, that invasive approach is not entirely without hazard.[14] Accordingly, application of that approach to the monitoring of patients with myocardial infarction is not likely to be as widespread as non-invasive ECG monitoring.

Criteria for the Selection of Patients for Specialized Invasive Hemodynamic Monitoring

Specialized invasive hemodynamic monitoring is considered to be indicated for the following patients:

1. Patients who manifest left ventricular failure and/or cardiogenic shock

2. Patients who require rapid infusion of intravenous fluids, including blood replacement

3. Patients who require drugs known to have potent depressive effects on myocardial contractility

4. Patients with risk factors that predispose them to left ventricular failure and cardiogenic shock; such factors include massive myocardial infarction, persisting ventricular tachyarrhythmias, and multiple previous myocardial infarctions.

Patients who develop cardiac pump complications tend to be older than those who do not develop pump complications. The average age of patients with left ventricular failure and/or shock following myocardial infarction is slightly more than 65 years.[15] Although shock occurs in any adult age group, it is not commonly seen before the sixth decade. The incidence of previous myocardial infarction as well as of hypertension seems to significantly affect the potential for development of left ventricular failure.[16] Moreover, anterior myocardial infarction and diabetes mellitus are particularly common in patients with cardiogenic shock.[17,18] In the absence of ECG evidence of transmural myocardial infarction and marked elevation in cardiac enzyme levels, left ventricular failure is unlikely.[19] However, subendocardial infarction affecting such vital areas as the papillary muscle may produce severe mitral regurgitation, resulting in congestive heart failure and shock. It has been our policy to expect severe left ventricular dysfunction in patients with acute myocardial infarction associated with the clinical circumstances just mentioned. Consequently, monitoring of the pulmonary artery pressure is employed whenever the patient has the clinical profile of pump failure.

The effectiveness and simplicity of the balloon-tipped catheter technique permit serial monitoring of the pulmonary artery wedge pressure. In addition to providing an index of left ventricular function, high-quality wedge tracings may disclose acute mitral regurgitation due, for example, to papillary muscle dysfunction. However, measurement of the central pulmonary artery pressure suffices for continuous monitoring of left ventricular pressure. In most circumstances the end-diastolic pulmonary artery pressure appears to approximate closely the left ventricular end-

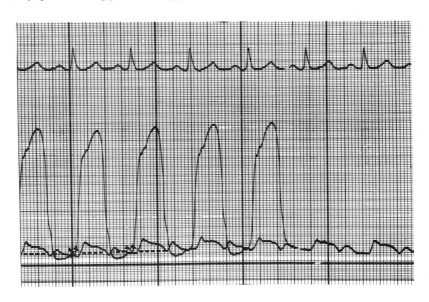

Figure 5–1. The pulmonary artery pressure and the left ventricular pressure are recorded simultaneously. Note that the end-diastolic pulmonary artery pressure and the end-diastolic left ventricular pressure are located at the same pressure level. In the last third of the tracing, the pulmonary artery pressure is recorded simultaneously from both transducers, indicating that the calibration and the sensitivity of each transducer are identical.

diastolic pressure (Fig. 5–1). When the central pulmonary artery is used, the hazard of pulmonary infarction resulting from continuous obstruction of the peripheral pulmonary artery (by the wedged catheter) is avoided.

The catheter insertion technique involves the isolation of a suitably sized antecubital vein. Since the wave forms must be recognized, fluid columns cannot be used. Appropriate strain gauges and display systems are necessary since proper guidance requires the recognition of sequential entry into the right atrium, right ventricle, and pulmonary artery. Because the method is invasive, surgical draping and sterile technique are mandatory. The catheter is prepared for monitoring by being filled from a pressurized fluid source through a flush system (Fig. 5–2). Physiologic saline with four units of heparin per ml is pressurized to 300 mm Hg in an air-free plastic bag. The continuous flow of 2 to 3 ml/hr allowed by the flush system through the catheter prevents clotting and consequent loss of catheter function. A rapid flush valve simplifies filling and flushing the system and permits dynamic response testing of the catheter transducer system.

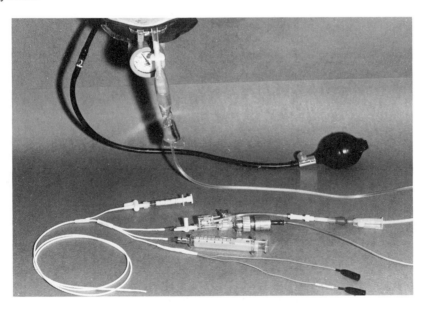

Figure 5–2.   Bedside setup for monitoring pulmonary artery pressure and cardiac output. The catheter terminates in four parts (top to bottom): (1) syringe and stopcock connected through a lumen to a distal balloon; (2) transducer connected through a controlled continuous-flush device (limiting flow to 2 to 3 ml/hr) to a distal-tip catheter opening sampling pulmonary artery pressure; (3) syringe for room-temperature saline injection (thermal dilution cardiac output) connected to a catheter lumen opening 20 cm proximal to the catheter tip; and (4) electric terminals from a distal-tip thermistor connecting to a Wheatstone bridge. (Catheter supplied through the courtesy of the American Catheter Corporation, Stokes Road, Medford, N.J. 08055.)

The principal complications of the use of the balloon-tipped catheter system include cardiac arrhythmias, pulmonary emboli and infarction, and infection. Because of the catheter's construction, cardiac arrhythmias are less frequent with its use than with other types of catheters. During insertion, the balloon-tipped surface tends to cushion the impact as the catheter is manipulated through the sensitive endocardial surfaces along the right ventricular outflow tract. Ventricular premature contractions are encountered only occasionally (in 11% of cases) during passage of the catheter.[14] Pulmonary emboli and infarction can be avoided by the use of low-dose heparin, a continuous flush system, and withdrawal of the catheter from the pulmonary artery wedge position after balloon inflation or during spontaneous advancement. The risk of serious infection can be reduced by the application of a topical antibiotic ointment (Neosporin) to the site of incision, sterile dressings, and removal of the catheter as soon as the patient's clinical condition warrants.

Determination of the Cardiac Output

Determination of the cardiac output provides an additional vital insight into the management of critically ill patients. The simultaneous measurement of the cardiac output and the left ventricular filling pressure provides an objective assessment of left ventricular function in the Frank-Starling framework. In acute myocardial infarction, the relationship of the left ventricular stroke work to the left ventricular end-diastolic pressure invariably shows the most pronounced depression of left ventricular function in patients experiencing cardiogenic shock. Similar but less profound changes are noted when myocardial infarction is complicated solely by the signs and symptoms of heart failure. The manipulation of preload by the rapid infusion of volume expanders in patients with normal or mildly elevated left ventricular filling pressures or the application of potent rapid diuretics when the left ventricular filling pressure is markedly elevated (>20 mm Hg) can establish an optimum left ventricular pressure on an individualized basis. Thus cardiac function may be measured in order to achieve the optimum cardiac output in a manner appropriate to the metabolic requirements of the body. Occasionally in cardiogenic shock the infarcted ventricle does not fully utilize its reserve capacity. In those cases, further increase in end-diastolic pressure can augment the stroke work and avert irreversible changes.

Cardiac output may be measured by central venous injection of Cardio-Green followed by densitometric determination made with blood sampled from a peripheral artery (in the dye dilution technique). However, that technique requires much equipment and technical expertise. An adequate and simple index of cardiac output may be obtained by sampling blood from the pulmonary artery. The close correlation between mixed

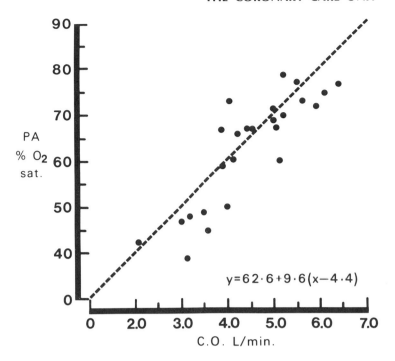

Figure 5–3.   Pulmonary artery (PA) oxygen saturation correlated with cardiac output (CO).

venous oxygen saturation and cardiac output measured by the dye dilution technique has been demonstrated (Fig. 5–3). Recently the balloon-tipped, flow-directed catheter has been modified to permit rapid and accurate measurement of the cardiac output by the thermal dilution technique. A thermistor system is balanced against a Wheatstone's bridge at the patient's body temperature. A 10-cc volume of physiologic saline solution or 5% solution of dextrose in water at room temperature is injected rapidly into the right atrium by means of the proximal lumen of a specially designed balloon-tipped catheter. The off-balance output from the Wheatstone's bridge caused by the change in pulmonary artery blood temperature is amplified and recorded. The area under the temperature-time curve may be determined by planimetry, calculated from the Stewart-Hamilton indicator dilution equipment or computed immediately with an analogue computer.

UNSTABLE ANGINA PECTORIS

Unstable angina pectoris is one of the many terms used to describe the prodromal syndrome of acute myocardial infarction. Other terms are impending myocardial infarction, pre-infarction angina pectoris, acute coronary insufficiency, crescendo angina pectoris, and the intermediate syndrome. Those terms are not necessarily synonymous. Pre-infarction angina pectoris and impending myocardial infarction are terms given to conditions in which myocardial infarction is expected to occur in the near future (zero to three months). Unfortunately, the predicted occurrence of acute myocardial infarction is subject to considerable variation, depending on the criteria applied. Impending myocardial infarction may appear in people who have not had clinical evidence of coronary heart disease, in people with previously stable angina pectoris, and in people who have remained asymptomatic after myocardial infarction. In people with previously stable angina pectoris, the changing anginal pattern is most specific. Two types of unstable angina pectoris are observed: accelerated (or crescendo) angina pectoris and rest angina pectoris. In accelerated angina pectoris, the discomfort is effort induced, easily provoked, intense and persistent, and it responds only hesitantly to nitroglycerine. In rest angina pectoris, on the other hand, the attack develops unpredictably, with no relation to physical or emotional stress, and it is often not relieved by rest or nitroglycerine. In either type, the phenomenon that commands attention is the departure from the previous form of angina. The ECG at rest may be normal. The most characteristic abnormality consists of repeated S–T segment depression and inverted T waves. No sustained ECG changes are evident. Serial cardiac enzyme studies are not indicative of myocardial necrosis.

The terms coronary insufficiency and the intermediate syndrome refer to unstable anginal conditions in which the angina pectoris may occur at rest or with activity but is sustained for periods in excess of 15 minutes. Those conditions appear to have a somewhat higher incidence of morbid complications. Recent evidence indicates that as many as 20% of patients experiencing sustained atypical resting angina pectoris may have Prinzmetal's variant angina pectoris. It has been confirmed that Prinzmetal's variant angina pectoris results from coronary artery spasm. It is cyclic in nature, relatively unresponsive to antiangina therapies, and often accompanied by tachyarrhythmias and bradyarrhythmias. Occasionally it results in myocardial infarction and sudden death.

HAZARDS OF THE CORONARY CARE UNIT

Treatment of acute myocardial infarction in the CCU has distinct advantages, but it also has certain limitations and even dangers.

The ECG as displayed on the oscilloscope is often difficult to interpret because of rapid sweep, baseline instability, 60-cycle interference, movement of the patient, and pacemaker artifacts.[20] The use of electronic filtering circuits, while minimizing those difficulties, often distorts the basic nature of the ECG wave forms. It is important for all staff members working in the CCU to be familiar with those problems so that the ECG will not be misinterpreted.

Leakage of electrical currents can result in ventricular fibrillation.[21] The moist skin under monitoring electrodes may provide a low-resistance pathway for current. Intravascular catheters and, in particular, artificial cardiac pacing catheters form a direct electrical pathway to the heart. Since the ischemic heart can be fibrillated by currents as low as 150 microamp, extreme care must be taken to protect patients from extraneous current leakage. For safety in the CCU, the following guidelines should be observed:

1. A defibrillator with all the necessary equipment and emergency drugs for cardiopulmonary resuscitation should be readily available whenever electrical devices are applied to the patient.

2. Electrical equipment should be checked before and after it is applied to the patient in order to prevent current leakage.

3. The equipment should be adequately grounded to avoid the vast majority of hazards.

4. The ground circuits should be tested periodically to ascertain that they lead to a common ground.

5. New equipment and wiring within the CCU should have properly isolated circuits.

ACCOMPLISHMENTS OF CORONARY CARE UNITS; FUTURE GOALS

It is clear, from statistics from coronary care units throughout the world, that the original plan in intensive coronary care has reached a point of maximum effectiveness. No further significant decrease in mortality can be expected from aggressive prophylactic management of cardiac arrhythmias. The residual 15 to 20% mortality reflects our inability to combat death from pump failure. Despite the system of management outlined here, once overt congestive heart failure develops, the mortality is approximately 40% and at least 80% of patients with true cardiogenic shock die.[15,22-24]

It is now widely agreed that pump failure in acute myocardial infarction is usually the result of extensive structural damage to the left ventricle.[25] Accordingly, management with potent inotropic drugs cannot be expected to provide sustained improvement once circulatory failure becomes fully developed. Recently the effectiveness of mechanical devices for support of the failing left ventricle has been demonstrated.[25] However, there is little reason to believe that once circulatory failure resulting from exten-sive progressive myocardial infarction becomes evident the ultimate outcome will be significantly altered. If a further reduction in mortality is to be achieved, it appears that the concept of aggressive management by prophylaxis must be extended to pump failure. Recent studies have offered some hope that the cause of pump failure can be identified.[27,28] Research into the cause of pump failure requires specialized myocardial metabolic studies that involve cardiac catheterization. It is hoped that subsequent correlations will permit the development of a bedside non-invasive clinical profile that will permit recognition of high-risk patients. Once the high- and low-risk categories are separated, the various medical and surgical methods of treatment can be applied in a more individualized and rational manner.

SUMMARY

1. A unified plan to reduce mortality from acute myocardial infarction has been considered.

2. The monitoring and treatment of cardiac arrhythmias that occur in the CCU are fundamental to reducing mortality.

3. It has been demonstrated that ventricular fibrillation and cardiac standstill are sometimes reversible and that with appropriate prophylactic treatment of premonitory arrhythmias they can often be prevented.

4. The current mortality of 15 to 20% will not be reduced further until the problem of pump failure is solved.

5. The next step in the battle against sudden death from acute myocardial infarction involves an extension of the concept of aggressive management by prophylactic means to include prophylaxis for circulatory failure.

6. The prehospital management of acute myocardial infarction (with the mobile coronary care unit) and the intermediate CCU are described in detail in Chapters 4 and 6.

REFERENCES

1. Bloom, B.S., and Peterson, O.L.: End results, costs, and productivity of coronary care units. N. Engl. J. Med. 288:72, 1973.
2. Mather, H.G., Pearson, N.G., and Read, K.L.Q.: Acute myocardial infarction: Home and hospital treatment. Br. Med. J. 3:334, 1971.
3. U.S. Department of Health, Education, and Welfare: Coronary Care Units. Public Health Service Publication No. 1250, 1966.
4. Grace, W.J., and Soscia, J.L.: Reducing mortality from acute myocardial infarction: Current ideas. Cardiol. Digest 4:29, 1969.
5. Lown, L., Vassaux, C., Hood, W.B., et al.: Unresolved problems in coronary care. Am. J. Cardiol. 20:494, 1967.
6. Meltzer, A.: The Current Status of Intensive Coronary Care. Symposium. New York, The Charles Press, 1966.
7. Oliver, M.F., Julian, D.G., and Donald, K.W.: Problems in evaluating coronary care units. Am. J. Cardiol. 20:465, 1967.

8. Killip, T., III, and Kimball, J.T.: Treatment of myocardial infarction in a coronary care unit. Am. J. Cardiol. 20:457, 1967.
9. Lown, B., Klein, M.D., and Hershberg, P.I.: Coronary and precoronary care. Am. J. Med. 46:705, 1969.
10. Lown, B., and Vassaux, C.: Lidocaine in acute myocardial infarction. Am. Heart J. 76:568, 1968.
11. Lown, B., Fakhro, A.M., Hood, W.B., Jr., and Thorn, G.W.: The coronary care unit: New perspectives and directions. J.A.M.A. 199:156, 1967.
12. Friedberg, C.K., Cohen, H., and Donoso, E.: Advanced heart block as a complication of acute myocardial infarction. Role of pacemaker therapy. Prog. Cardiovasc. Dis. 10:466, 1968.
13. Forrester, J.S., Diamond, G., McHugh, T.J., and Swan, H.J.C.: Filling pressures in the right and left side of the heart in acute myocardial infarction. N. Engl. J. Med. 285:190, 1971.
14. Swan, H.J.C., Ganz, W., Forrester, J., et al.: Catheterization of the heart in man with use of a flow-directed balloon-tipped catheter. N. Engl. J. Med. 283:447, 1970.
15. Scheidt, S., Aschein, R., and Killip, T., III: Shock after acute myocardial infarction. Am. J. Cardiol. 26:556, 1970.
16. Mintz, S.S., and Katz, L.N.: Recent myocardial infarction: An analysis of five hundred and seventy-two cases. Arch. Intern. Med. 80:205, 1947.
17. Norris, R.M., Brandt, P.W.T., Caughey, D.E., et al.: A new coronary progenetic index. Lancet i:274, 1969.
18. Stock, E.: Prognosis of myocardial infarction in a coronary care unit. Med. J. Aust. 2:377, 1967.
19. Wiener, L.: Rational therapeutic approach to cardiogenic shock. Cardiovasc. Clin. 6:223, 1973.
20. Arbeit, S.R., Rubin, I.L., and Gross, H: Dangers in interpreting the electrocardiogram from the oscilloscope monitor. J.A.M.A. 211:453, 1970.
21. Electrical charges can be dangerous. J.A.M.A. 201:27, 1967.
22. Gunnar, R.M., Cruz, A., Boswell, J., et al.: Myocardial infarction with shock: Hemodynamic studies and results of therapy. Circulation 33:753, 1966.
23. Wan, S.H., Thompson, P.L., Dowling, J.T., et al.: Cardiogenic shock. A review of one year's experience. Med. J. Aust. 1:1000, 1971.
24. Ratshin, R.A., Rackley, C.E., and Russell, R.O., Jr.: Hemodynamic evaluation of left ventricular function in shock complicating myocardial infarction. Circulation 45:127, 1972.
25. Page, D.L., Caulfield, J.B., Kastor, J.A., et al.: Myocardial changes associated with cardiogenic shock. N. Engl. J. Med. 285:133, 1971.
26. Mueller, H., Ayres, S.M., Gainnelli, S., Jr., et al.: Effect of isoproterenol, I-norepinephrine and intraaortic counter-pulsation on hemodynamics and myocardial metabolism in shock following acute myocardial infarction. Circulation 45:335, 1972.
27. Smullens, S.N., Wiener, L., Kasparian, H., et al.: Evaluation and surgical management of acute evolving myocardial infarction. J. Thorac. Cardiovasc. Surg. 64:495, 1972.
28. Wiener, L., Kasparian, H., Brest, A.N., and Templeton, J.Y., III: Surgical management of acute evolving myocardial infarction: A coronary circulatory, metabolic and angiographic profile. Am. J. Cardiol. 29:296, 1972.

Chapter 6

THE INTERMEDIATE CORONARY CARE UNIT

WILLIAM J. GRACE*
MICHAEL J. GULLOTTI
EDWARD K. CHUNG

GENERAL CONSIDERATIONS

The patients in the intermediate coronary care unit who have had a myocardial infarction (usually one that is a few days to two weeks old) should be treated in accordance with the following basic principles of coronary care:

1. The patients should be in one geographic area.
2. The patients should have continuous ECG monitoring.
3. The monitor should be kept under the constant "eyeball" surveillance of trained personnel.
4. Those in charge of the patients should have an aggressive attitude toward the control of cardiac arrhythmias.

Although the period of maximum risk to the patient is the first few days of hospitalization, death from a variety of possible cardiac causes may occur at any time during the hospital course.

*Deceased, 1977.

It is well known that the peak mortality occurs near the onset of myocardial infarction and recedes nearly exponentially thereafter, with 65% of the deaths occurring in the first three days and 85% of the deaths occurring within the first week.[1-3] Figure 6–1 shows data from St. Vincent's Hospital in New York that indicate that more than 31% of the deaths occur after the fifth day.[9] Data from several different institutions reveal that from 20 to 35% of the hospital deaths from acute transmural myocardial infarction occur after the patient's discharge from the coronary care unit (CCU).[4-8] Figure 6–2, which gives data from a series of almost 3000 patients, indicates that at the end of a week of hospitalization, only 75% of the deaths have been accounted for.[9] Although most such deaths appear to be related to left ventricular dysfunction, a sizable minority of those deaths are sudden and unexpected, usually occurring from ventricular tachyarrhythmias.[10,11] Thus it has become clear that the period of ECG monitoring must be extended beyond the traditional four or five days in the CCU if maximum benefit is to be derived for patients hospitalized for transmural or subendocardial myocardial infarctions.

The usual CCU is not ideal for prolonged patient stay since there is always a considerable demand for beds. Furthermore, good medical practice now demands that the patient be mobilized as soon as possible

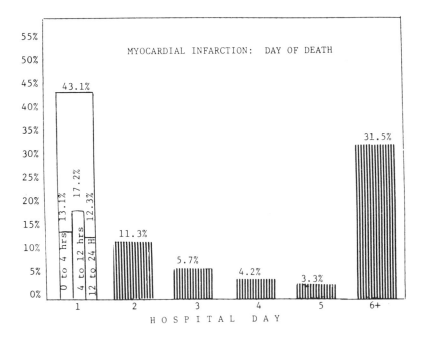

Figure 6–1.

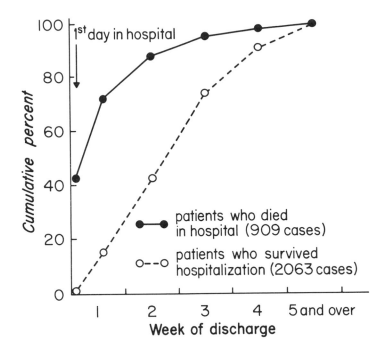

Figure 6–2.

after an acute myocardial infarction. The mobilization requires additional personnel and modifications of monitoring techniques that are usually difficult to make in the CCU. Some institutions have solved the problem by continuing to monitor the ECG beyond the fifth hospital day and through the tenth to fourteenth day while keeping the patient in the same bed. Other institutions, by increasing the size of the CCU, have been able to begin to mobilize the patient while he is still in the CCU. In some institutions, neither of those solutions has been possible because of space limitations. Our solution to the problem has been to establish a separate monitoring area, referred to as the intermediate coronary care unit (ICCU), where continuous ECG monitoring by telemetry is used for all patients.

The ICCU may accommodate any patient who does not have a recent myocardial infarction and whose cardiac disease (most commonly a cardiac rhythm problem) is serious enough to require continuous monitoring and immediate medical attention.

GOALS OF THE INTERMEDIATE CORONARY CARE UNIT

The ICCU should provide:

1. Continuous monitoring that allows immediate recognition of cardiac rhythm disturbances and prophylactic therapy for potentially dangerous arrhythmias

2. Improved survival rates (because prompt recognition of cardiac arrest allows for the successful use of cardiopulmonary resuscitation)

3. Nurses whose training is like that of the CCU nurses

4. Shorter hospital stays (because the ICCU permits the monitoring of patients during the progressive increases in their activity levels)

5. Definition of the individual patient's risk and early construction of plans for his continued care

6. Greater availability of CCU beds (because patients with acute myocardial infarctions or ischemic episodes can be transferred sooner from the CCU)

7. An efficient emergency call system

8. The ready availability of emergency equipment and medications

THE INTERMEDIATE CORONARY CARE UNIT AT THOMAS JEFFERSON UNIVERSITY HOSPITAL

At Thomas Jefferson University Hospital, all patients with an uncomplicated acute myocardial infarction are transferred to the ICCU after their fourth to fifth hospital day. Although all the medical patients admitted to the ICCU do not have acute myocardial infarctions, they do have one or more basic cardiovascular problems that require specialized care and ECG monitoring (e.g., severe congestive heart failure, suspected pacemaker malfunction, serious cardiac arrhythmias). The ICCU also accepts patients from the CCU who are recovering from open-heart surgery and thus need ECG surveillance postoperatively. Patients with pre-infarction angina (persistent chest pain without evidence of pathologic Q waves on the ECG) who need hemodynamic catheters or mechanical assistance devices are kept in the CCU until those indicators of instability are no longer needed.

Monitoring

In the ICCU, the "hard-wire" monitoring of the CCU is replaced by telemetry-system equipment attached to each patient. In both the CCU and the ICCU we use the same computer arrhythmia-monitoring system (Hewlett-Packard 78220A/B) to provide a continuity in the surveillance of each patient. With the telemetry equipment, the patient no longer needs to be confined to his bed or room. He can either be stationary or ambulatory anywhere in the ICCU area because his ECG is continuously transmitted to the central display screen at the nursing station as well as to two overhead display screens at each end of the ICCU.

In addition, there is an individual monitoring screen above and beside each patient's bed to allow for the visual surveillance of the patient's cardiac rate and rhythm by members of the medical or nursing staff while they are in the patient's room. A rhythm strip can be generated at the nursing station from each patient's console. Each rhythm strip produced is a 10-second record that is automatically labelled with the patient's name, room number, the date, and the time.

With the arrhythmia-monitoring system we can care for 15 ICCU patients simultaneously. There is a continuous display of each patient's heart rate and rhythm as well as his "on-line" QRS morphology. We also are able to graphically display the patient's heart rate and the frequency of ventricular premature contractions in the preceding 9-hour period, and to make a permanent record of those phenomena for the patient's chart.

It is of value to realize that any intervention prompted by information obtained through monitoring need not be of direct benefit to the patient, but as in the case of persistent sinus tachycardia, may have been unrecognized by physicians or nurses in their routine examination. However, we have noted that the occurrence of persistent sinus tachycardia is made more obvious when it is consistently recorded on the monitor screen and in the routine rhythm strips on the patient's chart from each nursing shift.

It should be emphasized that persistent sinus tachycardia usually indicates various cardiovascular problems, including impending congestive heart failure, pulmonary embolism, and the extension of recent myocardial infarction.

We believe that the continuous monitoring directs attention to certain clinical findings that might otherwise not be detected until later and that it may allow for the earlier and proper consideration of the diagnostic and therapeutic approaches.

Emergencies

The physical arrangement of our ICCU—it is separate from but contiguous with the CCU—permits the rapid availability of physicians and any other necessary aides in an emergency. In our hospital, each patient's room has an "emergency call" button that allows verbal communication between the patient's room and a central hospital operator. Thus the first person to arrive in a patient's room in an emergency can summon further assistance promptly and efficiently without leaving the patient.

The ICCU crashcart equipment is listed in Table 6–1, and the contents of the ICCU emergency kit are listed in Table 6–2.

Table 6–1. *List of the Crashcart Equipment at Thomas Jefferson University Hospital*

General

1. Emergency drug kit
2. Flat board
3. 4 S tubes (airways)
4. Flashlight
5. Electrical paste

Drawer 1

1. 2 NaHCO$_3$ injection syringes
2. 2 Epinephrine (Adrenalin) injection syringes
3. 2 Lidocaine (Xylocaine) 5 ml (20 mg/ml) injection syringes
4. 2 Lidocaine 25 ml (40 mg/ml) vials
5. 1 Epinephrine 1:1000 ampule
6. 5 Propranolol (Inderal) 1 mg ampules
7. 5 Edrophonium (Tensilon) 10 mg ampules
8. 5 Furosemide (Lasix) 10 ml, 10 mg/ml
9. 5 Digoxin 2 ml, 0.25 mg/ml
10. 4 Dopamine (Inotropin) 10 mg vials
11. 2 CaCl$_2$ vials
12. 2 Diazepam (Valium) 10 mg injectable syringes
13. 2 Solu-Medrol (Methylprednisolone Succinate) 125 mg vials
14. 1 Dexamethasone (Decadron) 5 cc (4 mg/cc) vials
15. 2 Vitamin K (Aquamephyton) vials
16. 2 Alpha-methyldopa (Aldomet) 250 mg/5 ml vials
17. 5 Heparin 10 ml (100 μ/ml) vials
18. 2 Dextrose 50% injection syringes
19. 5 Metaraminol (Aramine) vials
20. 5 Isoproterenol (Isuprel) vials
21. 5 Quinidine vials
22. 4 Atropine vials
23. 5 Aminophylline 10 ml (250/10 ml) vials
24. 3 Calcium gluconate 10 ml (1 g/10 ml) vials
25. 2 NaCl sterile 30 ml vials
26. 2 H$_2$O sterile 30 ml vials
27. Tongue blades
28. 2 Diphenylhydantoin (Dilantin) 2 ml (100 mg/2 ml)
29. 3 Diphenyhydramine (Benadryl) vials
30. Laryngoscope
31. Cardiac needles
    (9) 18 g × 3½ in
    (4) 20 g × 3½ in
    (1) 25 g × 3½ in
    (1) 22 g × 3½ in
32. Assorted needles
33. 2 Nalaxone (Narcon) 1 ml (0.4 mg/ml) vials
34. Alcohol swabs
35. 1 Protamine sulfate 50 mg vial

Drawer 2

1. Aterial blood gases measurement kit
2. Surgilube
3. Suture removal kit
4. 3 Culturettes

  5. Alligator clamp
  6. Longdwell intravenous catheters
       (2) 20 g
       (1) 18 g
       (1) 16 g
       (1) 14 g
  7. Tape
  8. Tourniquet
  9. Betadine ointment
 10. Vacutainer
 11. Assorted blood collection tubes (red, yellow, blue, lavender)
 12. 1 Procaine (Novocain) 2% vial
 13. Assorted suture material
 14. Sterile gloves

Drawer 3

  1. 5 D_5W 150 cc bags
  2. 2 D_5W 500 cc bags
  3. 2 Salt-poor albumin vials
  4. Minidrippers
  5. Solution administration sets
  6. Blood administration sets
  7. 3 Subclavian catheters (one 14 g; two 17 g)
  8. O_2 catheters (14 f)
  9. Betadine spray
 10. Syringes
       (3) 20 cc
       (5) 10 cc
       (5) 5 cc
       (5) 3 cc
       (5) T_3
       (2) Insulin
 11. 2 Three-way stopcocks
 12. 1 Four-way stopcock

Drawer 4

  1. 1 Foley bag
  2. 1 Bulb syringe
  3. 1 Urinary disposable catheterization tray
  4. 1 Cutdown tray
  5. Foley catheters (18 f, 16 f, 14 f, straight)
  6. Connecting tubing
  7. 1 Levine tube (16 f)
  8. Trays
       1 Phlebotomy
       1 Tracheostomy
       1 Lumbar puncture
       1 Thorocentesis
  9. 2 N-T suction catheters
 10. 2 N-T suction kits

Miscellaneous

E for M portable defibrillator that delivers 500 Wsec
Ambu bag
Assorted endotracheal tubes

Table 6–2.   *Contents of the Intermediate Coronary Care Unit Emergency Kit*

Administration sets
Atropine 1 ml (1 mg/ml)
CaCl$_2$ 1 g/10 cc vial
D$_5$W 500 cc bag
Epinephrine (Adrenalin) 10 cc (1:10,000) 18 g × 3½ in cardiac needle
Epinephrine 10 cc (1:10,000) 21 g × 1½ in cardiac needle
Isoproterenol (Isuprel) 1 mg/5 cc
Levarterenol (Levophed) 4 cc
Lidocaine (Xylocaine) 1 g (50 cc 2%)
Metaraminol (Aramine) 10 cc (10 mg/cc)
Needles 18 g × 1½ in
Procainamide (Pronestyl) 10 cc (100 mg/cc)
NaHCO$_3$ 44.6 mEq/50 cc
NaCl 0.9% 20 cc
Syringes (1 cc TB, 5 cc, 10 cc, 50 cc)

Convalescence

While the patient convalesces in the ICCU, the physician is able to make detailed observations on the patient's physical condition as his activity progressively increases. The presence of early congestive heart failure, cardiac arrhythmias, or chest discomfort may be detected more readily in the ICCU than in the general medical ward.

TRANSFER OF PATIENTS BACK TO THE CORONARY CARE UNIT

The decision to return a patient from the ICCU to the CCU is usually based on one of the following occurrences:

1. Recurrent severe chest pain, which would be presumed to be due to extension of acute myocardial infarction; it occurs in approximately 5% of our patients.

2. The onset of ventricular tachyarrhythmias.

3. The need for hemodynamic monitoring and/or control by the use of a pulmonary artery catheter, systemic arterial catheter, artificial pacemaker, or intra-aortic balloon pump.

At present, we are not able to monitor "on-line" hemodynamic values in the ICCU. Thus all patients who have indwelling catheters to measure those values are kept under observation in the CCU until the catheters are no longer needed.

TRANSFER OF PATIENTS FROM THE INTERMEDIATE CORONARY CARE UNIT TO THE GENERAL MEDICAL FLOOR

After the eighth to tenth hospital day (at times up to the fourteenth day), the patient with an uncomplicated acute myocardial infarction is transferred from the ICCU to the general medical floor, where he receives continuous medical care from his personal physician. Usually, the patient stays another four to six days in the hospital and is then discharged.

THE PHYSICIANS IN THE INTERMEDIATE CORONARY CARE UNIT

At Thomas Jefferson University Hospital, the smooth functioning of the ICCU is maintained by direct supervision by the unit's director and co-director. The director or co-director conducts regular teaching rounds on all medical patients and is always available for consultation with the ICCU house staff or nursing staff about diagnostic and therapeutic problems.

THE NURSES IN THE INTERMEDIATE CORONARY CARE UNIT
(See also Chapter 20)

The nurses assigned to the ICCU (and other intensive care units) must attend a rigorous four-week critical-care course before they are allowed to care for cardiac patients. The course, which is taught by physicians and by nurses with advanced training in cardiac care, aims to equip the staff of the ICCU with high-quality skills.

The ICCU nurses must be thoroughly familiar with coronary heart disease and its complications, the differential diagnosis and management of various cardiac arrhythmias, and the emergency procedures to be followed in patients with hemodynamic compromise. All hospital employees having contact with patients must be certified in cardiopulmonary resuscitation.

The ICCU nurses are actively involved in the formal cardiac rehabilitation program. They are interested in and capable of educating cardiac patients about their conditions—a vitally important job. (The patients in the ICCU also educate one another as they become acquainted.) Working closely with the patient's own physician, as well as with the ICCU director and co-director, the ICCU nurses and other health professionals instruct the patients about diet, medications, exercise, and the resumption of activity after myocardial infarction.

The ICCU nurses are responsible also for helping patients work through their periods of mental depression as they recover from myocardial infarction. The nurses are given time to provide the emotional support the patients and their families need to help them deal with the feelings of fear, unreality, and depersonalization so often experienced in a critical care environment.

RESULTS IN THE INTERMEDIATE CORONARY CARE UNIT

Most patients recovering from uncomplicated acute myocardial infarction do not need to be hospitalized beyond the second week.[12-14] Although most physicians with extensive CCU experience have had patients who have died on the twenty-first to twenty-fifth hospital day or as they were about to leave the hospital, such deaths are rare. Our experience in observing patients in the ICCU has enabled us to identify those patients recovering from myocardial infarction who are at risk for sudden death. Grayboys,[15] who retrospectively studied the course of 749 patients with acute myocardial infarction, identified a patient subgroup at high risk for sudden death. Those patients had one or more of the following conditions:

1. Persistent sinus tachycardia
2. Ventricular tachyarrhythmias early in their CCU stay
3. Acute atrial fibrillation or flutter
4. Acute intraventricular and AV conduction disturbances
5. Anterior wall myocardial infarction

It has been suggested that patients who have such a profile have their management changed to include a longer period of hospitalization in a monitored setting, a more liberal use of antiarrhythmic drugs after they have been discharged, and a greater use of permanent artificial pacemakers in specific conditions, particularly in acute intraventricular and/or AV conduction disturbances (see also Chapter 11).

SUMMARY

1. The continuous ECG monitoring of patients admitted to the hospital with acute myocardial infarction after their discharge from the CCU is an important and useful practice.

2. The benefit of continuous monitoring derives mainly from the added ability it gives the staff to recognize and effectively treat potentially lethal cardiac rhythm disturbances, 30% of which occur after the patient's discharge from the CCU.

3. The ICCU provides transitional care for patients after they leave the early intensive care of the CCU and before they begin mobilization prior to their hospital discharge.

4. In the ICCU, while the patient's rehabilitation is begun, his ECG is constantly monitored and he is attended by a staff able to diagnose and treat any cardiac rhythm and/or hemodynamic disturbances.

5. In our experience, ICCU monitoring has brought a reduction in the number of deaths following discharge from the CCU because it has enabled the staff to recognize and treat promptly potentially serious cardiac arrhythmias (such as multifocal or grouped ventricular premature contractions) so that life-threatening arrhythmias—ventricular tachycardia and fibrillation—can be prevented.

6. Lethal arrhythmias, particularly ventricular fibrillation, can be terminated immediately in the ICCU by direct current shock administered by members of the medical or nursing staff.

REFERENCES

1. Lown, B., and Wolf, M.: Approaches to sudden death from coronary artery disease. Circulation 44:130, 1971.
2. Lown, B., Klein, M.D., and Hershberg, P.I.: Coronary and precoronary care. Am. J. Med. 46:705, 1969.
3. Lown, B., Fakhro, A., and Hood, W.B.: The coronary care unit: New perspectives and directions. J.A.M.A. 199:188, 1967.
4. Grace, W.J., and Yarvote, P.M.: Acute myocardial infarction: The course of the illness following discharge from the coronary care unit. Chest 59:15, 1971.
5. Wilson, C., and Adgey, A.A.J.: Survival of patients with late ventricular fibrillation following acute myocardial infarction. Lancet II:124, 1974.
6. Yanowitz, F., and Fozzard, H.A.: A medical information system for the coronary care unit. Arch. Intern. Med. 134:93, 1974.
7. McGrive, L.B., and Krall, M.S.: Evaluation of cardiac care units and myocardial infarction. Arch. Intern. Med. 130:677, 1972.
8. Lindsay, J., and Gorfinkel, H.J.: Arrhythmias in the postcoronary care unit phase of myocardial infarction. Chest 72:571, 1977.
9. Most, A.S., and Peterson, D.R.: Myocardial infarction surveillance in a metropolitan community. J.A.M.A. 208:2433, 1969.
10. Wyman, M., Swan, H.J.C., and Rapaport, M.: Arrhythmia deaths in 15,000 acute myocardial infarction. Circulation (Suppl. IV) 48:40, 1973.
11. Gorfinkel, H.J., Kercher, L., and Lindsay, J.: ECG radiotelemetry in the early recuperative period of acute myocardial infarction. Chest 69:158, 1976.
12. Hutter, A.M., Jr., Sidel, V.W., Shine, K.I., and DeSanctis, R.W.: Early hospital discharge after myocardial infarction. N. Engl. J. Med. 288:1141, 1973.
13. Boyle, J.A., Lorimor, A.R., Brown, A., et al.: Early mobilization after uncomplicated myocardial infarction. Lancet, II:346, 1973.
14. Cannom, D., Levy, W., and Cohen, L.: The short- and long-term prognosis of patients with transmural and non-transmural myocardial infarction. Am. J. Med. 61:452, 1976.
15. Grayboys, T.B.: In-hospital sudden death after coronary care unit discharge. Arch. Intern. Med. 135:512, 1975.

Chapter 7

TACHYARRHYTHMIAS

EDWARD K. CHUNG

GENERAL CONSIDERATIONS

With the availability of direct current cardioverters and artificial pacemakers in the past two decades, the therapeutic results of the management of the various cardiac arrhythmias have improved appreciably. For the best therapeutic results, a precise diagnosis of the arrhythmia is necessary, because some drugs are more effective or even almost specific for certain arrhythmias.[1] For instance, digitalis is often the drug of choice for the treatment of various supraventricular tachyarrhythmias, especially atrial fibrillation with rapid ventricular response. Conversely, digitalis is ineffective or even contraindicated in the treatment of ventricular tachyarrhythmias.[2]

It is essential first to remove the cause of the arrhythmia if the cause is apparent. For instance, the first and most important step in the treatment of digitalis-induced arrhythmia is the immediate discontinuance of digitalis[2] (Chapter 16). In addition, underlying causative factors significantly affect the therapeutic result. For example, ventricular tachycardia associated with acute myocardial infarction is best treated with lidocaine (Xylocaine), whereas digitalis-induced ventricular tachycardia responds best to diphenylhydantoin (Dilantin) or potassium[1-3] (Chapter 16).

Because prevention of recurrence is important in the management of tachyarrhythmias, long-term maintenance therapy with digitalis and other antiarrhythmic drugs is often necessary. In such long-term therapy, quinidine is known to be best for preventing the recurrence of atrial fibrillation or flutter,[4] whereas procainamide (Pronestyl) is known to be best for the prevention of ventricular tachyarrhythmias.[5] Propranolol (Inderal) has been the most effective drug for the treatment of arrhythmias precipitated by exercise, emotional stress, or excessive sympathetic stimulation and of reciprocating tachycardia with normal QRS complexes due to the Wolff-Parkinson-White syndrome.[6,7] Bretylium tosylate, though still under investigation, reportedly is very effective in the treatment of refractory ventricular tachyarrhythmias.[8]

It is extremely important that the physician know the electropharmacologic effects of the various antiarrhythmic drugs before he prescribes one (Table 7–1). Information about the effects of various drugs on the

Table 7–1. *Effects of Cardiac Drugs on Conduction Time*

Drug	Effect on the A-H Interval (AV Nodal Conduction Time)	Effect on the H-V Interval (His-Purkinje Conduction Time)
Digitalis	Increase (slowing)	No change
Propranolol	Increase (slowing)	No change
Quinidine	Decrease (accelerating)	Increase (slowing)
Disopyramide	No change or increase (slowing)	No change
Procainamide	No change or increase (slowing)	Increase (slowing)
Diphenylhydantoin	Decrease (accelerating) or no change	No change
Lidocaine	No change	No change
Atropine	Decrease (accelerating)	No change
Isoproterenol	Decrease (accelerating)	No change or decrease (accelerating)

Table 7–2. *Effects of Drugs on the Refractory Periods of the Normal AV and the Anomalous Pathways*

Drug	Effective Refractory Period	
	AV Node	Accessory Pathway
Propranolol (Inderal)	Lengthened	No change
Digitalis	Lengthened	Shortened
Lidocaine (Xylocaine)	No change	Lengthened
Quinidine	Shortened	Lengthened
Procainamide (Pronestyl)	No change	Lengthened
Diphenylhydantoin (Dilantin)	Shortened	Variable
Amiodarone*	Lengthened	Lengthened
Ajmaline*	No change	Lengthened
Verapamil*	Lengthened	Variable

*Not available for clinical use in the United States.

refractory periods of the normal AV and anomalous pathways in the Wolff-Parkinson-White syndrome is summarized in Table 7–2. The physician should also be familiar with the therapeutic blood levels of common antiarrhythmic drugs (Table 7–3) so that he can prescribe the optimum dosage and prevent intoxication.

Carotid sinus stimulation is probably the simplest way of terminating tachyarrhythmias, particularly supraventricular tachycardia, and it is often effective[9] (Table 7–4).

Direct current shock is an extremely effective way of terminating the various acute tachyarrhythmias, including life-threatening ventricular

Table 7–3.   *Therapeutic Blood Levels of Antiarrhythmic Drugs*

Drug	Blood Level
Digoxin	0.5–2.5 ng/ml
Digitoxin	15–30 ng/ml
Quinidine	2–5 μg/ml
Disopyramide phosphate (Norpace)	2–4 μg/ml
Procainamide (Pronestyl)	3–10 μg/ml
Propranolol (Inderal)	20–200 ng/ml
Lidocaine (Xylocaine)	1–5 μg/ml
Diphenylhydantoin (Dilantin)	5–20 μg/ml

Table 7–4.   *Cardiac Arrhythmias: Various Responses to Carotid Sinus Stimulation*

Arrhythmia (or Other Phenomenon)	Response
Sinus tachycardia	1. Transient slowing of sinus (atrial) rate
	2. Varying degrees of AV block (less common)
Atrial tachycardia	1. Termination
	2. No response
	3. Slowing of ventricular rate due to increased AV block (less common)
	4. Increased atrial rate (less common)
Atrial fibrillation or flutter	Slowing of ventricular rate due to increased AV block
AV junctional tachycardia	
Paroxysmal	1. Termination
	2. No response
Nonparoxysmal	No response
Ventricular tachyarrhythmia	No response (with rare exceptions)
Wolff-Parkinson-White syndrome	Varies
Parasystole	Varies
Digitalis intoxication	Stimulation not recommended
Hypersensitivity	Stimulation not recommended

fibrillation. In addition, direct current shock is indispensable in terminating chronic atrial fibrillation or flutter that is refractory to various antiarrhythmic drugs.[10]

The primary indications for the insertion of an artificial pacemaker are the sick sinus syndrome (Chapter 9) and the Adams-Stokes syndrome due to complete AV block.[11,11a] In addition, the artificial pacemaker with an overdriving pacing rate is often lifesaving in the treatment of refractory tachyarrhythmias, particularly ventricular tachycardia.[11,12]

The use of various antiarrhythmic drugs combined with the direct current cardioverter and artificial pacemaker is not uncommon in the treatment of malignant cardiac arrhythmias.[1]

There are three major clinical categories of cardiac arrhythmias: brady-tachyarrhythmias, tachyarrhythmias, and bradyarrhythmias.

Brady-tachyarrhythmia is a combination of bradyarrhythmia and tachyarrhythmia (and it is often a late manifestation of the sick sinus syndrome—Chapter 9); it is best treated with an artificial pacemaker with a slightly overdriving pacing rate (80 to 100 beats/min).[1] Some people with the brady-tachyarrhythmia syndrome require one or more antiarrhythmic drugs in addition to artificial pacing (Chapter 9).

The therapeutic approaches differ greatly, depending on the origin, as well as the type, of the tachyarrhythmias.[3] Among the tachyarrhythmias encountered are premature (atrial, AV junctional, or ventricular) contractions (extrasystoles), atrial tachyarrhythmias (atrial tachycardia, flutter, and fibrillation), AV junctional tachyarrhythmias (paroxysmal and nonparoxysmal forms), and ventricular tachyarrhythmias (ventricular tachycardia, flutter, and fibrillation).[13]

MANAGEMENT OF THE VARIOUS TACHYARRHYTHMIAS

Premature Contractions (Extrasystoles)

The first step in the management of extrasystoles is to remove any obvious cause of the premature contractions, regardless of the origin of the ectopic impulses. For example, as mentioned, digitalis-induced premature contractions, particularly those that are ventricular in origin, are best treated by the discontinuance of digitalis.[2] Sedation is another important method of eliminating premature beats, especially in people who are high strung. Premature contractions are often eliminated by stopping heavy smoking or excessive coffee drinking.[1]

If the premature contractions are frequent (six or more beats per minute), particularly in such conditions as acute myocardial infarction, various antiarrhythmic drugs (Table 7–5) may be required.[3] Supraventricular (atrial or AV junctional) premature contractions are best treated with quinidine, but propranolol is almost equally effective. Digitalis is particularly effective when premature contractions are associated with heart failure.[2] Lidocaine is the drug of choice for the treatment of ventricular premature contractions associated with acute myocardial infarction or occurring during catheterization and cardiac surgery.[14,15]

Treatment. The treatment of ventricular premature contractions is indicated in the following situations[13] (Figs. 7–1 and 7–2):

1. Frequent ventricular premature contractions (six or more beats per minute)

2. The R–on–T phenomenon (a ventricular premature contraction superimposed on the top of the T wave of the preceding beat)

3. Multifocal ventricular premature contractions

4. Grouped or paired ventricular premature contractions

5. Mild exercise–induced (70% or less of the maximum heart rate) ventricular premature contractions[15a]

6. Ventricular premature contractions in acute myocardial infarction or any acute myocardial ischemic event

7. Ventricular premature contractions after the termination of ventricular tachycardia or fibrillation

For long-term therapy of the ventricular premature contractions, various drugs, such as propranolol, quinidine, procainamide, and disopyramide phosphate (Norpace), may be used.[5,15b] Diphenylhydantoin is probably the best drug for the treatment of digitalis-induced premature beats.[16]

Supraventricular Tachyarrhythmias

In supraventricular tachyarrhythmias, again the first step in management is the elimination of the cause if the cause is apparent. For instance, atrial fibrillation associated with thyrotoxicosis cannot be treated satisfactorily unless the thyroid function returns to a euthyroid level.

Carotid sinus stimulation is often effective in terminating paroxysmal atrial or AV junctional tachycardia.[9] Of the antiarrhythmic drugs, digitalis is usually the drug of choice in the treatment of various supraventricular tachyarrhythmias, especially atrial fibrillation (Fig. 7–3). Needless to say, in digitalis-induced supraventricular tachyarrhythmias, digitalis must be discontinued immediately.[2] Diphenylhydantoin or potassium has been found to be effective in terminating digitalis-induced supraventricular tachyarrhythmias[2,16] (Chapter 16). Quinidine is the best drug for preventing the recurrence of atrial fibrillation or flutter.[4] Propranolol is the most effective drug for the treatment of arrhythmias precipitated by exercise, emotional distress, or excessive sympathetic stimulation (Fig. 7–4), as

Table 7-5. Common Antitachyarrhythmic Drugs

Drug	Full Dosage	Maintenance Dosage	Onset of Action	Maximum Effect	Duration of Action	Indications	Side Effects and Toxicity Dosage-Dependent	Dosage-Independent
Digoxin (Lanoxin)	0.5–1 mg IV initially, then 0.25–0.5 mg q̄ 2 hr as needed (total: 1–2.5 mg)	0.125–0.75 mg (average: 0.25 mg) daily (PO)	10–30 min	2–3 hr	3–6 days	SV tachyarrhythmias (AF, AFl, AT, AV JT)	Almost all known arrhythmias, aggravation of CHF, anorexia, nausea, vomiting, color vision, blurring vision, headache, dizziness, confusion	Allergic manifestations (urticaria, eosinophilia), idiosyncrasy, thrombocytopenia, GI hemorrhage and necrosis
Deslanoside (Cedilanid-D)	0.8–1.6 mg IV initially, then 0.4 mg q̄ 2 hr as needed (total: 1.2–2 mg)	—	10–30 min	2–3 hr	3–6 days	As above	As above	As above
Ouabain (G-Strophanthin)	0.25–0.5 mg IV initially, then 0.1 mg q̄ ½ hr as needed (total: 0.5–1.2 mg)	—	3–10 min	30 min–1 hr	12 hr–3 days	As above	As above	As above
Lidocaine (Xylocaine)	75–100 mg direct IV q̄ 10–20 min as needed (total: 750 mg) or 200–250 mg IM q̄ 10–20 min as needed	1–5 mg/min IV infusion	At once	At once	Minutes	Primary: V tachyarrhythmias Secondary: SV tachyarrhythmias	Dizziness, drowsiness, confusion, muscle twitching, disorientation, euphoria, cardiac and respiratory depression, convulsion, hypotension, AV and IV block	—
Procainamide (Pronestyl)	1–2 g/200 cc 5% D/W IV drip, 100 mg q̄ 2–4 min (1 g in 30 min–1 hr) (total: 2 g) or 1 g PO initially, then 0.5 g q̄ 2–3 hr (total: 3.5 g)	0.25–0.5 g q̄ 3–6 hr (PO)	At once Rapid	Minutes 1–2 hr	6 hr 6–8 hr	Primary: V tachyarrhythmias Secondary: SV tachyarrhythmias	AV and IV block, ventricular arrhythmias, LE, nausea, vomiting, lymphadenopathy, hypotension, convulsion	Allergic manifestations (eosinophilia, urticaria), agranulocytosis

Quinidine gluconate	0.8 g/200 cc 5% D/W IV drip, 25 mg/min or 0.4–0.6 g IM initially then 0.4 g q̄ 2–4 hr (total: 2.6 g)	—	10–15 min	Not immediate	6–8 hr	Primary: SV tachyarrhythmias Secondary: V tachyarrhythmias	AV, IV block, nausea, vomiting, photophobia, diplopia, headache, tinnitus, diarrhea, ventricular arrhythmias	Respiratory depression, hypotension, convulsion, rashes (macular or papular), thrombocytopenic purpura, thrombocytopenia, hemolytic anemia
Quinidine sulfate	Oral route (see text, p. 72)	0.3–0.4 g q̄ 6 hr (PO)	—	2–3 hr	6–8 hr	—	—	—
Disopyramide phosphate (Norpace)	300 mg (PO) initially, then 150 mg q̄ 6 hr	100–150 mg q̄ 6 hr (PO)	30 min–3 hr	2 hr	6–7 hr	Ventricular arrhythmias	Urinary retention, frequency, urgency, abdominal pain, nausea, anorexia, constipation, blurred vision, dryness of nose, eyes, and throat, dry mouth, headache, rash, edema, weight gain, IV block, prolonged Q–T interval and sinus node depression	—
Diphenylhydantoin (Dilantin)	125–250 mg IV q̄ 10–20 min as needed (total: 750 mg/hr)	100–200 mg q̄ 6 hr (PO)	At once	Minutes	4–8 hr	Primary: Digitalis-induced arrhythmias Secondary: Nondigitalis induced arrhythmias (ventricular)	Cardiac depression, hypotension, AV, SA block, sinus bradycardia, ataxia, tremor, gingival hyperplasia	Allergic manifestations (urticaria, purpura, eosinophilia)
Propranolol (Inderal)	1–3 mg IV initially, then second dose may be repeated after 2 min. Additional medication should not be given less than 4 hr (total: 10 mg)	10–30 mg q̄ 6 hr (PO)	At once	Minutes	3–6 hr	Various tachyarrhythmias	SA, AV block, CHF, nausea, vomiting, diarrhea, asthma, cardiogenic shock	Erythematous rashes, paresthesias of hands and fever

IV: intravenous injection; IM: intramuscular injection; q̄: every; D/W: dextrose in water; PO: orally; IV block: intraventricular block; LE: lupus erythematosus; CHF: congestive heart failure; GI: gastrointestinal; AF: atrial fibrillation; AFl: atrial flutter; AT: atrial tachycardia; AV JT: AV junctional tachycardia; SV tachyarrhythmias: supraventricular tachyarrhythmias; V tachyarrhythmias: ventricular tachyarrhythmias.

Source: Slightly adapted from Chung.[3]

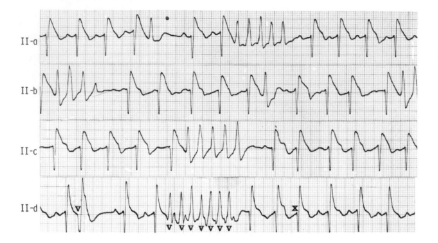

Figure 7–1.   The ECGs shown in Figures 7–1 and 7–2 were obtained from the same patient. In Figure 7–1, leads II-a,b,c, and d are continuous. The basic rhythm is sinus with first-degree AV block (P–R interval: 0.24 sec). Note the frequent ventricular premature beats with short runs of ventricular tachycardia (marked V) initiated by the R–on–T phenomenon. Also there are occasional supraventricular premature beats (marked X).

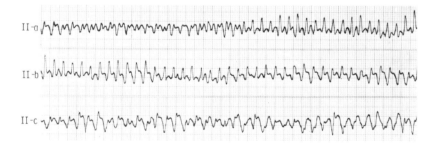

Figure 7–2.   Leads II-a,b, and c are continuous. Ventricular fibrillation.

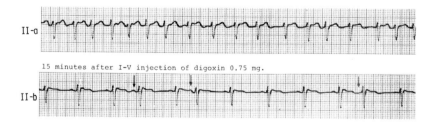

Figure 7–3.   Leads II-a and b are not continuous. Atrial fibrillation (lead II-a) has been converted to sinus rhythm (lead II-b) by digitalization. Note the occasional atrial premature beats (indicated by arrows).

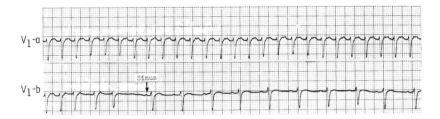

Figure 7–4.   Leads V_1-a and b are continuous. Paroxysmal supraventricular (most likely atrial) tachycardia (187 beats per minute) has been converted to sinus rhythm (indicated by arrow) by the intravenous injection of 1 mg of propranolol (Inderal).

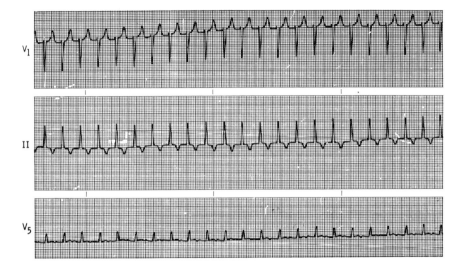

Figure 7–5.   Reciprocating tachycardia (148 beats per minute) with normal QRS complexes in the Wolff-Parkinson-White syndrome.

well as for the treatment of reciprocating tachycardia with normal QRS complexes due to the Wolff-Parkinson-White syndrome (Fig. 7–5).[16a] Procainamide is less commonly used for the treatment of supraventricular tachyarrhythmias, and lidocaine is rarely used in that condition.[14] On the other hand, lidocaine is the drug of choice for the treatment of various supraventricular tachyarrhythmias, particularly atrial fibrillation with anomalous AV conduction in the Wolff-Parkinson-White syndrome (Table 7–2 and Figs. 7 6 and 7–7).[16a]

Direct current shock is often very effective in terminating various acute supraventricular tachyarrhythmias[10] (Fig. 7–8). Elective cardioversion

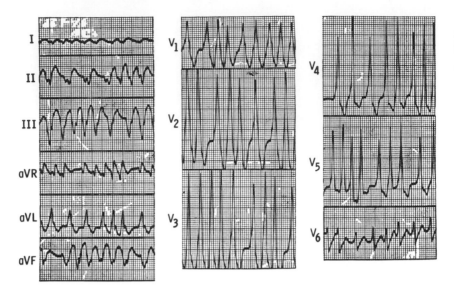

Figure 7–6. The ECGs shown in Figures 7–6, 7–7, and 7–14 were obtained from a 24-year-old man who had had repetitive episodes of palpitations ever since childhood. His 12-lead ECG taken during one of the episodes of palpitations shown in Figure 7–6 reveals atrial fibrillation with a very rapid ventricular rate (180 to 280 beats per minute) and anomalous AV conduction in the Wolff-Parkinson-White syndrome, type A.

is another important means of terminating chronic atrial fibrillation or flutter.[10]

Artificial pacemakers with an overdriving pacing rate are occasionally needed in the suppression of the various supraventricular tachyarrhythmias (Fig. 7–9) that are refractory to antiarrhythmic drugs and to direct current shock.[11] (Direct current shock and artificial pacemakers are discussed in detail in Chapters 10 and 11.) Sedation, in conjunction with other therapeutic measures, is often beneficial in the treatment of supraventricular tachyarrhythmias.

Ventricular Tachyarrhythmias

In ventricular tachyarrhythmias, once again the first step in management is the elimination of the cause if the cause is apparent. Digitalis should be stopped immediately when ventricular tachyarrhythmias are due to digitalis intoxication[2] (Chapter 16).

Direct current shock is the most effective way of terminating ventricular tachycardia, fibrillation and flutter[10] (Fig. 7–10). Defibrillation, in

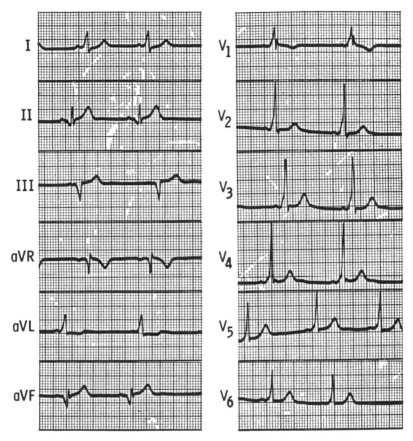

Figure 7–7. The tracing, which was obtained following termination of atrial fibrillation (Fig. 7–6) by direct current shock, reveals sinus arrhythmia and the Wolff-Parkinson-White syndrome, type A.

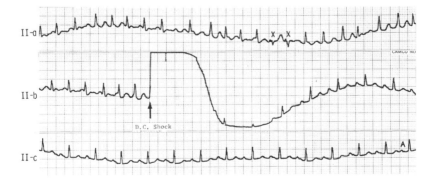

Figure 7–8. Leads II-a,b, and c are continuous. Atrial fibrillation has been converted to sinus rhythm by direct current shock. Note the occasional aberrant ventricular conduction (marked X) and the one atrial premature beat (marked A).

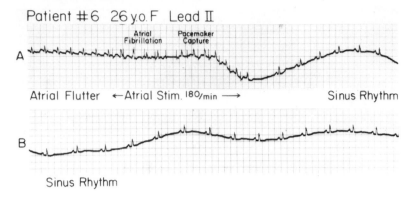

Figure 7–9.   The rhythm strips A and B are not continuous. Atrial flutter is terminated by the atrial stimulation (180 beats per minute), and the sinus rhythm is restored. (Reprinted with permission from Chung.[3])

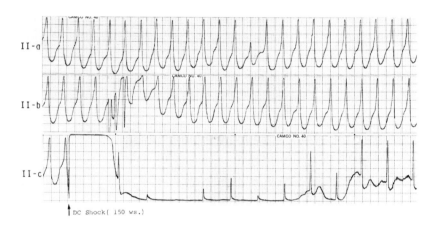

Figure 7–10.   Leads II-a, b, and c are continuous. Ventricular tachycardia (150 beats per minute) is terminated by direct current shock (150 Wsec).

addition to cardiopulmonary resuscitation if that is needed, should be carried out immediately for the treatment of ventricular fibrillation or flutter (Fig. 7–11). However, direct current shock should be avoided in digitalis-induced ventricular tachycardia,[2] because in that condition direct current shock often produces new cardiac arrhythmias, particularly ventricular fibrillation (Chapter 16).

Lidocaine is the drug of choice for the treatment of ventricular tachycardia associated with acute myocardial infarction or arising during anesthesia and cardiac catheterization[14,15,17] (Fig. 7–12). Procainamide is probably the next most commonly used drug in that situation.[17] Quinidine, propranolol, and disopyramide phosphate may be used in place of procainamide. Diphenylhydantoin is the best drug for the

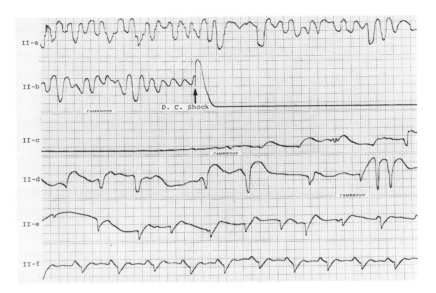

Figure 7–11. Leads II-a,b,c,d,e, and f are continuous. Ventricular fibrillation is terminated by direct current shock, and sinus rhythm is restored. Note that there are ventricular premature contractions and unstable AV junctional escape rhythms in leads II-d and e before sinus rhythm is established.

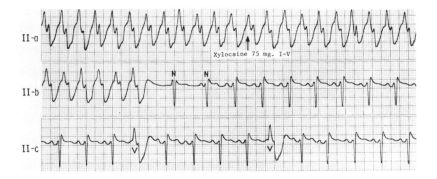

Figure 7–12. Leads II-a and b are continuous. Ventricular tachycardia is terminated by the intravenous injection of 75 mg of lidocaine. Note the occasional AV junctional premature beats (marked N) and the ventricular premature contractions (marked V). The configurations of the isolated ventricular premature beat and the tachycardia beats are identical.

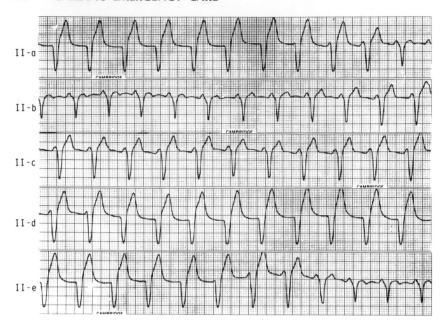

Figure 7–13.   Leads II-a,b,c,d, and e are continuous. These rhythm strips show sinus rhythm with nonparoxysmal ventricular tachycardia (76 beats per minute), causing isorhythmic AV dissociation. Note the many ventricular fusion beats, a result of similar sinus and ectopic rates.

treatment of digitalis-induced ventricular tachycardia.[2,16] Bretylium tosylate, which is still under investigation, has been reported to be very effective in the treatment of refractory ventricular tachycardia.[8]

When ventricular tachyarrhythmias are refractory to antiarrhythmic drugs and/or direct current shock, an artificial pacemaker with an overdriving pacing rate (100 to 120 beats per minute) is often lifesaving.[11]

It should be noted that no treatment is indicated for nonparoxysmal ventricular (idioventricular) tachycardia (accelerated ventricular rhythm) or parasystolic ventricular tachycardia because those arrhythmias are usually self limited (Fig. 7–13).

ANTITACHYARRHYTHMIC DRUGS (See also Table 7–5)

Digitalis

A Guide to Digitalization. Digitalis is one of the oldest and most valuable drugs. However, digitalis intoxication is often unavoidable because the margin between the therapeutic dose and the toxic dose is relatively narrow.[2] The margin is further reduced in elderly and seriously ill patients who have various modifying conditions, such as renal insufficiency, hypokalemia, and hypoxia. It has been shown that the therapeutic dose is approximately 60% of the toxic dose.[2]

Before the physician attempts to digitalize a patient, he must consider the following guidelines:[2]

1. The physician should be sure that digitalis is indicated. He should know whether the patient is suffering from congestive heart failure and/or supraventricular tachyarrhythmias. Needless to say, two major indications for digitalis therapy are congestive heart failure and various supraventricular tachyarrhythmias, except those that are digitalis induced.

In addition, the physician should be aware that the only absolute contraindication to digitalization is digitalis intoxication. A probable contraindication to digitalization is idiopathic hypertrophic subaortic stenosis; because digitalis improves the contractile state of the left ventricular myocardium, which further reduces the left ventricular outflow tract. Deterioration induced by digitalization in that condition usually improves when the digitalis is withdrawn. Digitalis should be avoided also when supraventricular tachyarrhythmias are present, particularly atrial fibrillation with anomalous AV conduction in the Wolff-Parkinson-White syndrome (Figs. 7–6 and 7–7). The reason is that the conduction via an accessory pathway may be enhanced by digitalis (Table 7–2) so that the clinical condition often deteriorates, and sudden death may occur as a result of digitalis-induced ventricular fibrillation (Fig. 7–14).

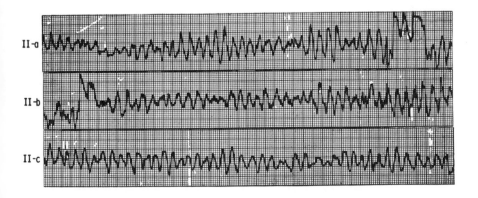

Figure 7–14. Leads II-a, b, and c are continuous. Ventricular fibrillation was provoked by digitalis for atrial fibrillation with anomalous AV conduction in the Wolff-Parkinson-White syndrome (Fig. 7–6).

2. The physician should attempt to obtain precise information about any previous digitalization of the patient, particularly information about any digitalization within three to four weeks. Exact information about not only the duration of digitalization but also the preparation, dosage, and route of administration is indispensable.

If the clinical symptoms are rather mild and information about previous digitalization is unclear, I prefer not to give any digitalis until a definite indication for digitalization is present. Determination of the serum digitalis level by radioimmunoassay is extremely valuable when information about previous digitalization is unclear.

3. A control ECG must be done immediately before digitalization, regardless of the patient's clinical condition, except when the patient has an unusually acute condition. The most important reason for taking the ECG is to determine the fundamental mechanism of the cardiac rhythm so that any cardiac arrhythmia that develops after digitalization will be clearly evident. Any new cardiac arrhythmia that develops during or after digitalization strongly suggests digitalis intoxication since almost every known type of rhythm disturbance may be induced by digitalis (Chapter 16). A control ECG also reveals any unexpected abnormalities, such as acute myocardial infarction or hypokalemia, that directly affect the efficacy of digitalis therapy and the probability of digitalis intoxication. In addition to the control ECG, frequent follow-up ECG tracings are needed until the patient is fully digitalized. The ECG should be taken as soon as any change in cardiac rhythm is detected by physical examination or if digitalis intoxication is suspected. To confirm the current cardiac mechanism, long strips of leads II and V_1 are adequate.

4. The preparation and method of digitalization directly and indirectly affect the efficacy of digitalis and the development of digitalis intoxication. In an emergency, such as acute pulmonary edema, particularly that associated with supraventricular tachyarrhythmias, a short-acting preparation, such as deslanoside or digoxin, should be given intravenously. If there are any modifying factors, short-acting preparations are always preferable. If the patient's clinical condition is not urgent, oral administration with a slower method is advisable. Every physician should be thoroughly familiar with the preparation he has chosen. He should know the precise oral and parenteral dosages, as well as the advantages and disadvantages of the particular preparation. Every physician should also be thoroughly familar with at least one preparation for intravenous use for very rapid digitalization and one preparation for oral use for slow digitalization.

I believe that in most clinical situations digoxin has been proved to be the most useful preparation. There is no point in changing from one preparation to another unless a definite advantage can be gained by the change or unless an allergy to the original preparation is discovered.

5. Modifying factors, such as hypokalemia, and various cardiac and noncardiac diseases, directly affect the efficacy of the drug and the development of digitalis intoxication.

6. In the past 15 years, several methods[18,19] have been developed for determining the serum digitalis level in order to establish an optimum therapeutic dosage and to diagnose digitalis intoxication. The clinical importance of determining the serum digitalis level lies in the fact that there is reasonably close correlation between the digitalis content of blood or cardiac tissue and that of other tissue, so that the blood levels reflect total body and myocardial concentrations (Chapter 16).

At present, it is generally agreed that patients with obvious digitalis intoxication have significantly higher serum or plasma levels of digoxin or digitoxin than have non-intoxicated patients. Nevertheless, there is a substantial overlap between toxic and nontoxic serum or plasma cardiac glycoside levels. The overlap is a problem, particularly in patients who suffer from intractable congestive heart failure or various complex cardiac arrhythmias. It is extremely important to remember that the dosage of digitalis varies not only from patient to patient but also from time to time in the same patient. Similarly, toxic and nontoxic serum or plasma digitalis levels may differ from patient to patient, depending largely on various modifying factors. In general, serum digoxin levels of 2 ng/ml or below and serum digitoxin levels of 20 ng/ml or below are considered to be nontoxic although intoxicated patients may have serum levels within that range.[18,19] Determination of the levels of serum digitalis by radioimmunoassay is extremely valuable when those levels are interpreted in conjunction with the total clinical picture and the ECG findings.

7. Refractory congestive heart failure requires careful evaluation to determine whether the patient needs more digitalis or whether digitalis must be discontinued. The presence of any modifying factors and the reevaluation of the initial diagnosis are additional factors to be considered in treating refractory congestive heart failure. It should be emphasized again that digitalis intoxication is an important cause of refractory congestive heart failure (Chapter 16).

8. At times, digitalis-induced arrhythmias may be so complex that experienced electrocardiographers disagree about the mechanism of the cardiac rhythm. A given tracing may suggest a variety of mechanisms, and the cardiac rhythm may change form every few seconds or minutes. It may be reasonable to state that disagreement about the mechanism of the cardiac rhythm during digitalization is in itself often sufficient reason to suspect digitalis intoxication.

Methods of Digitalization[2] (See also Table 7–6). The digitalis preparation and the method of digitalization directly affect the therapeutic results of digitalis and the incidence of digitalis intoxication In most clinical situations there are five methods of digitalization: (1) very rapid parenteral

Table 7-6. *Methods of Digitalization*

	Very Rapid Digitalization (Within 12 Hr)	Rapid Digitalization (Within 24 Hr)	Moderately Rapid Digitalization (Within 2–3 Days)	Slow Digitalization (Within 5–8 Days)	Digitalization With Daily Oral Maintenance Dosage
Digoxin	0.5–1 mg IV initially, then 0.25–0.5 mg q̄ 2–4 hr as needed	1–1.5 mg by mouth initially, then 0.5 mg q̄ 6 hr until digitalized	0.5 mg t.i.d. by mouth for 2–3 days until digitalized	0.25 mg t.i.d. by mouth for 5–8 days until digitalized	0.25 mg daily by mouth
Deslanoside	0.8–1.6 mg IV initially, then 0.4 mg q̄ 2–4 hr as needed	—	—	—	—
Ouabain	0.25–0.5 mg IV initially, then 0.1 mg q̄ ½ hr as needed	—	—	—	—
Digitoxin	—	0.8 mg by mouth initially, then 0.2 mg q̄ 6 hr until digitalized	0.2 mg t.i.d. by mouth for 2–3 days until digitalized	0.1 mg t.i.d. by mouth for 5–8 days until digitalized	0.1 mg daily by mouth
Digitalis leaf	—	0.8 g by mouth initially, then 0.2 g q̄ 6 hr until digitalized	0.2 g t.i.d. by mouth for 2–3 days until digitalized	0.1 g t.i.d. by mouth for 5–8 days until digitalized	0.1 g daily by mouth

Source: Chung.[2]

digitalization (within 12 hours), (2) rapid oral digitalization (within 24 to 48 hours), (3) moderately rapid oral digitalization (within 2 to 3 days), (4) slow oral digitalization (within 5 to 8 days), and (5) digitalization with daily maintenance dosage. The choice depends on the degree of urgency, the nature of the underlying heart disease, and the presence or absence of cardiac arrhythmias.

Very Rapid Parenteral Digitalization (Within 12 Hours). For urgent situations, such as acute pulmonary edema due to left ventricular failure and supraventricular tachyarrhythmias, very rapid parenteral digitalization is indicated. Short-acting preparations, such as digoxin (Lanoxin), deslanoside (Cedilanid-D), or ouabain (G-Strophanthin) are commonly used.

1. *Digoxin.* The usual initial dose of digoxin is 0.5 mg to 1 mg intravenously, followed by 0.25 mg to 0.5 mg every 2 to 4 hours as needed.

2. *Deslanoside.* The usual initial dose of deslanoside is 0.8 mg to 1.6 mg intravenously, followed by 0.4 mg every 2 to 4 hours as needed.

3. *Ouabain.* The usual initial dose is 0.25 mg to 0.5 mg intravenously, followed by 0.1 mg every 30 minutes as needed.

Rapid Oral Digitalization (Within 24 Hours). Rapid oral digitalization may be used when patients are suffering from acute congestive heart failure or supraventricular tachyarrhythmias and when the clinical situation is not urgent enough to require very rapid parenteral digitalization. In those situations, a therapeutic effect is reached in 24 to 48 hours.

1. *Digoxin.* The preparation of choice for rapid oral digitalization is digoxin. The usual initial dose of digoxin is 1 mg to 1.5 mg orally, followed by 0.5 mg every 6 hours until the patient is digitalized.

2. *Digitoxin.* When digitoxin is used, the initial dose is 0.8 mg orally, followed by 0.2 mg every 6 hours until the patient is digitalized.

3. *Digitalis leaf.* Digitalis leaf is now seldom used for rapid oral digitalization.

Moderately Rapid Oral Digitalization (Within Two to Three Days). Moderately rapid oral digitalization is the preferred method when the patient shows well-developed but not acute signs of congestive heart failure. It is not usually recommended when congestive heart failure is associated with or due to supraventricular tachyarrhythmias. The method can be used in either the hospital or the outpatient clinic.

1. *Digoxin.* When digoxin is used, full digitalization can be accomplished with a dosage schedule of 0.5 mg three times a day for 2 to 3 days until the patient is digitalized. If I give digoxin to an ambulatory patient either at a clinic or in my office, I prefer to see the patient after he has received a total of 3 mg in 48 hours rather than to prescribe routinely. I do so in order to prevent digitalis intoxication. I do not prescribe more

digitalis until I have made a careful evaluation of the patient, including an evaluation of his ECGs.

2. *Digitoxin.* When digitoxin is used, 0.2 mg may be given in the manner described for digoxin.

3. *Digitalis leaf.* Digitalis leaf is now seldom used for moderately rapid oral digitalization.

Slow Oral Digitalization (Within Five to Eight Days). Slow oral digitalization is very useful for patients with mild congestive heart failure without any acute symptoms and without supraventricular tachyarrhythmias. The method is frequently used for ambulatory patients at clinics or in private offices. It can, of course, be used in the hospital as well.

1. *Digoxin.* I often use digoxin in the dosage of 0.25 mg 3 times a day for 5 to 8 days. I prefer to see the patient after five days of digitalization. At that point, I prescribe additional digoxin as required after I have made a full evaluation of the clinical and ECG findings. The method is quite safe for the treatment of uncomplicated mild congestive heart failure.

2. *Digitoxin.* If digitoxin is used, 0.1 mg may be given in the manner described for digoxin.

3. *Digitalis leaf.* Digitalis leaf is now seldom used for slow oral digitalization.

Digitalization with a Daily Oral Maintenance Dosage. Recently it has been well demonstrated that slow digitalization can be successfully carried out by a daily oral maintenance dosage for mild congestive heart failure. The method is rather popular for outpatients.

1. *Digoxin.* The usual maintenance dosage of digoxin is 0.25 mg a day, but in some patients, 0.125 mg a day may be sufficient. On the other hand, 0.375 mg or 0.5 mg may be necessary as a maintenance dose for some patients.

2. *Digitoxin.* Most patients require 0.1 mg of digitoxin as a maintenance dose, although some may need 0.05 mg or 0.2 mg as a daily maintenance dose.

3. *Digitalis leaf.* I now seldom use digitalis leaf in my daily practice. When I do use it, I usually prescribe 0.1 gm as a daily maintenance dose.

Full Digitalization and Maintenance Doses (See also Table 7–7). Although the dosage differs markedly for different people and even in the same person at different times, I have set guidelines (based on extensive clinical experience) for average doses, full digitalization doses, and maintenance doses.

1. *Digoxin.* The average parenteral full digitalizing dose is 1.5 mg, with a usual range of 1 to 2.5 mg. The average oral full digitalizing dose is approximately 2.5 mg, with a usual range of 1.5 to 4 mg. The usual maintenance dose of digoxin is 0.25 mg, but some patients may require as little as 0.125 mg or as much as 0.75 mg a day as a maintenance dose.

Table 7-7. *Full Digitalization and Maintenance Doses*

| | Digitalizing Doses Within 24–48 hr | | | | Maintenance Doses | |
| | IV or IM Administration | | Oral Administration | | | |
	Average	Usual Range	Average	Usual Range	Average	Usual Range
Digoxin	1.5 mg	1–2.5 mg	2.5 mg	1.5–4 mg	0.25 mg	0.125–0.75 mg
Deslanoside	1.6 mg	1.2–2 mg	—	—	—	—
Ouabain	1 mg	0.5–1.2 mg	—	—		
Digitoxin	1.2 mg	1–2 mg	1.5 mg	1.2–2 mg	0.1 mg	0.05–0.2 mg
Digitalis leaf	—	—	1.5 g	1.2–2 g	0.1 g	0.05–0.2 g

Source: Chung.[2]

2. *Deslanoside*. The average full digitalizing dose is 1.6 mg, with a usual range of 1.2 to 2 mg.

3. *Ouabain*. The average full digitalizing dose is 1 mg, with a usual range of 0.5 to 1.2 mg.

4. *Digitoxin*. The average parenteral full digitalizing dose is 1.2 mg, with a usual range of 1 to 2 mg. The average oral digitalizing dose is 1.5 mg, with a usual range of 1.2 to 2 mg. The average maintenance dose is 0.1 mg, with a usual range of 0.05 to 0.2 mg.

5. *Digitalis leaf*. Digitalis leaf is seldom used because it is inferior to the many other digitalis preparations.

Digitalis in Children. With a few exceptions, the fundamental principles, indications, and contraindications regarding the digitalization of children are essentially the same as those regarding the digitalization of adults.[20-22] The initial dose of the cardiac glycosides varies markedly according to the patient's age. For example, patients under two years of age require significantly different amounts of digitalis than do patients over two years of age.[20-22] The manifestations of digitalis intoxication in children are somewhat different from those in adults.[20-22] Ventricular premature contractions, the most common digitalis-induced arrhythmias in adults, are rather uncommon in children;[2,20-22] instead, AV block, SA block, and marked sinus arrhythmia are commonly found. A detailed dosage schedule for the parenteral and oral digitalization with digoxin, the preparation most often used in children is as follows:

Parenteral (Intravenous) Digitalization with Digoxin. 1. *Initial dosage.* One-fourth to one-half of the estimated total digitalizing dosage, which is (a) 0.02 to 0.03 mg/lb for children under two years of age and (b) 0.01 to 0.02 mg/lb for children over two years of age.

2. *Full digitalizing dosage.* The initial dose is followed by one-fourth of the estimated total digitalizing dose every 8 to 12 hours until the child is digitalized.

Oral Digitalization with Digoxin. 1. *Initial dosage.* One-fourth to one-half of the estimated total digitalizing dose, which is (a) 0.03 to 0.04 mg/lb for children under two years of age and (b) 0.02 to 0.03 mg/lb for children over two years of age.

2. *Full digitalizing dosage.* The initital dose is followed by one-fourth of the estimated total digitalizing dose every 6 to 8 hours until the child is digitalized.

3. *Maintenance dosage.* One-fourth of the total digitalizing dose.

Quinidine

For more than 50 years, quinidine has been the most valuable antitachyarrhythmic drug available. Quinidine has two major effects, a direct one and an indirect one.[1] The direct effect is on the cell membrane, and the indirect effect is anticholinergic. The net clinical result of the anticholinergic effect and the direct effect is marked prolongation of the refractory period in the atria and a lesser degree of prolongation in the ventricles. Quinidine also induces a shortening of the refractory period in the AV junction. The sinus rate tends to be slowed by the direct effect of quinidine, but the indirect (vagolytic) effect tends to counteract that effect. As a result, the sinus rate may not be altered significantly by quinidine, or it may even be accelerated.

Indications. The primary use of quinidine has been to convert atrial fibrillation or flutter to sinus rhythm. Before direct current cardioverters were available, large amounts of quinidine sulfate were necessary to restore sinus rhythm, but the drug is now used for that purpose only when a direct current cardioverter is not available. At present, quinidine is used largely to prevent the recurrence of atrial fibrillation or flutter after restoration of sinus rhythm by either digitalization or direct current shock.[1] It is also useful in the treatment of various acute supraventricular and ventricular tachyarrhythmias. Quinidine is often effective in the treatment of atrial fibrillation or flutter with anomalous AV conduction in the Wolff-Parkinson-White syndrome (Fig. 7–6).[1,16a] In the treatment of acute tachyarrhythmias, quinidine is found to be more effective in supraventricular tachyarrhythmias than in ventricular ones. Quinidine is also useful for the suppression of premature beats that are supraventricular or ventricular in origin.

Full Dosage. For the treatment of acute tachyarrhythmias, quinidine gluconate, 0.8 g diluted in 200 cc of a 5% solution of dextrose in water may be given intravenously at a rate of about 25 mg per minute under continuous ECG monitoring. The intramuscular administration of quinidine gluconate may be carried out by giving 0.4 to 0.6 g initially, followed by 0.4 g every 2 to 4 hours as needed. The total dosage by intramuscular route should not exceed 2.4 g.

Maintenance Dosage. The usual maintenance dosage of quinidine sulfate for the prevention of recurrence of various arrhythmias is 0.3 to 0.4 g every 6 hours.

Side Effects and Toxicity. The mild toxic manifestations include nausea, vomiting, diarrhea, tinnitus, a slight impairment of hearing and vision, and a slight widening of the QRS complex. When quinidine intoxication increases, those manifestations become more severe. Thus the patient may develop blurring vision, disturbed color perception, photophobia, diplopia, abdominal pain, headache, confusion, and ventricular tachyarrhythmias. If the patient has an unusual sensitivity or idiosyncratic reaction to quinidine, respiratory depression, hypotension, convulsion, urticaria, macular or papular rashes, fever, thrombocytopenia, hemolytic anemia, and even sudden death may result.[1]

One of the most serious untoward effects of quinidine is the so-called

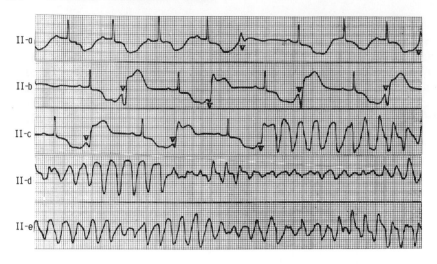

Figure 7–15.   Leads II-a,b,c,d, and e are continuous. The basic rhythm is sinus with first-degree AV block. Note that ventricular fibrillation is provoked by ventricular premature contractions (marked V), with the R–on–T phenomenon as a result of a markedly prolonged Q–T interval with a broad T wave due to quinidine.

quinidine syncope, or sudden death during quinidine therapy. It has been shown that ventricular fibrillation is often provoked by a ventricular premature contraction with the R–on–T phenomenon as a result of a markedly prolonged Q–T interval and a broad T wave due to quinidine (Fig. 7–15).[16b] Sudden death may occur from quinidine-induced ventricular fibrillation.

Lidocaine

The discovery of the antiarrhythmic properties of lidocaine is probably the most important addition to the therapy of cardiac arrhythmias. The structure of lidocaine is similar to that of quinidine and procainamide (pp. 123 and 125), but its electrophysiologic properties are quite different.[14,15,17] Since it has little effect on the atria, lidocaine is of little use in the treatment of atrial tachyarrhythmias. Lidocaine depresses diastolic depolarization and automaticity in the ventricles. It is of interest that lidocaine in standard doses has no effect on the conduction velocity, and it generally shortens both the action potential and the refractory period. Approximately 90% of an administered dose of the drug is metabolized in the liver, and the remaining 10% is excreted unchanged through the kidneys. The action of lidocaine is more transient than that of procainamide, and it also penetrates the cardiac tissues more rapidly than does procainamide.[14,15,17]

Indications. Lidocaine is widely used, primarily for the treatment of ventricular tachyarrhythmias and ventricular premature contractions associated with acute myocardial infarction, cardiac surgery, and cardiac catheterization (Fig. 7–12).[14,15,17] In the past decade, lidocaine has gradually replaced procainamide for parenteral use because of its greater effectiveness and the infrequency with which it produces hypotension when it is given properly. In addition, lidocaine is extremely useful in the treatment of supraventricular tachyarrhythmias, particularly atrial fibrillation or flutter with anomalous AV conduction in the Wolff-Parkinson-White syndrome (Fig. 7–6), because the drug can depress anomalous AV conduction (Table 7–2).[16a]

Administration.[14,15,17] For the initiation of therapy, direct injection of 75 mg to 100 mg of lidocaine (1 to 1.5 mg/kg) is given slowly; the same dose may be repeated every 5 to 10 minutes until the ventricular tachyarrhythmias are terminated. In general, the total dose should not exceed 750 mg, and it is advisable that no more than 300 mg be administered during a one-hour period. When intravenous injection is not feasible, 200 to 250 mg of lidocaine may be given intramuscularly, and the same dose may be repeated once or twice every 10 to 20 minutes. It is recommended that lidocaine be administered under continuous ECG monitoring. Following the termination of ventricular tachyarrhythmia, in most cases continuous intravenous infusion at a rate of 1 to 5 mg/min is needed for 24 to 72 hours to prevent recurrence of the arrhythmia. If ventricular tachyarrhythmias do not recur, lidocaine may be replaced gradually with oral procainamide. The oral use of lidocaine in clinical practice needs further investigation.

Side Effects and Toxicity. Toxicity with the use of lidocaine is relatively uncommon, but the drug may produce dizziness, drowsiness, confusion, muscle twitching, disorientation, euphoria, cardiac and respiratory depression, convulsions, and hypotension. Caution should be exercised in the repeated use of lidocaine in patients with severe liver or renal disease because an accumulation may lead to intoxication.

Propranolol

Propranolol is a beta-adrenergic blocking drug that has been widely used for the management of various tachyarrhythmias, including those induced by digitalis and those resistant to digitalis.[6,7] The antiarrhythmic actions of propranolol are produced in two ways: (1) by inhibition of the adrenergic stimulation of the heart and (2) by direct alteration of the electrophysiologic properties of the cardiac tissue. Thus the overall effects of propranolol usually result in the reduction of automaticity, including the reduction of the sinus rate and the prolongation of the atrial and the AV conduction times.[6,7]

Indications. Propranolol is effective in terminating various tachyarrhythmias. The direct membrane actions of propranolol are primarily responsible for its effectiveness in the treatment of digitalis-induced tachyarrhythmias.[6,7] In addition, propranolol is very effective in the treatment of catecholamine-induced tachyarrhythmias, such as the arrhythmias precipitated by exercise, emotional distress, or excessive sympathetic stimulation, and in the treatment of reciprocating tachycardia with normal QRS complexes due to the Wolff-Parkinson-White syndrome.[6,7,16a] In particular, propranolol is considered to be the drug of choice in the treatment of catecholamine-induced arrhythmias and reciprocating tachycardia with normal QRS complexes associated with the Wolff-Parkinson-White syndrome in young people without demonstrable heart disease (Figs. 7–4 and 7–5).[16a] In some cases of hyperthyroidism, tachyarrhythmias may be terminated by propranolol, but often a large dosage is required.[6,7] Propranolol is contraindicated in patients with bronchial asthma, allergic rhinitis, marked sinus bradycardia, second- or third-degree AV block, SA block, sinus arrest, cardiogenic shock, and congestive heart failure.

Full Dosage. Propranolol should be administered slowly by intravenous injection, and the rate of administration should be 1 to 3 mg per minute under ECG monitoring. The second dose may be repeated after two minutes if needed. Additional medication should be withheld for at least four hours, and the total dosage should not exceed 10 mg.

Maintenance Dosage. In non-urgent situations, propranolol may be given orally in doses ranging from 10 to 30 mg 3 to 4 times a day before meals and at bedtime. The same dosage is also recommended for long-term use or for prophylactic purposes.

Side Effects and Toxicity. The side effects or toxic manifestations of propranolol include nausea, vomiting, lightheadedness, diarrhea, constipation, mental depression, asthma, hypotension, bradycardia, precipitation of congestive heart failure, and cardiogenic shock. In some patients, allergic manifestations, such as erythematous rashes, paresthesias of the hands, and fever, may be observed. It has been demonstrated that cardiopulmonary resuscitation is often difficult during major cardiac surgery when the patient has been taking large amounts of propranolol prior to the surgery. Thus it is highly recommended that propranolol be discontinued for at least several days before major cardiac surgery if the patient's clinical condition permits.[16b]

Procainamide

Procainamide had been the drug of choice for the treatment of ventricular tachycardia until the past decade, when lidocaine was proved to be a safer and more effective drug.[5,14,15] Large amounts of procainamide were often used in the treatment of ventricular tachycardia, especially before direct current cardioverters became readily available.

The electrophysiologic effects of procainamide are very similar to those of quinidine. Procainamide slows electrical conduction, increases the refractory period, and depresses diastolic depolarization and automaticity.[5,14,15] Procainamide has an indirect vagolytic action, and in low doses it may improve AV conduction. However, the direct effect of procainamide given in higher doses is depression of AV conduction. The therapeutic levels are easily achieved by oral administration since procainamide is almost completely absorbed from the gastrointestinal tract.[5,14,15] Procainamide should be administered with caution to patients with significant renal disease, because it is excreted primarily by the kidneys in unchanged form.

Indications. Although the electrophysiologic actions of procainamide are very similar to those of quinidine, procainamide has been used primarily for the treatment of ventricular tachyarrhythmias (Fig. 7–16). At present, the primary indication for procainamide is prevention of the recurrence of ventricular tachyarrhythmias after they have been terminated by direct current shock or intravenous lidocaine.[14,15] Procainamide is also effective for the treatment of supraventricular tachyarrhythmias although it is not the drug of choice. Procainamide has been used in place of quinidine when the patient is unable to tolerate quinidine. At present, a large dosage of parenteral procainamide is used only when a direct current

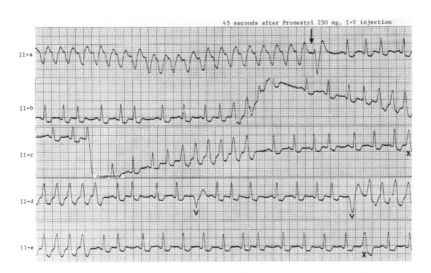

Figure 7–16.   Leads II-a,b,c,d, and e are continuous. Bidirectional ventricular tachycardia is terminated by the intravenous injection of 250 mg of procainamide. Note the frequent ventricular premature contractions (marked V and X).

cardioverter is not available and lidocaine has been found to be ineffective. Procainamide is very effective in suppressing ventricular premature beats. It is also useful for the prevention of various supraventricular tachyarrhythmias, particularly atrial fibrillation with anomalous AV conduction in the Wolff-Parkinson-White syndrome (Table 7–2 and Figs. 7–6 and 7–7).[16a]

Full Dosage. When intravenous procainamide must be used, 1 to 2 g of the drug diluted in 200 cc of a 5% solution of dextrose in water is administered by continuous drip at a rate of 100 mg every 2 to 4 minutes under continuous ECG monitoring. The total intravenous dosage should not exceed 2 g. When the clinical situation is not urgent, procainamide may be given orally. Initially, 1 g of procainamide may be given orally followed by 0.5 g every 2 to 3 hours as needed. The total oral dosage should not exceed 3.5 g.

Maintenance Dosage. Since the half-life of procainamide is relatively short, the ideal maintenance oral dosage has been reported to be 250 to 500 mg every 3 hours.[5] However, simply because of the inconvenience such a dosage would cause the patient, many physicians prescribe a maintenance dose of procainamide of 250 to 500 mg every 4 to 6 hours orally.

Side Effects and Toxicity. The toxic manifestations of procainamide include nausea, vomiting, fever, leukopenia, lymphadenopathy, lupus erythematosus–like syndrome, convulsion, AV and intraventricular block of varying degrees, ventricular tachyarrhythmias, and hypotension.[5,14,15] In some patients who are sensitive to procainamide, allergic manifestations, such as eosinophilia, urticaria, and agranulocytosis, may be observed.

Diphenylhydantoin

The discovery of the antiarrhythmic properties of diphenylhydantoin provided another important tool for the management of various cardiac arrhythmias, particularly those induced by digitalis.[2,16] Diphenylhydantoin has a structure similar to that of the barbiturates, but its electrophysiologic properties are quite different from those of other antiarrhythmic drugs. Atrial conduction velocity is accelerated by diphenylhydantoin as a result of a faster depolarization of the atria while the sinus rate is usually unaffected. While the AV conduction may not be affected by diphenylhydantoin, it is often accelerated by the action of the drug. As a rule, intraventricular conduction is not altered significantly by diphenylhydantoin. One of the most important aspects of the drug is that it counteracts the depressant effect on the AV conduction induced by digitalis and procainamide. In addition, diphenylhydantoin depresses diastolic depolarization and automaticity and shortens the duration of the action potential and the effective refractory period.[2,16]

Indications. At present, diphenylhydantoin is considered to be the drug of choice in the treatment of various tachyarrhythmias induced by digitalis,[2,16] especially digitalis-induced ventricular tachycardia (Chapter 16). It is also a very useful substitute for procainamide or lidocaine when those drugs are found to be ineffective.[1] In addition, diphenylhydantoin has value in preventing postcardioversion arrhythmias, especially when the patient is taking any amount of digitalis. Usually, a 125 to 250 mg intravenous injection of diphenylhydantoin is sufficient for the purpose.[16b]

Full Dosage. The initial dose of diphenylhydantoin is from 125 to 250 mg intravenously for 1 to 3 minutes under ECG monitoring. Most patients respond in three seconds to five minutes. The same dose may be repeated every 10 to 20 minutes as needed, but the total dose should not exceed 750 mg per hour. Continuous intravenous drip is not practicable because diphenylhydantoin easily precipitates with various commonly used intravenous solutions. When the situation is not urgent, 200 mg of diphenylhydantoin may be given orally as an initial dose, followed by 100 mg every 4 to 6 hours as needed.[1]

Maintenance Dosage. After termination of the tachyarrhythmias, a maintenance dose of diphenylhydantoin, 100 mg 3 to 4 times a day, is often needed; the duration depends on the clinical situation. Oral diphenylhydantoin is often useful in place of procainamide or quinidine for long-term therapy.[1]

Side Effects and Toxicity. The toxic manifestations or side effects of diphenylhydantoin include respiratory and cardiac depression, skin reactions, such as urticaria and purpura, eosinophilia, drowsiness, ataxia, tremor, depression, nervousness, arthralgia, gingival hyperplasia, hypotension, and AV block of varying degree.[2,16] Fortunately, these manifestations are rare.

Disopyramide Phosphate

Disopyramide phosphate (Norpace) has been recently introduced in clinical medicine as a class 1 antiarrhythmic drug similar to procainamide and quinidine.[15b] Norpace has been shown to be effective for various ventricular tachyarrhythmias, particularly ventricular premature contractions. Norpace is available only for oral clinical use in the United States[15b] although it is already available for parenteral use in many European countries (e.g., disopyramide—Rythmodan, Roussel Laboratories, Ltd., the United Kingdom).[22a]

Chemically, Norpace is unique among the antiarrhythmic drugs, but in its pharmacologic actions it is related to quinidine and procainamide.[15b] In animal studies, the drug has been shown to reduce the rate of diastolic depolarization (phase 4) and to decrease the upstroke velocity (phase 0) in cells with augmented automaticity and to increase the action potential duration of normal cardiac cells. Norpace has had no effect on alpha- or beta-adrenergic receptors in animal studies.[15b] Electrophysiologic studies in humans have shown prolongation of conduction in accessory pathway.[15b]

Hemodynamically, Norpace rarely produces significant alterations of the blood pressure at the recommended oral doses.[15b] The mean plasma half-life of Norpace in healthy humans is shown to be 6.7 hours, with a range of 4 to 10 hours. Information about the onset of action, maximum effect, and duration of action of Norpace is given in Table 7–5.

In regard to the metabolism of Norpace, the orally administered drug is almost completely absorbed; 80% is excreted in the urine (50% unchanged) and 10% is excreted in the feces.[15b]

Indications. Norpace is indicated for various ventricular tachyarrhythmias, including ventricular premature contractions and ventricular tachycardia.[15b] In my experience, several patients responded to Norpace when refractory ventricular premature contractions were resistant to other commonly used drugs, including procainamide, quinidine, diphenylhydantoin, and propranolol. In Europe, disopyramide (Rythmodan) has been used with varying success[22b] for various supraventricular tachyarrhythmias, including those associated with the Wolff-Parkinson-White syndrome.

Full Dosage. Norpace is supplied as 100 mg and 150 mg capsules; the usual oral adult loading dose is 300 mg. In adults of small stature or with moderate-to-severe renal insufficiency, hepatic insufficiency, cardiomyopathy, and significant congestive heart failure, the loading dose should be reduced to 200 mg.

In Europe, a single intravenous dose of between 50 and 150 mg (Rythmodan) was given for various cardiac arrhythmias associated with myocardial infarction in 85 patients.[22a] In that study, successful and rapid termination of ventricular arrhythmias was observed in 78%, whereas the drug was effective in only 42% of supraventricular arrhythmias.

Maintenance Dosage. The usual recommended adult dosage is 400 to 800 mg a day in divided doses following an initial loading dose.[15b] In most clinical situations, the drug is given orally in the dosage of 150 mg every 6 hours. Again, in smaller adults or in people with renal or hepatic insufficiency and significant congestive heart failure, the dosage should be reduced to 100 mg every 6 hours.

Side Effects and Toxicity. The side effects of Norpace have been reported to be usually mild and to be anticholinergic. The most common untoward side effects include dry mouth (reported in 40% of patients) and urinary hesitancy (reported in 16%).[15b] In addition, the drug may produce anorexia, nausea, vomiting, bloating, gas, diarrhea, constipation, blurred vision, dry nose, eyes, or throat, urinary frequency or retention, dizziness, fatigue, muscle weakness, headache, edema, weight gain, hypotension, cardiac conduction disturbances (varying degrees of AV block and intraventricular block), nervousness, and generalized rash.[15b]

Norpace is contraindicated in the presence of cardiogenic shock, second-degree or complete AV block, severe congestive heart failure, glaucoma, and known hypersensitivity to the drug. In addition, Norpace should be administered with caution to patients with the sick sinus syndrome, the Wolff-Parkinson-White syndrome, intraventricular block and severe renal or hepatic insufficiency.

Miscellaneous Drugs

Various antiarrhythmic drugs, including verapamil, amiodarone, and ajmaline, are available in many European countries for clinical use.[16a,22b] Those drugs have been shown to be very effective in the prevention and treatment of various tachyarrhythmias associated with the Wolff-Parkinson-White syndrome (Table 7-2). (The clinical availability of intravenous disopyramide—Rythmodan—in Europe was discussed on p. 130.[22a])

CAROTID SINUS STIMULATION

Carotid sinus stimulation is indicated for two major purposes—therapy and diagnosis.[9]

Therapy

Carotid sinus stimulation is extremely valuable in terminating paroxysmal atrial as well as AV junctional tachycardia. In addition, regular and rapid tachycardia (160 to 250 beats per minute) is often terminated by carotid sinus stimulation even if the exact location of the ectopic focus is uncertain. Carotid sinus stimulation may be effective whether the QRS complex is normal or wide.

It should be noted, however, that a person with a hypersensitive reaction to carotid sinus stimulation may develop near syncope or syncope following the procedure as a result of a long ventricular standstill (Fig. 7-17). As described on p. 104, carotid sinus syncope is one of the important manifestations of the sick sinus syndrome (Chapter 9).

The various responses of the tachyarrhythmias to carotid sinus stimulation are summarized in Table 7-4. It has been shown that the responses to

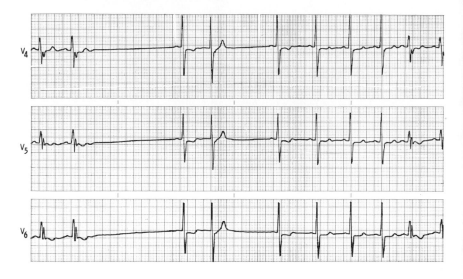

Figure 7–17.   Marked slowing of sinus rate (sinus arrest) was produced by carotid sinus stimulation. Note the disappearance of the left bundle branch block during slow rate.

carotid sinus stimulation, in terms of the development of varying degrees of AV block, are usually exaggerated by various drugs, such as digitalis, propranolol, and methyldopa (Aldomet).[16b]

Diagnosis

It has been known for years that carotid sinus stimulation is extremely useful in differentiating various tachyarrhythmias (Fig. 7–18), particularly regular ectopic tachycardia and wide QRS complex (Fig. 7–19). It should be emphasized that applying carotid sinus stimulation to patients with digitalis intoxication is dangerous; it may induce ventricular fibrillation (Chapter 16).

Depending on the type and nature of the tachyarrhythmias,[4] various responses to carotid sinus stimulation may be observed, as discussed in the following paragraphs.

1. Sinus tachycardia. In general, it is not necessary to apply carotid sinus stimulation either diagnostically or therapeutically in cases of sinus tachycardia. However, the procedure is occasionally useful when the rate of sinus tachycardia is very rapid (around 150 to 160 beats per minute) and differentiation from atrial tachycardia is needed. Sinus tachycardia slows only transiently in response to carotid sinus stimulation (Figs. 7–18 and 7–19). On rare occasions, carotid sinus stimulation may cause varying

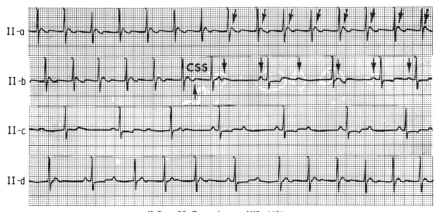

M.B., 62 F. - ACUTE AMI (#2)
(RESPONSE TO CAROTID SINUS STIMULATION)

Figure 7–18.   Leads II-a,b,c, and d are continuous. The basic rhythm before carotid sinus stimulation (CSS) shows sinus rhythm with markedly prolonged P–R intervals (the arrows indicate sinus P waves). The sinus P waves become clearly discernible by CSS as the ventricular rate is reduced as a result of increased AV block.

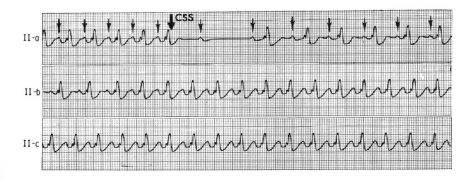

Figure 7–19.   The arrows indicate sinus P waves. Leads II-a,b, and c are continuous. Note clearly identifiable P waves (indicated by arrows) by carotid sinus stimulation (CSS) as the result of increased AV block. The cardiac rhythm before CSS is sinus tachycardia with first-degree AV block and left bundle branch block.

degrees of AV block leading to slow ventricular rate (Figs. 7–18 and 7–19).

2. Atrial tachycardia. Carotid sinus stimulation is extremely valuable in terminating paroxysmal atrial tachycardia (Fig. 7–20). The response of atrial tachycardia to carotid sinus stimulation may be one of the following: (a) termination, (b) slowing of ventricular rate due to increased AV block,

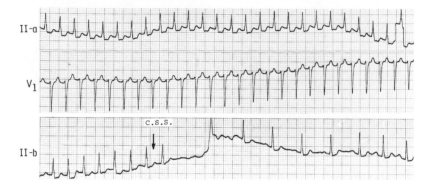

Figure 7–20.   Leads II-a and b are not continuous. Supraventricular (probably atrial) tachycardia (187 beats per minute) is terminated by carotid sinus stimulation (indicated by arrow).

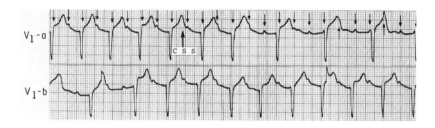

Figure 7–21.   Leads V₁-a and b are continuous. The arrows indicate P waves. Note a transient slowing of the ventricular rate in atrial tachycardia by carotid sinus stimulation (indicated by CSS). Atrial tachycardia (atrial rate: 190 beats per minute) in this case is considered to have been induced by digitalis.

and (c) increased atrial rate, or (d) there may be no response. When slowing of the ventricular rate occurs in atrial tachycardia because of increased AV block, the underlying cause is usually digitalis intoxication (Fig. 7–21).

3. Atrial fibrillation or flutter. When carotid sinus pressure is applied to patients with atrial fibrillation or flutter, the ventricular rate invariably slows because of the increased AV block. Occasionally a long ventricular standstill may result when carotid sinus pressure is applied to an elderly patient with atrial fibrillation or flutter.

4. AV junctional tachycardia. It is often difficult (at times impossible) to distinguish paroxysmal atrial tachycardia from paroxysmal AV junctional tachycardia when only conventional ECGs are available. The P wave may be superimposed on the S–T segment, T wave, QRS complex,

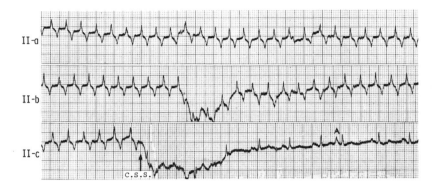

Figure 7–22.   Leads II-a,b, and c are continuous. AV junctional tachycardia is terminated by carotid sinus stimulation (indicated by arrow). Note the one atrial premature beat (marked A) in lead II-c.

or the preceding or succeeding beat. Therefore the term, supraventricular tachycardia is often used to describe the condition. It is believed that the response to carotid sinus stimulation is similar in paroxysmal atrial tachycardia and paroxysmal AV junctional tachycardia.

Paroxysmal AV junctional tachycardia may convert to sinus rhythm (Fig. 7–22) or it may not respond to carotid sinus stimulation. On the other hand, nonparoxysmal AV junctional tachycardia is usually unresponsive to carotid sinus stimulation, but ventricular fibrillation may ensue if the underlying cause is digitalis intoxication. Thus carotid sinus stimulation is not recommended in the presence of nonparoxysmal AV junctional tachycardia, which is a common sign of digitalis intoxication (Chapter 16).

5. Ventricular tachyarrhythmias. Carotid sinus stimulation is often used to distinguish ventricular tachycardia from supraventricular tachycardia, especially when the QRS complex is wide and bizarre. Unlike supraventricular tachyarrhythmias, ventricular tachycardia does not respond to carotid sinus stimulation. Therefore any response to the procedure rules out ventricular tachycardia.

DIRECT CURRENT SHOCK

The two major uses of direct current cardioversion are in the treatment of (1) acute tachyarrhythmias and (2) chronic atrial fibrillation and flutter (by elective cardioversion).

Direct Current Cardioversion for Acute Tachyarrhythmias

In various supraventricular (atrial and AV junctional) and ventricular tachyarrhythmias with an acute onset, direct current cardioversion is often lifesaving. When the clinical situation is extremely urgent, as in the case of ventricular tachycardia or fibrillation (Figs. 7–10 and 7–11), premedication for transient amnesia or anesthesia is not needed. Thus 100 to 200 Wsec of direct current shock can be applied directly. If the arrhythmia persists, direct current shock of increased energy (200 to 400 Wsec) should be repeated immediately. On the other hand, if the clinical situation is not extremely urgent, small amounts of thiopental sodium or diazepam may be administered before the application of direct current shock. Premedication may not be indicated when only a small energy discharge is required, particularly in the treatment of atrial flutter. Following the termination of ventricular tachyarrhythmias, a continuous intravenous infusion of lidocaine (less commonly procainamide) is usually indicated and followed by oral maintenance therapy with procainamide, diphenylhydantoin, or quinidine. When atrial flutter or fibrillation is terminated by direct current shock (Fig. 7–8), maintenance doses of oral quinidine after digitalization are needed in most instances. Direct current shock is often effective in terminating any tachyarrhythmia associated with the Wolff-Parkinson-White syndrome (Fig. 7–23).

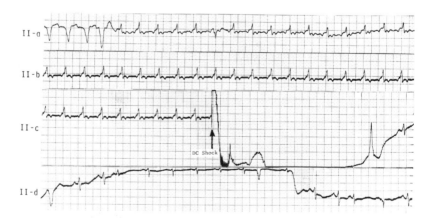

Figure 7–23.   Leads II-a,b,c, and d are continuous. Atrial flutter with 2:1 AV response in the Wolff-Parkinson-White syndrome is terminated by direct current shock (indicated by arrow). Note the two types of anomalous AV conduction during atrial flutter. There are occasional atrial as well as ventricular premature contractions.

Elective Cardioversion

Elective cardioversion is indicated for the treatment of chronic tachyarrhythmias, primarily atrial fibrillation or flutter, when restoration of sinus rhythm is considered to be beneficial. Less commonly, elective cardioversion is used to terminate other tachyarrhythmias, such as atrial or AV junctional tachycardia.

Direct current shock is discussed in detail in Chapter 10.

ARTIFICIAL PACEMAKERS

Although the primary use of the artificial pacemaker is in the treatment of slow rhythms, particularly the sick sinus syndrome and complete AV block, artificial pacemakers may also be indicated for terminating and preventing drug-resistant refractory tachyarrhythmias.[11] In these circumstances, the overdriving pacing rate is needed to suppress ectopic tachycardia. The primary indication for the use of the overdriving pacing rate (about 100 to 120 beats per minute) is in the management of refractory ventricular tachyarrhythmias[11] (Figs. 7–24 and 7–25).

The overdriving pacing rate is also extremely useful in the treatment of the brady-tachyarrhythmia syndrome (Figs. 7–26 and 7–27). In that condition, only a slight overdriving pacing rate (about 80 to 100 beats per minute) may be sufficient. Occasionally, the overdriving pacing rate is indicated in the treatment of refractory supraventricular tachyarrhythmias (Fig. 7–9).

Artificial pacemakers are discussed in detail in Chapter 11.

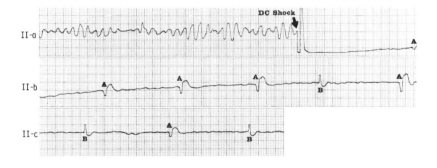

Figure 7–24. Figures 7–24 and 7–25 were obtained from the same patient on different occasions. In Figure 7–24, leads II-a,b, and c are continuous. Ventricular fibrillation is terminated by direct current shock (indicated by arrow). However, following direct current shock, ventricular escape rhythms (idioventricular rhythms) originating from two foci (marked A and B) are observed in the presence of atrial fibrillation due to complete AV block. That ECG finding reflects a type of the brady-tachyarrhythmia syndrome.

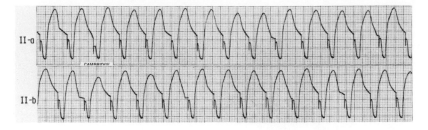

Figure 7–25.   Leads II-a and b are continuous. These rhythm strips were obtained after the insertion of a temporary artificial pacemaker with an overdriving pacing rate (98 beats per minute).

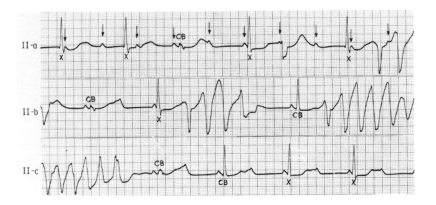

Figure 7–26.   The ECGs shown in Figures 7–26 and 7–27 were obtained from the same patient on different occasions. In Figure 7–26, leads II-a, b, and c are continuous. The tracing shows sinus rhythm with intermittent ventricular escape rhythm (marked X) due to high-degree AV block and frequent ventricular premature contractions with short runs of ventricular tachycardia. Note the occasional ventricular captured beats (marked CB). That type of arrhythmia is called the brady-tachyarrhythmia syndrome.

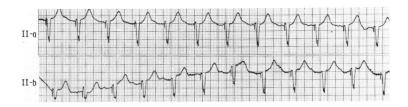

Figure 7–27.   Leads II-a and b are continuous. These rhythm strips were obtained after the insertion of a temporary artificial pacemaker with a slightly overdriving pacing rate (75 beats per minute).

SURGICAL APPROACHES

In the past several years, various surgical approaches to the management of drug-resistant refractory tachyarrhythmias have been developed.[23–28] Surgical management has been restricted primarily to the treatment of the life-threatening ventricular tachyarrhythmias associated with coronary heart disease[23,24] and the drug-resistant supraventricular tachyarrhythmias associated with the Wolff-Parkinson-White syndrome.[25–28]

Recently, very favorable surgical results were reported in a study of eight patients with drug-resistant life-threatening ventricular tachyarrhythmias associated with documented coronary heart disease.[23] The surgical procedures in the study included a resection of the ventricular aneurysm or localized hypokinetic area in six patients and aortocoronary bypass grafting to at least one major coronary artery in all eight patients.

But surgical management of drug-resistant supraventricular tachyarrhythmias associated with the Wolff-Parkinson-White syndrome has not been always successful.[25–28] The surgical procedures include a ligation of the AV bundle and a surgical interruption of the anomalous pathway following an epicardial mapping study.[25–28] The surgical approaches to the Wolff-Parkinson-White syndrome require further investigation.

The surgical approaches to the management of refractory tachyarrhythmias are discussed in detail in Chapter 18.

SUMMARY

1. The best therapeutic results can be obtained when a precise diagnosis of the tachyarrhythmia is made.

2. In addition, underlying causative factors also significantly affect the therapeutic result.

3. The first step in management is to eliminate the cause of the tachyarrhythmia if the cause is apparent.

4. Prevention of the recurrence of tachyarrhythmias is another important aspect of management. Many patients require maintenance therapy with digitalis or another antiarrhythmic drug for long periods, perhaps indefinitely. After the tachyarrhythmia has been terminated by carotid sinus stimulation or direct current shock, the use of one or more drugs may be indicated to prevent a recurrence of the arrhythmia.

5. Digitalis is often the drug of choice in the treatment of supraventricular tachyarrhythmias, particularly atrial fibrillation or flutter with rapid ventricular response.

6. But digitalis is contraindicated in supraventricular tachyar-

rhythmias, particularly atrial fibrillation with anomalous AV conduction in Wolff-Parkinson-White syndrome.

7. Propranolol is the drug of choice in the treatment and prevention of catecholamine-induced tachyarrhythmias and reciprocating tachycardia with normal QRS complexes associated with the Wolff-Parkinson-White syndrome, especially in young people without demonstrable heart disease.

8. Lidocaine is the drug of choice in the treatment of supraventricular tachyarrhythmias, particularly atrial fibrillation or flutter with anomalous AV conduction in the Wolff-Parkinson-White syndrome.

9. Lidocaine is the drug of choice in the treatment of ventricular tachyarrhythmias in almost all clinical conditions, particularly in acute myocardial infarction.

10. For digitalis-induced tachyarrhythmias, however, potassium or diphenylhydantoin is the drug of choice. Diphenylhydantoin is especially valuable in the treatment of digitalis-induced ventricular tachycardia.

11. At present, the primary use for quinidine is in the prevention of atrial fibrillation or flutter by oral administration following a restoration of sinus rhythm by digitalization or direct current shock.

12. Similarly, the main use of procainamide is in the prevention of ventricular tachyarrhythmias by oral administration after termination of the arrhythmia by lidocaine or direct current shock.

13. Norpace is a new antiarrhythmic drug that has been found to be effective for various ventricular tachyarrhythmias.

14. In urgent situations, particularly in ventricular tachyarrhythmias, direct current shock should be applied immediately.

15. In refractory tachyarrhythmias, the use of an artificial pacemaker with an overdriving pacing rate is often lifesaving.

16. Carotid sinus stimulation is the simplest and often the most effective way of terminating supraventricular tachycardia when it is applied properly. The procedure is also extremely valuable in the differential diagnosis of various tachyarrhythmias.

17. In refractory ventricular tachyarrhythmias, especially in the presence of coronary heart disease, surgical procedures may be indicated in selected cases.

REFERENCES

1. Chung, E.K.: Cardiac Arrhythmias: Management. Baltimore, Williams & Wilkins Co., 1973.
2. Chung, E.K.: Digitalis Intoxication. Baltimore, Williams & Wilkins Co., 1969.
3. Chung, E.K.: Clinical Electrocardiography. 7. Drug Therapy for Cardiac Arrhythmias. New York, Medcom, Inc., 1977.

4. Hurst, J.W., Paulk, E.A., Jr., Proctor, H.D., and Schlant, R.C.: Management of patients with atrial fibrillation. Am. J. Med. 37:728, 1964.
5. Koch-Weser, J., and Klein, S.W.: Procainamide dosage schedules, plasma concentrations, and clinical effects. J.A.M.A. 125:1454, 1971.
6. Gibson, D., and Sowton, E.: The use of beta-adrenergic receptor blocking drugs in dysrhythmias. Prog. Cardiovasc. Dis. 12:16, 1969.
7. Kosman, M.E.: Current status of propranolol hydrochloride (Inderal). J.A.M.A. 225:1380, 1973.
8. Day, H.W., and Bacaner, M.: Use of bretylium tosylate in the management of acute myocardial infarction. Am. J. Cardiol. 27:177, 1971.
9. Chung, E.K.: Use and abuse of carotid sinus stimulation. Postgrad. Med. 51:190, 1972.
10. Chung, E.K.: Use and abuse of direct current shock. Cardiology 55:310, 1970.
11. Furman, S., and Escher, D.J.W.: Principles and Techniques of Cardiac Pacing. Hagerstown, Md., Harper & Row, 1970.
11a. Chung, E.K.: Artificial Cardiac Pacing: Practical Approach. Baltimore, Williams & Wilkins Co., 1979.
12. Lister, J.W., Cohen, L.S., Bernstein, W.H., and Samet, P.: Treatment of supraventricular tachycardia by rapid atrial stimulation. Circulation 38:1044, 1968.
13. Chung, E.K.: Electrocardiography: Practical Applications with Vectorial Principles. Hagerstown, Md., Harper & Row, 1974.
14. Bigger, J.T., Jr., and Heissenbuttel, R.H.: The use of procaine amide and lidocaine in the treatment of cardiac arrhythmias. Prog. Cardiovasc. Dis. 11:515, 1969.
15. Harrison, D.C., Sprouse, J.H., and Morrow, A.G.: The antiarrhythmic properties of lidocaine and procaine amide. Circulation 28:486, 1963.
15a. Chung, E.K.: Exercise Electrocardiography: Practical Approach. Baltimore, Williams & Wilkins Co., 1979.
15b. A Clinical Profile—Norpace. G.D. Searle & Co., 1977.
16. Damato, A.N.: Diphenylhydantoin: Pharmacological and clinical use. Prog. Cardiovasc. Dis. 12:1, 1969.
16a. Chung, E.K.: Wolff-Parkinson-White syndrome: Current views. Am. J. Med. 62:252, 1977.
16b. Chung, E.K.: Principles of Cardiac Arrhythmias, 2nd ed. Baltimore, Williams & Wilkins Co., 1977.
17. Wyman, M.G., and Hammersmith, L.: Comprehensive treatment plan for the prevention of primary ventricular fibrillation in acute myocardial infarction. Am. J. Cardiol. 33:661, 1974.
18. Beller, G.A., Smith, T.W., Abelman, W.H. et al.: Digitalis intoxication. A prospective study with serum level correlations. N. Engl. J. Med. 284:989, 1971.
19. Doherty, J.E.: The clinical pharmacology of digitalis glycosides: A review. Am. J. Med. Sci. 255:382, 1968.
20. Hauck, A.J., Ongley, P.A., and Nadas, A.S.: The use of digoxin in infants and children. Am. Heart J. 56:443, 1958.
21. Levine, O.R., and Blumenthal, S.: Digoxin dosage in premature infants. Pediatrics 29:18, 1962.
22. Neill, C.A.: The use of digitalis in infants and children. Prog. Cardiovasc. Dis. 7:399, 1965.
22a. Ankier, S.I., and Woodings, D.F.: Disopyramide (Rythmodan) Seminar, St. John's College, Cambridge, England, 1977.
22b. Krikler, D.: Verapamil in cardiology. Eur. J. Cardiol. 2:3, 1974.
23. Graham, A.F., Miller, D.C., Stinson, E.B., et al.: Surgical treatment of refractory life-threatening ventricular tachycardia. Am. J. Cardiol. 32:909, 1973.
24. Welch, T.G., Fontana, M.E., and Vasko, J.S.: Aneurysmectomy for recurrent ventricular tachyarrhythmias. Am. Heart J. 85:685, 1973.
25. Neutze, J.M., Kerr, A.R., and Whitlock, R.M.L.: Epicardial mapping in a variant of type A Wolff-Parkinson-White syndrome. Circulation 48:662, 1973.

26. Dreifus, L.S., Nichols, H., Morse, D., Watanabe, Y., and Truex, R.: Control of recurrent tachycardia of Wolff-Parkinson-White syndrome by surgical ligation of the A-V bundle. Circulation 38:1030, 1968.
27. Linsay, A.E., Nelson, R.M., Abildskov, J.A., and Wyatt, R.: Attempted surgical division of the preexcitation pathway in the Wolff-Parkinson-White syndrome. Am. J. Cardiol. 28:581, 1971.
28. Cole, D.D., Wills, R.E., Winterscheid, L.C., Reichenback, D.D., and Blackmon, J.R.: The Wolff-Parkinson-White syndrome. Problems in evaluation and surgical therapy. Circulation 42:111, 1970.

Chapter 8

BRADYARRHYTHMIAS

EDWARD K. CHUNG

Bradyarrhythmia is defined as slow cardiac rhythm (usually fewer than 60 beats per minute) that is due to various fundamental mechanisms.[1] Bradyarrhythmias may be divided into two major categories:

1. Disturbances of sinus impulse formation and conduction (sinus bradycardia, sinus arrest, and sinoatrial block)

2. Atrioventricular (AV) block of various degrees.

The therapeutic approaches to bradyarrhythmia vary markedly, depending on the fundamental mechanism responsible for the production of bradyarrhythmias, the ventricular rate, the underlying cause, and the symptoms, if present.[2]

DISTURBANCES OF SINUS IMPULSE FORMATION AND CONDUCTION

Mild sinus bradycardia (50 to 59 beats per minute) is not uncommon in healthy people, especially in young athletes and elderly people. When the sinus rate is 40 to 50 beats per minute, there may be some symptoms. Marked sinus bradycardia (fewer than 40 beats per minute) often produces significant hemodynamic alterations, especially when it is associated with acute myocardial infarction.[2,3] Among the most common causes of sinus bradycardia are the therapeutic or toxic effects of various drugs, including digitalis, propranolol, reserpine, and guanethidine, and acute diaphragmatic myocardial infarction.[1-4] Drug-induced sinus bradycardia,

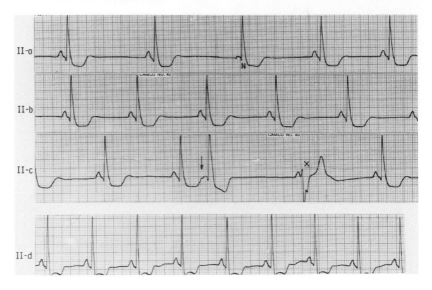

Figure 8–1.   Leads II-a,b, and c are continuous. The first three rhythm strips show marked sinus bradycardia (30 to 35 beats per minute), with AV junctional and ventricular escape beats (marked N and X, respectively). Note the single atrial premature beat (indicated by arrow). The sinus rate has increased (56 beats per minute) immediately following the intravenous injection of 0.4 mg of atropine (lead II-d).

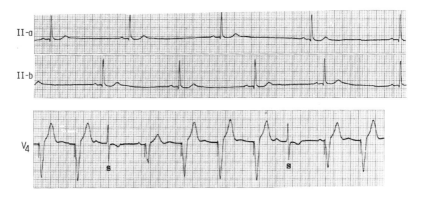

Figure 8–2.   Leads II-a and b are continuous. The tracing shows sinus arrhythmia with marked sinus bradycardia (27 to 33 beats per minute). Because of symptomatic and drug-resistant sinus bradycardia due to the sick sinus syndrome, a permanent artificial (demand) pacemaker is implanted (lead V_4). In lead V_4, there are two sinus beats with long P–R intervals (0.28 sec) in the presence of artificial pacemaker-induced ventricular rhythm (68 beats per minute). The patient shows definite evidence of the sick sinus syndrome, in which a markedly slow sinus mechanism fails to respond to any drug.

sinus arrest, or sinoatrial (SA) block is best treated by discontinuing administration of that particular drug.[4]

Active treatment is indicated when marked sinus bradycardia persists and becomes symptomatic, and especially when it is associated with acute myocardial infarction (Fig. 8–1). The treatment of choice in that case is atropine, and the next commonly used drug is isoproterenol (Isuprel).[2,3] Essentially the same therapeutic approach may be used in the treatment of symptomatic sinus arrest and SA block.

In drug-resistant sinus bradycardia, sinus arrest, or SA block, the diagnosis of the sick sinus syndrome is strongly suggested. The implantation of a permanent artificial pacemaker is recommended for every patient with significant sick sinus syndrome (Fig. 8–2).[5,6] The sick sinus syndrome is discussed in detail in Chapter 9.

ATRIOVENTRICULAR (AV) BLOCK

It is important to remember that AV block per se does not require treatment. Whether the treatment of AV block is indicated depends primarily on the degree and the cause of the AV block, the ventricular rate, and the presence or absence of symptoms.[2]

First-degree AV block usually requires no particular treatment, except that any apparent direct cause, such as digitalis intoxication, may be eliminated.[4] It has been reported that atropine is effective in abolishing digitalis-induced first- and second-degree AV block. Isoproterenol may be effective, but it often produces untoward reactions, such as increased ventricular irritability.

Wenckebach (Mobitz type I) AV block (Fig. 8–3) usually does not

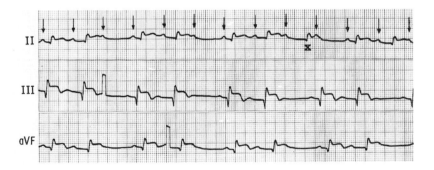

Figure 8–3.   The arrows indicate sinus P waves. The tracing shows sinus rhythm (atrial rate: 98 beats per minute) with predominantly 3:2 Wenckebach AV block associated with acute diaphragmatic myocardial infarction. The unexpectedly conducted beat with a long P–R interval (marked X) is considered to represent a supernormal AV conduction.

require active treatment unless significant symptoms are produced. On the other hand, Mobitz type II AV block often requires an artificial pacemaker, because it is considered to be a precursor of complete AV block due to trifascicular block.[7]

In complete AV block, the therapeutic approach depends on the ventricular rate and the magnitude of the symptoms. Unless there are symptoms, active treatment is usually not indicated when the ventricular rate is relatively rapid (50 to 60 beats per minute) in AV junctional escape rhythm due to complete AV block (Fig. 8–4), such as seen in acute diaphragmatic myocardial infarction. On the other hand, a temporary or often a permanent artificial pacemaker is indicated when the ventricular rate is slow (fewer than 40 beats per minute) in ventricular escape (idioventricular) rhythm due to complete AV block, as is seen in acute anterior myocardial infarction or in elderly people with degenerative changes in the conduction system[5,6,8] (Fig. 8–4). Bilateral bundle branch block (bifascicular and trifascicular block) of varying degrees often requires a permanent artificial pacemaker[7] (Fig. 8–5).

In urgent situations before the insertion of an artificial pacemaker, various drugs, such as isoproterenol or epinephrine (Adrenalin), may be tried, particularly in ventricular standstill (Fig. 8–6). Extremely slow rhythm may be produced when an artificial pacemaker malfunctions, especially when the newer demand models are used.[5,6] The slow pacemaker rhythm is often associated with irregular pacing (Fig. 8–7). When a malfunction of the pacemaker is diagnosed, needless to say, that pacemaker should be replaced immediately by a normally functioning pacemaker.[5,6]

Chapter 11 discusses artificial pacemakers in detail.

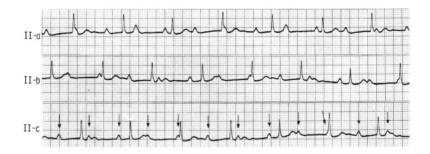

Figure 8–4. Leads II-a,b,c, and d are continuous. The arrows indicate P waves. The tracing reveals sinus rhythm (atrial rate: 87 beats per minute) with AV junctional escape rhythm (ventricular rate: 55 beats per minute) due to complete AV block.

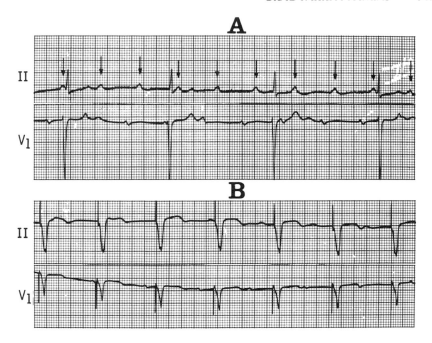

Figure 8–5. Tracings A and B were obtained from the same patient, who had the Adams-Stokes syndrome. In tracing A, the arrows indicate P waves. The tracing A shows sinus rhythm (atrial rate: 89 beats per minute) with ventricular escape (idioventricular) rhythm (35 beats per minute) due to complete AV block. Tracing B, taken after implantation of a permanent pacemaker, reveals artificial pacemaker-induced ventricular rhythm (ventricular rate: 63 beats per minute).

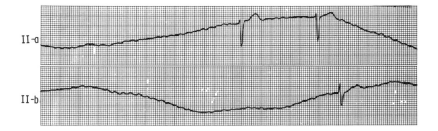

Figure 8–6. Leads II-a and b are *not* continuous. The rhythm is atrial fibrillation with areas of ventricular standstill.

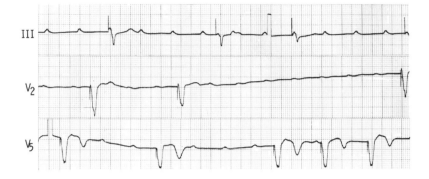

Figure 8–7. Sinus rhythm with markedly irregular and slow artificial pacemaker-induced ventricular rhythm due to a malfunctioning unit.

ANTIBRADYARRHYTHMIC DRUGS (See also Table 8–1)

Because of the ready availability of artificial pacemakers, the various antibradyarrhythmic drugs have been much less commonly used in the past decade. Nevertheless, those drugs are valuable for the management of milder forms of slow rhythms, such as marked sinus bradycardia and SA block.[9–12] In addition, antibradyarrhythmic drugs are extremely useful for urgent situations, such as in the Adams-Stokes syndrome, when artificial pacemakers are not immediately available.[9–12] Of the antibradyarrhythmic drugs, those most commonly used are probably atropine sulfate and isoproterenol.[2]

Atropine Sulfate[2,9–12]

Indications. Atropine is used primarily to accelerate the sinus rate by vagal inhibition. Thus it is the drug of choice for marked symptomatic sinus bradycardia (Fig. 8–1). Atropine is also effective in the treatment of sinus arrest or SA block. In first- or second-degree AV block (usually the Wenckebach type), especially in acute diaphragmatic myocardial infarction or digitalis intoxication, atropine may also be used. It is usually not effective in the treatment of high-degree or complete AV block.

Administration. Atropine is best administered intravenously in a dose of 0.3 to 1 mg (up to 2 mg), and a similar dose may be repeated every 10 to 15 minutes as needed. When the optimal dose is determined, it may be repeated every 4 to 6 hours, but the total dosage of atropine should not exceed 4 mg. The effect of the drug is usually prompt. Atropine may be given subcutaneously if it is not feasible to use the intravenous route.

Atropine has been administered orally, but the effectiveness of oral atropine is less predictable.

Side Effects and Toxicity. Serious toxic effects of atropine are uncommon, but ventricular premature contractions or ventricular tachyarrhythmias may be induced. Common side effects include a dry mouth, urinary retention, exacerbation of glaucoma, hallucinations, hyperpyrexia, and marked sinus tachycardia.

Isoproterenol[2,9-12]

Before artificial pacemakers were available for clinical use, the treatment of choice for complete AV block was the administration of isoproterenol. The drug is still very useful in the emergency treatment of Adams-Stokes syndrome or as a temporary measure until an artificial pacemaker can be implanted. Thus isoproterenol is still the drug of choice in the treatment of the Adams-Stokes syndrome due to bradyarrhythmias, primarily complete AV block and ventricular standstill. Isoproterenol is capable of accelerating both the supraventricular and the ventricular pacemakers and of improving AV conduction. The drug has a potent inotropic action that increases the stroke volume, the amplitude of myocardial contraction, and the coronary blood flow.

Indications. The primary indication for isoproterenol is in the treatment of the Adams-Stokes syndrome due to complete AV block or ventricular standstill (Fig. 8–6) until an artificial pacemaker is inserted. Isoproterenol may also be used in place of atropine in the treatment of symptomatic sinus bradycardia, sinus arrest, and SA block.

Administration. Isoproterenol can be given by direct intracardiac, intravenous, intramuscular, or subcutaneous injection, or it may be given by intravenous infusion.

In an emergency, such as in severe Adams-Stokes syndrome or ventricular standstill, isoproterenol can be given by intracardiac or intravenous injection. The usual dose is 0.02 mg to 0.05 mg, but up to 0.1 mg may be administered. Otherwise, the drug can be given subcutaneously or intramuscularly in a dosage of 0.1 mg to 0.4 mg every 2 to 6 hours as needed. Continuous intravenous infusion of isoproterenol is indicated in severe cases to maintain the ventricular rate around 50 to 60 beats per minute until an artificial pacemaker can be inserted. The usual method is to dilute 0.1 mg of isoproterenol in 200 cc of 5% solution of dextrose in water, and the initial infusion rate is 1 μg to 4 μg per minute. The infusion rate may be increased to 5 μg to 10 μg per minute, and up to 40 μg per minute may occasionally be required to maintain an ideal ventricular rate.

The most popular route of administration of this drug is the sublingual route, and the usual dosage is 10 to 30 mg every 1 to 6 hours. The drug can be given as often as every 30 minutes if needed.

Table 8–1. *Antibradyarrhythmic Drugs*

Drugs	Dosage	Onset of Action	Maximum Effect	Duration of Action	Indications	Side Effects and Toxicity
Atropine sulfate	0.3–2 mg q̄ 4–6 hr IV inj. as needed or the same dose may be given by SC inj. (total: 4 mg) or 0.4–0.8 mg q̄ 4–6 hr PO for mild form	1–5 min	Few minutes to 30 min	4–6 hr	Primary: Sinus bradycardia, sinus arrest, SA block Secondary: First-degree and occasionally second-degree AV block	Dry mouth, urinary retention, exacerbation of glaucoma, hallucinations, hyperpyrexia, postural hypotension, sinus tachycardia, VPC, ventricular tachycardia
Isoproterenol (Isuprel)	0.02–0.05 mg (up to 0.1 mg) IC or IV inj., or 0.1–0.4 mg SC or IM inj. q̄ 2–6 hr as needed or 1 mg/200 cc 5% D/W IV infusion, 1–4 μg/min initially and may increase to 5–10 μg/min as needed. 10–30 mg sublingually q̄ 1–6 hr (for mild cases)	At once Irregular	At once Irregular	Minutes Irregular	Ventricular standstill, severe AS syndrome Primary: High-degree or complete AV block Secondary: Sinus bradycardia, sinus arrest, and SA block	Tremor, nausea, nervousness, sweating, weakness, dizziness, headache, palpitation, VPC, ventricular tachycardia and fibrillation, hypotension

Epinephrine hydrochloride (Adrenalin)	0.3–0.6 cc of 1:1000 solution IV, IM, SC, or IC inj., or 0.5–1 mg/250 cc 5% D/W IV infusion, 1–4 μg/min initially and may increase to 4–8	At once	At once	Very short	High degree or complete AV block and ventricular standstill	Trembling, pallor, nervousness, hypertension, VPC, ventricular tachycardia and fibrillation
Ephedrine	30–60 mg PO q̄ 2–4 hr	—	—	—	High-degree or complete AV block	Urinary retention, nervousness, vertigo, insomnia, hypertension, ventricular tachyarrhythmias
Corticosteroids	Hydrocortisone IV inj. 200–600 mg for 24 hr or Solu-Medrol 80 mg daily by IM inj. or Prednisone 40–60 mg daily PO	—	—	—	Primary: AV block with acute onset Secondary: Chronic AV block	Prolonged steroid therapy may induce sodium retention, Cushing's syndrome, dissemination of TB, aggravation of diabetes mellitus, glaucoma, and psychosis
Molar sodium lactate	5–7 cc/kg IV infusion over periods of hours. If urgent, 25–50 cc rapid IV drip initially	—	—	—	AV block in the presence of acidosis or hyperkalemia	Precipitation of CHF, alkalosis, hypokalemia, ventricular tachyarrhythmias
Chlorothiazide	0.5–2 g daily (PO) for 6–8 weeks	—	—	—	Sinus rhythm with intermittent AV block	Hypokalemia, precipitation of gout, predispose to digitalis toxicity

q̄: every; IV: intravenous; SC: subcutaneous; IC: intracardiac; IM: intramuscular; D/W: dextrose in water; PO: by mouth; AS syndrome: Adams-Stokes syndrome; VPC: ventricular premature contraction; TB: tuberculosis; CHF: congestive heart failure.

Side Effects and Toxicity. The side effects of isoproterenol include tremor, nervousness, sweating, nausea, weakness, headache, dizziness, palpitation, and hypotension. A serious toxic effect is the production of ventricular tachyarrhythmias, a danger that is not dose dependent.

Epinephrine Hydrochloride[2,9-12]

Epinephrine has been almost as popular as isoproterenol in the treatment of the Adams-Stokes syndrome. However, epinephrine is considered to be definitely inferior to isoproterenol because it produces significant hypertension and is likely to provoke ventricular irritability, particularly ventricular fibrillation.

Epinephrine is capable of accelerating the atrial rate as well as the ventricular rate. The degree of acceleration of the atrial rate has no relationship to the initial atrial rate, whereas the degree of acceleration of the idioventricular rate is closely related to the initial ventricular rate. Thus the degree of acceleration of the idioventricular rate is greatest when the initial ventricular rate is very slow, and the enhancement of the ventricular rate is insignificant when the initial ventricular rate is relatively rapid.

Indications. The primary indication for epinephrine is in the treatment of ventricular standstill, particularly that associated with acute myocardial infarction. It is also indicated in the treatment of the Adams-Stokes syndrome due to complete AV block until an artificial pacemaker is implanted.

Administration. In urgent situations, such as ventricular standstill, 0.3 cc to 0.6 cc of a 1:1000 solution of epinephrine may be given by intravenous, intramuscular, subcutaneous, or even intracardiac injection. Slow injection over a period of several minutes under ECG monitoring is recommended, and the rate of injection should be regulated according to the patient's response. For long-term therapy, 0.5 mg to 1 mg of a 1:1000 solution of epinephrine diluted in 250 cc of a 5% solution of dextrose in water can be given by a continuous intravenous infusion. The initial rate of the intravenous drip is usually 1 μg to 4 μg per minute, and the rate may be increased to 4 μg to 8 μg per minute according to the patient's response.

Side Effects and Toxicity. The side effects of epinephrine include nervousness, trembling, pallor, and hypertension. A serious toxic effect is the production of ventricular tachycardia and fibrillation.

In general, the usefulness of epinephrine in the treatment of the Adams-Stokes syndrome is limited by its serious toxic effects and its ineffectiveness in some cases.

Other Drugs

The other drugs listed in Table 8–1 (ephedrine, corticosteroids, molar sodium lactate, and chlorothiazide) are now little used in antibradyarrhythmic therapy.

ARTIFICIAL PACEMAKERS

Although artificial pacemakers are discussed in detail in Chapter 11, the indications for short-term and long-term pacing are briefly discussed here.

Indications for Short-Term Pacing

The precise criteria for use of a temporary or a permanent pacemaker vary slightly from institution to institution, but the following conditions are generally accepted as indications for short-term pacing.[2,5,6,8,13,14]

1. Symptomatic second- or third-degree AV block (Fig. 8–5), especially during acute myocardial infarction requires a temporary pacing. It should be noted that AV block per se does not require artificial pacing.

2. Symptomatic and drug-resistant sinus arrhythmias, including sinus bradycardia (Fig. 8–1), sinus arrest, and SA block.

3. Newly developed left bundle branch block and bilateral bundle branch block (bifascicular and trifascicular block) due to acute anterior myocardial infarction. Short-term pacing is usually required because those findings are often followed by a slow ventricular escape rhythm due to complete AV block.

4. Emergency treatment for the Adams-Stokes syndrome and symptomatic bilateral bundle branch block.

5. Before or during implantation of a permanent pacemaker.

6. Therapeutic trial for intractable congestive heart failure, cardiogenic shock, or cerebral or renal insufficiency.

7. Prophylactic pacing during major surgery when the Adams-Stokes syndrome is anticipated.

8. Drug-resistant tachyarrhythmias, which may be corrected by overdriving pacing rate.

9. The symptomatic sick sinus syndrome and the bradytachyarrhythmia syndrome before the implantation of a permanent pacemaker.

Indications for Long-Term Pacing

The decision about using long-term pacing should not be made lightly, because the patient must live with an artificial pacemaker all his life, taking the necessary precautions and caring for it daily. In addition, the battery should be changed every 18 to 24 months (30 to 36 months in some newer models), depending on the model. One of the most serious problems following permanent pacemaker implantation is malfunction of the unit, which may be fatal. At times, it is difficult to judge whether a permanent artificial pacemaker is required. In general, long-term pacing is considered to be indicated in the following situations.[2,5,6,8,13,14]

1. Symptomatic, chronic second-degree (usually Mobitz type II or 2:1 AV block) or third-degree AV block

2. Symptomatic, chronic, and drug-resistant sinus arrhythmias, including sinus bradycardia (Fig. 8–1), sinus arrest, and SA block due to the sick sinus syndrome

3. Complete AV block in acute myocardial infarction (usually anterior wall involvement) lasting more than two to three weeks

4. Symptomatic bilateral bundle branch block (bifascicular and trifascicular block)

5. Recurrent Adams-Stokes syndrome due to various causes

6. Intractable congestive heart failure or cerebral or renal insufficiency definitely benefited by temporary pacing

7. Recurrent drug-resistant tachyarrhythmias benefited by temporary pacing

SUMMARY

1. Bradyarrhythmias may be due to various fundamental mechanisms, and they may be found in many different clinical backgrounds.

2. The therapeutic approaches vary markedly, depending on the fundamental mechanism responsible for the production of bradyarrhythmia, the ventricular rate, the underlying cause, and the presence or absence of symptoms and their seriousness.

3. It should be reemphasized that ECG abnormality alone is not cause for treatment.

4. Because of the ready availability of artificial pacemakers, antibradyarrhythmic drugs are much less used now than in the past. The most commonly used antibradyarrhythmic drug is atropine sulfate, particularly for the treatment of a marked sinus bradycardia associated with acute myocardial infarction. Isoproterenol is the next most commonly used drug for the treatment of bradyarrhythmias.

5. When complete AV block is due to a block below the His bundle (infranodal block), a permanent artificial pacemaker is nearly always indicated. On the other hand, complete AV block associated with acute diaphragmatic (inferior) myocardial infarction usually does not require pacing because the ventricular rate is relatively fast (50 to 60 beats per

minute) and the patient is often asymptomatic. Complete AV block associated with anterior myocardial infarction usually requires a permanent pacemaker, because the AV block is considered to be due to complete bilateral bundle branch block.

6. Bradyarrhythmia induced by various drugs, particularly digitalis, is best treated by eliminating the direct causative agent.

7. Antiarrhythmic drugs alone are usually not effective in the treatment of the sick sinus syndrome and the brady-tachyarrhythmia syndrome, and artificial pacing is considered to be the treatment of choice in that circumstance. In some patients with the brady-tachyarrhythmia syndrome, one or more antitachyarrhythmic drugs (e.g., quinidine, propranolol, or procainamide) and/or digitalis are indicated in addition to the artificial pacing. However, pacing with a slightly overdriving rate (80 to 100 beats per minute) alone is often effective treatment for the brady-tachyarrhythmia syndrome.

REFERENCES

1. Chung, E.K.: Electrocardiography: Practical Applications with Vectorial Principles. Hagerstown, Md., Harper & Row, 1974.
2. Chung, E.K.: Cardiac Arrhythmias: Management. Baltimore, Williams & Wilkins Co., 1973.
3. Rotman, M., Wagner, G.S., and Wallace, A.G.: Bradyarrhythmias in acute myocardial infarction. Circulation 45:703, 1972.
4. Chung, E.K.: Digitalis Intoxication. Baltimore, Williams & Wilkins Co., 1969.
5. Siddons, H., and Sowton, E.: Cardiac Pacemakers. Springfield, Ill., Charles C Thomas, 1967.
6. Furman, S., and Escher, D.J.W.: Principles and Techniques of Cardiac Pacing. Hagerstown, Md., Harper & Row, 1970.
7. Rosenbaum, M.B., Elizari, M.V., and Lazzari, J.O.: The Hemiblocks. Oldsmar, Fla., Tampa Tracings, 1970.
8. Cosby, R.S., and Bilitch, M.: Heart Block. New York, McGraw-Hill, 1972.
9. Gregory, J.J., and Grace, W.J.: The management of bradycardia, nodal rhythm and heart block for the prevention of cardiac arrest in acute myocardial infarction. Prog. Cardiovasc. Dis. 10:505, 1968.
10. Shillingford, J., and Thomas, M.: Treatment of bradycardia and hypotension syndrome with acute myocardial infarction. Am. Heart J. 75: 843, 1968.
11. Adgey, A.A.J., Geddes, J.S., Mulholland, H.C., Keegan, D.A.J., and Pantridge, J.F.: Incidence, significance and management of early bradyarrhythmias complicating acute myocardial infarction. Lancet ii:1097, 1968.
12. Yu, P.N.: Prehospital care of acute myocardial infarction. Circulation 45:189, 1972.
13. Kaplan, B.M., Langendorf, R., Lev, M., and Pick, A.: Tachycardia-bradycardia syndrome (so-called "sick sinus syndrome"). Am. J. Cardiol. 31:497, 1973.
14. Chung, E.K.: Artificial Cardiac Pacing: Practical Approach. Baltimore, Williams & Wilkins Co., 1979.

Chapter 9

THE SICK SINUS SYNDROME AND THE BRADY-TACHYARRHYTHMIA SYNDROME

EDWARD K. CHUNG

GENERAL CONSIDERATIONS

There has been an increasing awareness of the clinical entity known as the sick sinus syndrome (SSS) in the past decade because the syndrome is found relatively commonly among our cardiac patients, particularly among elderly patients, and because in most cases it can be successfully treated with artificial cardiac pacing. The term SSS has been used to cover a broad spectrum of clinical manifestations (e.g., near syncope, syncope, dizziness, increased congestive heart failure, and/or angina pectoris and palpitations) that result from a dysfunctioning sinus node. The ECG manifestations of the SSS may include[1-12] (1) persistent and marked sinus bradycardia, (2) sinoatrial (SA) block, (3) sinus arrest, (4) a long pause following an atrial premature contraction (APC), (5) chronic atrial fibrillation or flutter with a slow ventricular rate, (6) carotid sinus hypersensitivity, (7) lack of a stable sinus rhythm after cardioversion, (8) AV junctional escape rhythm with or without slow and unstable sinus activity, and (9) the brady-tachyarrhythmia syndrome (BTS). Those ECG findings in SSS are *not* drug induced.

Besides the sick sinus syndrome, other terms have been used to describe those phenomena; the terms include sinoatrial syncope, sluggish sinus node syndrome, inadequate sinus mechanism, sick sinus node, and lazy sinus node.[1-16] When tachyarrhythmia components are present intermittently or periodically during slow rhythm, various terms, such as brady-tachyarrhythmia syndrome, brady-tachy syndrome, and tachycardia-bradycardia syndrome, have been used.[1,12,17,18] Although some investigators use the terms SSS and BTS interchangeably, the BTS is one of the common manifestations of the SSS.

As can be expected, the degree of the sinus node dysfunction may be so minimal that the SSS may be manifested only by a slight sinus bradycardia. In such a case, the patient is usually asymptomatic. On the other hand, the sinus node may be severely diseased, leading to complete generator failure—prolonged sinus arrest or atrial fibrillation with a slow ventricular rate. The advanced SSS is nearly always symptomatic. Any symptoms in the SSS are usually related to the cardiac or the cerebral dysfunction. That is, the perfusion deficit in the heart or brain causes the production of various symptoms in the SSS. Near-syncope or syncope is the most common clinical manifestation of the SSS.

ANATOMY AND ELECTROPHYSIOLOGY

The sinus node was discovered by Keith and Flack in 1907,[19] and the electrophysiologic property of the sinus node as cardiac pacemaker was first described by Wybouw[20] and by Lewis and his co-workers[21] in 1910. The term sinus node is probably the most popular and appropriate one because embryologic studies have shown that the ultimate cardiac pacemaker is derived from the sinus venosus and not from the atria.[22] Furthermore, the terms sinoatrial node and sinoauricular node are incorrect from a precise anatomic viewpoint since the node extends from the auriculocaval junction back to the atriocaval junction.[23] Thus sinus node (Walmsley's term) is the most accurate one, and it has been accepted as the standard name for the natural (primary) pacemaker of the heart.[24]

The electrophysiologic event known as spontaneous phase 4 depolarization is the factor that distinguishes the pacemaker cells from the other cells. The sinus node is the dominant pacemaker because the sinus node cells possess the fastest spontaneous depolarization. The spontaneous sinus node depolarization can be altered by parasympathetic and sympathetic influences. For example, vagal stimulation of acetylcholine can slow the automaticity of the sinus node by reducing the slope of phase 4 depolarization as well as by hyperpolarizing the cells.[31-33] On the other hand, sympathetic stimulation or catecholamine infusion enhances the spontaneous sinus node discharge rate, primarily as a result of an increase in the rate of phase 4 depolarization.[31-33] The sinus node has both sympathetic and parasympathetic (vagal) innervation but the parasympathetic innervation is richer in the AV node.[23,26,34,35]

Various investigative studies have confirmed that the sinus node is the primary pacemaker in the heart. Since the sinus node's inherent rate is faster than that of any other cardiac pacemaker, sinus rhythm is present in most healthy people. In the SSS, when the sinus node produces the cardiac impulses more slowly than usual (sinus bradycardia), or when it fails to produce any impulse (sinus arrest), or when the sinus impulse is not conducted to the atria because of SA block, the subsidiary pacemaker (commonly the AV junction) takes over the ventricular activity as an escape mechanism.[25] On the other hand, the chronic generator failure (sinus arrest) not uncommonly leads to the establishment of chronic atrial fibrillation (often with a slow ventricular rate).[25]

There is considerable variation in the shape, size, and location of the sinus node. The exact location of the node depends on how the sinus artery encircles the base of the superior vena cava. In the human heart, the sinus node is generally located in the sulcus terminalis near the junction of the superior vena cava and the right atrium.[23,25-27] The node is somewhat elongated along the axis of the sulcus terminalis, and its anterior margin is a few millimeters posterior to a crest formed by the junction of the right atrial appendage with the superior vena cava. The sinus node is located more anteriorly when the caval encirclement by the node artery is clockwise (viewed from above) than when encirclement is counterclockwise. The size of the sinus node varies considerably, and it is not closely proportional to the size of the heart. In general, its size is approximately 15 mm in length, 5 to 7 mm in width, and 1.5 to 2 mm in thickness.[23,25-27] The shape of the sinus node varies, but by and large it resembles an extended snail with its shell, which misleads one to think of the node as having a head, a body, and a tail.[23,25-27] Since the sinus node is situated at a position that is less than 1 mm beneath the epicardial surface, the sinus node is vulnerable to many disease processes, including trauma (e.g., that of pericarditis).[28] The superficial anatomical location of the sinus node may be directly or indirectly responsible for the development of the SSS in many cases.

In the human heart, the sinus node artery is commonly located near the center of the sinus node, but its location may be eccentric. In approximately 55 to 60% of human hearts, the sinus node artery arises from the proximal 2 to 3 cm of the right coronary artery, whereas in 40 to 45% of human hearts, it arises from the proximal 1 cm of the left circumflex coronary artery.[23,29] Other origins of the sinus node artery are rare; they account for about 2% of the total. At times, there are two branches of the sinus node artery of equal size. The sinus node artery, regardless of whether it arises from the right or left coronary artery, courses along the anteromedial atrial wall of the base of the superior vena cava, which it encircles.[23,29] The artery anastomoses with other atrial arteries of both ipsilateral and contralateral origin. Generally, the primary arterial supply of the sinus node is almost always unilateral in origin. Smaller branches of the artery are distributed throughout the sinus node.

Small veins are commonly found throughout the sinus node, whereas large veins are present infrequently.[23,29]

Microscopically, the sinus node is composed of three types of cells, including P cells, transitional cells, and working cells.[30] The term P cells has been used because the cells are pale and thus resemble primitive myocardial cells. The P cells are thought to be responsible for sinus node pacemaker function.

The Purkinje-like fibers, the "internodal pathways" that connect from the sinus node to the specialized atrial conduction tissue have been described: the anterior, middle, and posterior internodal tracts.[36,37] By electrophysiologic studies it has been demonstrated that the cardiac impulse from the sinus node reaches the AV node more rapidly than it would if it were conducted through the ordinary myocardium.[36] Although any one of three internodal pathways may be responsible for intra-atrial conduction, in most normal hearts the conduction is thought to be carried out preferentially via the anterior tract.[36] That theory is not universally accepted, however.

UNDERLYING DISORDERS

Although various drugs, such as digitalis, propranolol, and quinidine, frequently cause dysfunction of the sinus node, their functionally reversible effects on the sinus node are not considered part of the SSS. The basic underlying causes of the SSS are anatomic, with physiologic consequences that produce a long-standing and often irreversible process in the sinus node.

Coronary Artery Disease

Coronary heart disease, particularly myocardial infarction, has been reported to be the most common underlying disease that produces the SSS.[1-4,38-41] In one study, dysfunction of the sinus node was reported to occur in approximately 5% of patients with acute myocardial infarction.[42] In addition, the sinus node dysfunction can be expected to be present in over 50% of patients with diaphragmatic myocardial infarction.[43] In one study, 31 out of 32 patients with diseased sinus node were found to have diaphragmatic myocardial infarction.[42] Dysfunction of the sinus node is usually observed during the first four days of diaphragmatic myocardial infarction.[4,42] Commonly, the sinus node dysfunction is manifested by a progressive sinus bradycardia followed by various supraventricular arrhythmias, including atrial fibrillation or flutter and AV junctional escape rhythm with a periodic restoration of sinus bradycardia and intermittent sinus arrest or SA block. Atrial myocardial infarction may cause the sinus node dysfunction on rare occasions. Atrial damage, including sinus node dysfunction, is very common as a result of occlusions of the main right coronary artery (causing diaphragmatic myocardial infarction) and occlusions of the left circumflex artery (causing anterolateral myocardial infarction).[38-43]

Idiopathic Disorders (Sclerotic-Degenerative Process)

When one eliminates coronary heart disease as a cause of the SSS, the majority of the remaining cases show no clear evidence of clinical heart disease as a cause of the SSS. In those latter cases, a sclerotic-degenerative process involving the sinus node is usually considered to be the cause of the SSS. Pathologic studies revealed that severe fibrosis involving the sinus node and SA junction was the main feature of the SSS.[44-46] In some cases of the SSS, amyloid infiltration involving the sinus node was demonstrated.[12,45]

Miscellaneous Disorders

Other underlying causes of the SSS may be (1) rheumatic heart disease, (2) cardiomyopathies, (3) congenital heart disease, (4) surgical trauma, (5) hypertension, (6) pericarditis or myocarditis, (7) amyloidosis, (8) systemic lupus erythematosus, (9) muscular dystrophy, (10) Friedreich's ataxia, (11) malignancy, (12) hemochromatosis, and (13) diphtheria.[1,12,46-52]

Familial incidence of the SSS has been reported,[53-55] and its association with the long Q–T syndrome also has been described.[56-60] Recently, the SSS associated with systemic embolism[61] and the mitral valve prolapse syndrome has been reported.[62-64]

ELECTROCARDIOGRAPHIC MANIFESTATIONS[1-12]

Depending on the degree of the sinus node dysfunction, various ECG abnormalities may be produced in the SSS (Table 9–1). Persistent and severe sinus bradycardia (not due to drugs) is the most common (75 to 80% of all patients with the SSS) and the earliest manifestation of the SSS, and it is followed by various other ECG abnormalities as the syndrome progresses. In a long-standing SSS, atrial fibrillation is the commonest

Table 9–1.   *The Sick Sinus Syndrome: Electrocardiographic Manifestations*

Marked and persisting sinus bradycardia
Sinus arrest and/or SA block
Drug-resistant (e.g., to atropine or isoproterenol) sinus bradyarrhythmias
Long pause following an atrial premature contraction
Prolonged sinus node recovery time determined by atrial pacing
Chronic atrial fibrillation or the repetitive occurrrence of atrial fibrillation (less commonly atrial
    flutter). (a) with slow ventricular rate (b) preceded or followed by sinus bradycardia, sinus
    arrest, or SA block
AV junctional escape rhythm (with or without slow and unstable sinus activity)
Carotid sinus syncope
Failure of restoration of sinus rhythm following cardioversion
Brady-tachyarrhythmia syndrome
Common coexisting AV block and/or intraventricular block
Any combination of the above

---

underlying rhythm. When the SSS is far advanced, it is manifested by the BTS, in which a variety of cardiac rhythms are observed in many cases. In addition, AV conduction disturbances as well as intraventricular blocks often coexist in many persons with advanced SSS.

Sinus Bradycardia

Although some degree of sinus bradycardia is very common in healthy people, especially in athletes,[65] a persistent and marked sinus bradycardia (one not due to drugs) deserves medical investigation. The SSS should be strongly suspected when chronic sinus bradycardia shows a rate slower than 45 beats per minute (Fig. 9–1), with or without symptoms. Of course, marked sinus bradycardia frequently produces symptoms, such as light-headedness, near syncope, and syncope. It should be certain that the sinus bradycardia is not due to a drug, such as propranolol (Inderal) digitalis, reserpine (Serpasil), guanethidine (Ismelin), or methyldopa (Aldomet). On the other hand, the SSS may be "unmasked" by small amounts of drugs, particularly digitalis or propranolol. In other words, marked sinus bradycardia following the administration of small amounts of those drugs strongly suggests the SSS, especially in elderly people.

When sinus bradycardia is marked, one or more AV junctional or ventricular escape beats may occur, and incomplete AV dissociation is often produced (Fig. 9–2). At times, marked sinus bradycardia may lead to AV junctional escape bigeminy, in which sinus beats and AV junctional escape beats occur on every other beat. When the AV node as well as the sinus node is diseased—a common occurrence—the AV junctional escape rhythm also produces a markedly slow rate or ventricular escape beats appear because the AV node fails to produce any escape impulse (Fig. 9–2).

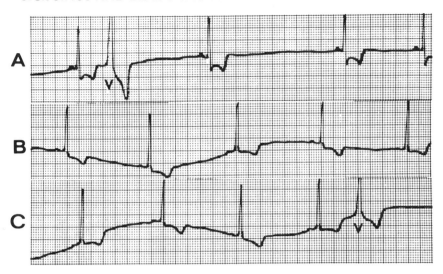

Figure 9–1.   The Holter monitor ECG rhythm strips A, B, and C are *not* continuous. The sick sinus syndrome is manifested by marked sinus bradycardia and arrhythmia (43 to 46 beats per minute) with a ventricular premature contraction (VPC).

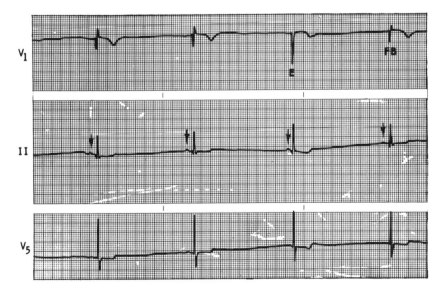

Figure 9–2.   These rhythm strips are those of an 85-year-old man who had had a diaphragmatic myocardial infarction two months previously. He complained of frequent dizzy spells. His slow heart rate failed to respond to atropine or isoproterenol. The rhythm is marked sinus bradycardia (28 beats per minute) and a ventricular escape beat (in the third QRS complex). Note also the ventricular fusion beat (in the last QRS complex). That rhythm disorder is a manifestation of the sick sinus syndrome. In this tracing, the expected AV junctional escape beat failed to appear, and as a result a ventricular escape beat occurred, a phenomenon that indicates coexisting AV node disease. A permanent demand ventricular pacemaker was implanted in the patient.

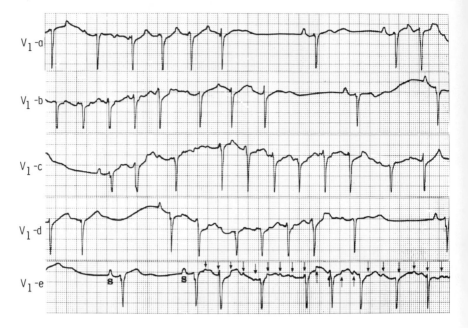

Figure 9–3. Leads V_1-a, b, c, d, and e are continuous. The arrows indicate ectopic atrial activities. The sick sinus syndrome is manifested by marked sinus bradycardia (marked S) with first-degree AV block and paroxysmal atrial fibrillation, flutter, and tachycardia. Digitalis is given to the patient, in addition to the implantation of a permanent demand ventricular pacemaker.

Marked sinus bradycardia is often irregular, and it may be followed by atrial or ventricular tachyarrhythmias (Figs. 9–1 and 9–3). First-degree AV block (in which the P–R interval is 0.28 sec or more) also commonly coexists (Fig. 9–3).

Sinus Arrest and/or Sinoatrial Block

When the SSS further progresses, the sinus node fails to produce any cardiac impulse, leading to sinus arrest (Fig. 9–4). The long P–P interval due to sinus arrest has no relationship to the basic P–P cycle.[25] During sinus arrest, it is common to observe one or more AV junctional (less commonly ventricular) escape beats to control the ventricular activity. In some other persons with SSS, SA block may be observed. In SA block, the sinus impulse is unable to conduct to the atria as a result of a block at the SA junction. SA block has two forms—Mobitz types I and II. Mobitz type II SA block is characterized by the intermittent absence of the expected P wave(s) in which the long P–P interval is a multiple of the

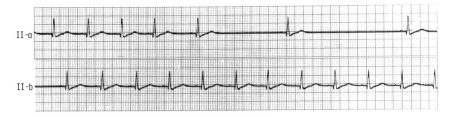

Figure 9–4.   Leads II-a and b are continuous. The sick sinus syndrome is manifested by sinus arrest.

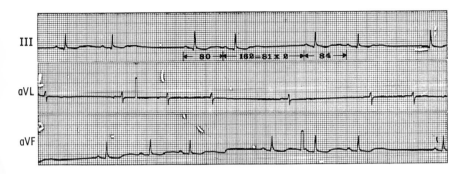

Figure 9–5.   The sick sinus syndrome is manifested by intermittent Mobitz type II and 2:1 SA block. (The numbers represent hundredths of a second.)

basic P–P cycle (Fig. 9–5).[25] On the other hand, Mobitz type I (Wenckebach) SA block produces a progressive shortening of the P–P cycles until a pause occurs.[25] Mobitz type I (Wenckebach) SA block is analogous to Mobitz type I (Wenckebach) AV block, whereas Mobitz type II SA block is analogous to Mobitz type II AV block.[25] In cases of far-advanced SA block or sinus arrest, the sinus activity is almost completely absent (at times, entirely absent), leading to atrial standstill.[25] When the basic sinus cycle is irregular, it is impossible to distinguish sinus arrest from SA block.

Drug-Resistant Sinus Bradyarrhythmias

When the sinus bradyarrhythmias fail to respond to atropine or isoproterenol, the presence of the SSS is almost certain (Figs. 9–1 and 9–2). The presence of the SSS is usually considered if the sinus rate is not accelerated beyond 90 beats per minute by the intravenous injection of atropine sulfate (1 to 2 mg).[66] For a similar reason, the SSS can be diagnosed when intravenous isoproterenol (1 to 2 mg/min) fails to enhance the sinus rate beyond 90 to 100 beats per minute in sinus bradycardia. It should be noted that the administration of isoproterenol may provoke ventricular tachyarrhythmias.

Long Pause Following an Atrial Premature Contraction

In general, an atrial premature contraction (APC) is *not* followed by a full compensatory pause because the sinus node is passively activated by the ectopic atrial impulse. Thus the automaticity of the sinus node is momentarily disturbed by the ectopic atrial impulse.[25] Occasionally, an APC is followed by a full compensatory pause when an APC occurs during late cardiac cycle so that the sinus node impulse formation is not disturbed. In such a case, the interference (collision) between the sinus impulse and the ectopic atrial impulse occurs at the SA junction, in the atria, or at the AV junction.[25] Extremely rarely, an APC may be interpolated.[25]

Although a post-ectopic pause following an APC is *not* fully compensatory, the returning cycle (the interval from the ectopic P wave to the first sinus P wave) is usually longer than the basic sinus P–P cycle because of a transient suppression of the sinus node by the ectopic atrial impulse—a physiologic phenomenon.[25] When the returning cycle is longer than usual, however, an abnormally prolonged refractory period of the sinus node is suspected. In cases of a markedly prolonged sinus node recovery time due to the SSS, a single APC may be sufficient to produce sinus arrest, leading to absence of the sinus P waves for a long period of time. In such a case, AV junctional or ventricular escape rhythm frequently appears to activate the ventricles.

Prolonged Sinus Node Recovery Time Determined by Atrial Pacing[66–68]

The prolonged sinus node recovery time determined by a rapid atrial pacing (120 to 150 beats per minute) is a reliable indicator for the SSS. The rapid atrial pacing is particularly valuable when the ECG manifestations of the SSS are not obvious and when the clinical symptoms of the syndrome are vague. Detailed descriptions of the determination and usefulness of the sinus node recovery time are given on page 177.

Chronic Atrial Fibrillation or Repetitive Occurrence of Atrial Fibrillation (Less Commonly, of Atrial Flutter)

Chronic atrial fibrillation (AF) is the most common underlying rhythm in patients with far-advanced SSS, in which the sinus node is no longer capable of producing the cardiac impulse. In such a case, AF or flutter is

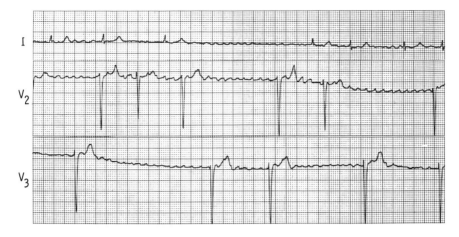

Figure 9–6.   The sick sinus syndrome is manifested by atrial flutter-fibrillattion with a very slow ventricular rate (15 to 30 beats per minute) due to advanced AV block.

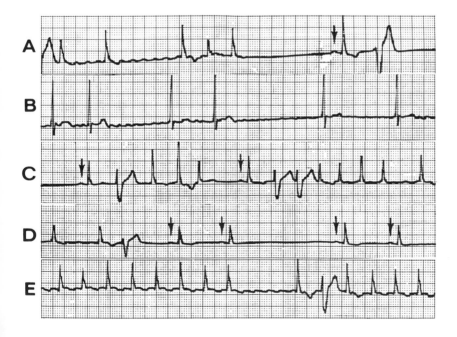

Figure 9–7.   Holter monitor ECG strips A, B, C, D, and E are *not* continuous. The arrows indicate sinus P waves. The sick sinus syndrome is manifested by sinus bradycardia and areas of atrial fibrillation, atrial flutter with a 2:1 AV response, and occasional ventricular premature contractions, as well as by aberrant ventricular conduction, producing the brady-tachyarrhythmia syndrome.

often associated with a slow ventricular rate (30 to 50 beats per minute) as a result of advanced AV block, and one or more AV junctional (less commonly, ventricular) escape beats may occur (Fig. 9–6). Until AF or flutter is well established as chronic, it is often preceded or followed by marked sinus bradycardia, sinus arrest, or SA block, with or without first-degree AV block (a P–R interval of more than 0.28 sec; Figs. 9–3 and 9–7). In some people with the SSS, however, the ventricular rate is relatively fast in AF or flutter, leading to the BTS (Fig. 9–7).

AV Junctional Escape Rhythm (with or without Slow and Unstable Sinus Activity)

When marked sinus bradycardia becomes worse, it is often followed by sinus arrest, and AV junctional escape rhythm may become the underlying rhythm with or without unstable sinus activity (Fig. 9–8). The AV junctional escape rhythm is commonly irregular until it becomes well established as chronic. In chronic AV junctional escape rhythm, the cycle is usually regular (Fig. 9–8). In such a case, retrograde P waves may be preceded or followed by the QRS complexes (Fig. 9–8), and at times no P wave is discernible.

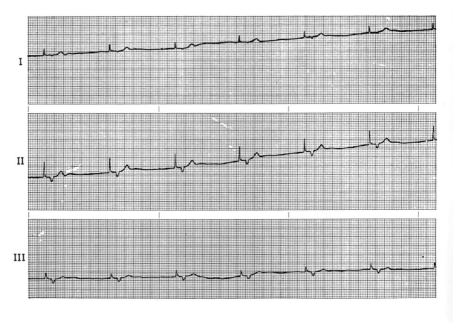

Figure 9–8.   The sick sinus syndrome is manifested by AV junctional escape rhythm (40 beats per minute). Note the retrograde P waves following each QRS complex.

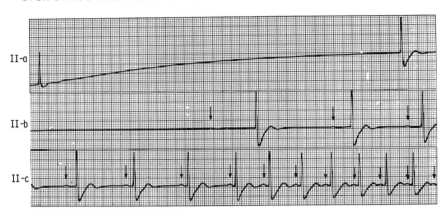

Figure 9–9.   Leads II-a, b, and c are continuous. The arrows indicate sinus P waves. A long period of sinus arrest with a long ventricular standstill (7.86 sec) is produced as a result of a hypersensitive reaction to carotid sinus stimulation (CSS).

Carotid Sinus Syncope[1,6,11,69,70]

It has been reported that the sudden development of sinus arrest by carotid sinus stimulation lasting more than three seconds is highly suggestive of inappropriate sinus responsiveness—the SSS (Fig. 9–9). Similarly, the appearance of a long ventricular standstill in chronic AF or flutter induced by carotid sinus stimulation probably has the same clinical significance.

Failure to Restore Sinus Rhythm Following Cardioversion[1,3,4,6,9,16]

The SSS is strongly suspected when the heart is unable to restore a stable sinus rhythm for a long period of time following the termination of any ectopic tachyarrhythmias by direct current shock (Fig. 9–10), particularly following the termination of AF or flutter. In that circumstance, the AV junctional escape rhythm often becomes the dominant rhythm, with or without unstable sinus P waves. In far-advanced SSS, AF may persist, with unstable AV junctional or ventricular escape rhythm following the termination of ventricular tachyarrhythmias by direct current shock.

The Brady-Tachyarrhythmia Syndrome

Although some investigators use the terms BTS and SSS interchangeably, the conditions are by no means identical. As mentioned, the BTS is one of the common manifestations of advanced SSS. In the BTS, the

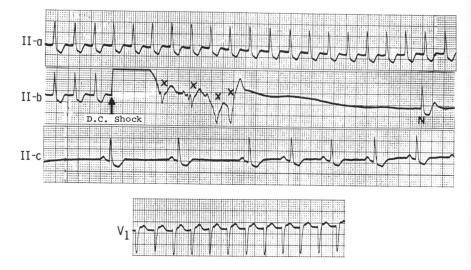

Figure 9–10.   Leads II-a, b, and c are continuous. Direct current (D.C.) shock was applied for supraventricular tachycardia (indicated by arrow). Note the long ventricular standstill and frequent ventricular premature contractions (marked X) with group beats and an AV junctional escape beat (marked N) until sinus rhythm is restored.

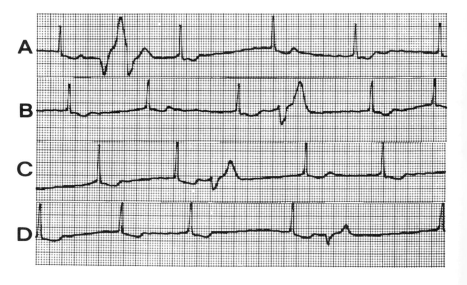

Figure 9–11.   Holter monitor ECG strips A, B, C, and D are *not* continuous. The sick sinus syndrome is manifested by atrial fibrillation with advanced AV block causing slow ventricular rate (30 to 42 beats per minute) and frequent ventricular premature contractions with group beats—the brady-tachyarrhythmia syndrome.

bradyarrhythmia component is commonly marked sinus bradycardia (Figs. 9–1, 9–3, and 9–7) and less commonly chronic atrial fibrillation with a slow ventricular rate (Fig. 9–11). The tachyarrhythmia component in the BTS is most commonly AF or flutter-fibrillation with rapid ventricular response (Fig. 9–3) and less commonly atrial flutter with rapid (often 2:1) ventricular response (Fig. 9–7). Paroxysmal atrial tachycardia (PAT) or AV junctional tachycardia as a tachyarrhythmia component in the BTS is not too common. The incidence of ventricular tachyarrhythmia in the BTS (Figs. 9–11 and 9–12) has been reported by different authors to be 8 to 10%.

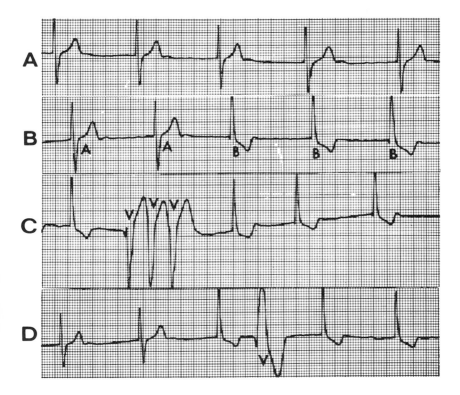

Figure 9–12.   Holter monitor ECG rhythm strips A, B, C, and D are *not* continuous. The rhythm is atrial fibrillation with escape rhythms from two foci (marked A and B) due to advanced AV block and frequent multifocal ventricular premature contractions (marked V) with ventricular group beats. Those ECG findings represent the brady-tachyarrhythmia syndrome as a manifestation of the sick sinus syndrome.

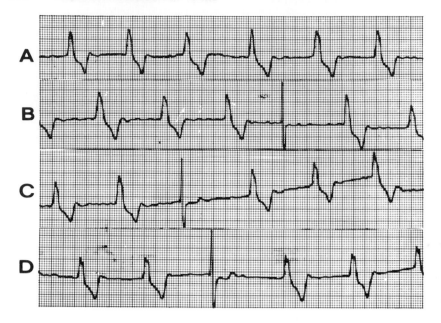

Figure 9–13.   Holter monitor ECG strips A, B, C, and D are *not* continuous. The sick sinus syndrome is manifested by atrial fibrillation with advanced AV block causing slow ventricular rate. Broad QRS complexes in the tracing probably represent coexisting left bundle branch block.

Common Coexisting Atrioventricular Block and/or Intraventricular Block

Although AV block or intraventricular block per se is *not* a part of the SSS, either condition often coexists with the SSS because the same underlying disease process—degenerative-sclerotic change—may diffusely involve the entire conduction system. That is why advanced or even complete AV block often occurs in chronic AF or flutter, leading to a very slow ventricular rate in advanced SSS (Figs. 9–6, 9–7, 9–11, and 9–12). In addition, first-degree AV block (a P-R interval greater than 0.24 sec) is extremely common in the BTS (Fig. 9–3), and it is often preceded or followed by AF with a slow ventricular rate (Fig. 9–3). Furthermore, various forms of intraventricular block frequently coexist with the SSS (Fig. 9–13).

Any Combination of the above Electrocardiographic Manifestations

As can be expected, various ECG manifestations of the SSS itself may be present, or common ECG abnormalities (e.g., AV block, intraventricular block, and AV junctional or ventricular escape rhythm) may coexist with the SSS. For example, an ECG tracing in advanced SSS may show marked sinus bradycardia, sinus arrest, AV junctional and ventricular escape beats, paroxysmal AF, and ventricular premature contractions. Another ECG may show sinus bradycardia, intermittent SA block, marked first-degree AV block, and AV junctional escape beats.

CLINICAL CONSIDERATIONS[1-12]

Laslett made the original report on the syncopal attacks associated with bradycardia (in 1909).[71] There has been increasing interest and awareness of the therapeutic problems regarding the SSS and the BTS among physicians since Short described the therapeutic dilemma in patients presenting with sinus bradycardia and tachyarrhythmia associated with syncope.[17] The clinical manifestations in patients with the SSS are fundamentally due to hypoperfusion of the vital organs, particularly the brain, heart, and kidney as a result of a markedly slow ventricular rate that may or may not be associated with tachyarrhythmias.

Sex and Age

There is no particular sexual preponderance in the SSS, but the syndrome has been reported more frequently among elderly women than among men. The SSS may involve any age group although it is primarily a disease of the elderly. The incidence of the SSS has been reported to reach a peak in people in their 60s and 70s. It has been suggested that the SSS may be the cause of sudden death in some young athletes.[4] Another recent report described eight Africans with the SSS; all of them were 32 years of age or younger.[72] The life expectancy in the different parts of the world seems to greatly affect the peak incidence of the SSS.

Underlying Heart Diseases

As described on page 160, the most common underlying heart disease in the SSS has been reported to be coronary heart disease (the incidence is about 50%). The next most common underlying disease process seems to be idiopathic, namely, sclerotic-degenerative change in the sinus node and other conduction system (the incidence is about 30 to 35%). Of course, many patients with the SSS may have more than one underlying cardiac disease. The less common underlying diseases of the SSS are rheumatic heart disease, congenital heart disease, hypertension, cardiomyopathy, amyloidosis, hemochromatosis, surgical injury, myocarditis, pericarditis, Friedreich's ataxia, progressive muscular dystrophy, collagen disease, and metastatic disease.

Clinical Manifestations

The clinical manifestations of the SSS may be multifaceted, and they may occur only intermittently. The most common manifestations of the advanced SSS are lightheadedness and near syncope or syncope. But in mild cases, the patient may be totally asymptomatic; and in the early stage, the condition may be extremely difficult to recognize or evaluate.

Cerebral Manifestations. In mild cases or in the early stage of the SSS, diminished cerebral arterial blood flow may be manifested by generalized fatigue, muscle ache, or slight personality changes, including irritability, intermittent memory loss, and insomnia. When the SSS progresses, the cerebral manifestations may be slurred speech, pareses, erroneous judgment, lightheadedness, and near syncope followed by syncope. Several of the cerebral manifestations, such as near syncope and syncope, are almost always due to a marked slowing of the heart rate or to cardiac arrest; the tachycardia component seldom produces significant cerebral symptoms.

Since the SSS is primarily a disease of the elderly, the various cerebral manifestations are frequently misinterpreted as cerebrovascular accidents or simply as "senility." Near syncope or syncope has been reported to occur in 40 to 70% of patients with the SSS.[1-12] Dizziness was reported to occur in 6 to 7% of patients with the SSS.[1-12]

Cardiac Manifestations. As can be expected, the various cardiac manifestations are the second most common finding in the SSS. In the early stage of mild SSS, the cardiac manifestations may be completely absent except for a slow heart rate or a mixture of slow and rapid cardiac rhythms. The three most common cardiac manifestations in the SSS are palpitations, increased signs of congestive heart failure, and increased angina pectoris. In some instances, a sudden occurrence of acute pulmonary edema or episodic acute pulmonary edema may be the first sign of the SSS because the patient may not seek medical attention during the mild stage of the syndrome. The feeling of palpitations may be due to an extremely slow rhythm itself (e.g., sinus bradycardia or AF with advanced AV block), irregular rhythm, or a mixture of slow and rapid rhythms (the BTS). Most patients experience palpitations when the cardiac rhythm suddenly changes—from slow rhythm to rapid rhythm, or vice versa. The three most common cardiac manifestations (palpitations, increased signs of congestive heart failure, and angina pectoris) of the SSS are closely interrelated, and one symptom frequently aggravates the others. In my experience, palpitations have been the most common cardiac manifestation of the SSS although Moss and Davis found that increased signs of congestive heart failure was the most common cardiac manifestation (occurring in 22% of cases).[1] Moss and Davis found also that the incidence of palpitations or an increase in angina pectoris was about equal (each symptom occurring in 15% of cases).[1]

In far-advanced cases of the SSS, the patients may develop prolonged cardiac arrest or ventricular fibrillation leading to death.

Other Manifestations. Various nonspecific manifestations, such as oliguria and gastrointestinal distress, are not uncommon in the SSS, but those manifestations are usually secondary to hypoperfusion of the heart itself.

DIAGNOSTIC APPROACH[1-12] (See also Table 9–2)

In mild cases of the SSS, it is not always easy to make a definitive diagnosis. The physician often needs a high index of suspicion to arrive at the diagnosis during the early stage of the SSS. The presence of a marked and persistent sinus bradycardia (that is not due to drugs) should always raise the possibility of the SSS, even in totally asymptomatic young people, including athletes.

Clinical Manifestations

The diagnosis of the SSS cannot be made definitively on the basis of the clinical manifestations alone. However, the SSS must be included in the differential diagnosis when the patient has a history of near syncope or syncope. Similarly, the SSS should be considered as an underlying disorder in any person with unexplainable pulmonary edema, palpitations, or angina pectoris, particularly when those manifestations (singly or together) are associated with a slow heart rate that is not due to drugs (e.g., digitalis and propranolol).

Table 9–2.   *The Sick Sinus Syndrome: Diagnostic Approach*

Clinical manifestations
Routine 12-lead ECG
Ambulatory (Holter monitor) ECG
Carotid sinus stimulation and Valsalva maneuver
Cardioversion
Exercise (stress) ECG test
Drugs (e.g., atropine, isoproterenol)
Electrophysiologic studies
Determination of sinus node recovery time by atrial pacing
Determination of SA conduction time by atrial extrastimulus technique
His bundle electrocardiography

Routine 12-Lead ECG

The diagnosis of the advanced SSS can be confirmed by the typical ECG findings shown on a routine 12-lead ECG or long rhythm strips (Figs. 9–2 to 9–6; 9–8).

Ambulatory (Holter Monitor) ECG[1,73]

When the typical ECG findings of the SSS are not documented on the routine 12-lead ECG because the findings occur intermittently, the Holter monitor ECG is the best diagnostic tool (Figs. 9–1, 9–7, 9–11 to 9–13).

Carotid Sinus Stimulation and the Valsalva Maneuver

Sinus arrest lasting more than three seconds with carotid sinus stimulation strongly suggests inappropriate sinus node responsiveness—the SSS (Fig. 9–9).[1,2,6,68,69] The response to the Valsalva maneuver may also be useful in demonstrating the sinus node dysfunction. The Valsalva maneuver produces the expected changes in the aortic pulse pressure but causes little or no change in the pulse rate. In contrast, the physiologic bradycardia of the elderly demonstrates the expected acceleration of the heart rate during the strain phase (phase 2) and the subsequent slowing of the heart rate during the blood pressure overshoot (phase 4). However, carotid sinus stimulation and the Valsalva maneuver do not provide direct diagnostic evidence of the sinus node disease; they give a clue to the functional status of the sinus node. Further investigation is indicated in many cases.

Cardioversion

Needless to say, cardioversion is *not* a diagnostic method for the SSS. However, failure to restore sinus rhythm following the termination of any ectopic tachyarrhythmia by cardioversion strongly suggests the SSS (Fig. 9–10).

The Exercise ECG Test[2]

When the sinus rate is not increased significantly by the standard exercise ECG (e.g., the treadmill) protocol, the SSS may be suspected provided that the inappropriate sinus rate change is *not* related to a drug (e.g., propranolol). Of course, people in good physical condition (e.g., runners and other athletes) may not show a significant increase in the heart rate with the exercise ECG protocol simply because the exercise load is insufficient, not because they have a sinus node dysfunction.

Drugs[1,2,4,6,66,74,75]

The SSS is often suspected when anyone, particularly an elderly person, develops marked sinus bradycardia following the administration of a small amount of digitalis or propranolol; the SSS may be "unmasked" by the drug. However, that finding is not always reliable in the diagnosis of the SSS. Recently, atropine has been used frequently to evaluate the response of the sinus node. Physiologic sinus bradycardia responds to the intravenous administration of atropine by a normal or exaggerated acceleration of the sinus rate. On the other hand, no significant increment of the sinus rate is observed in the SSS following the administration of atropine. It has been suggested that when intravenous atropine sulfate (1 to 2 mg) fails to increase the sinus rate beyond 90 beats per minute in sinus bradycardia and when the sinus node recovery time remains prolonged by rapid (120 to 140 beats per minute for 2 to 4 minutes) atrial pacing after atropine injection, the diagnosis of the SSS can be made. Similarly, the presence of the SSS may be considered when the sinus rate does not increase beyond 90 to 100 beats per minute in sinus bradycardia following the intravenous administration of isoproterenol (1 to 2 mg/min).

Electrophysiologic Studies[1,2,4,6,67-69,76-83]

Determination of Sinus Node Recovery Time by Atrial Pacing. Of the various electrophysiologic studies, the determination of the sinus node recovery time (post-pacing pause) by rapid atrial pacing is the most reliable provocative test to uncover indirect evidence of the SSS. The determination can be made by the use of a pervenous right atrial pacing catheter and the conventional ECG recordings. The artificial pacing can be performed by placing the pacing catheter either within the coronary sinus or at the junction of the superior vena cava and right atrium, whichever location permits the most effective and consecutive atrial capture. The initial pacing rate is usually 90 beats per minute, and it is progressively increased by 10 beats every 2 to 4 minutes, up to 150 beats per minute. The pacing is terminated suddenly at the end of each period, and the post-pacing pause (the interval from the last pacing spike to the onset of the next sinus P wave) is measured. When there is complete absence of sinus P wave (atrial standstill) following the termination of pacing, the first AV junctional escape interval (the interval from the last pacing spike to the first AV junctional escape beat) is measured. However, to avoid syncope, atrial pacing must be restarted immediately when there has been complete cardiac arrest for four seconds.

The post-pacing pause is expected to occur in people with normal sinus nodes as well as in those with diseased sinus nodes, it is comparable to the post-tachyarrhythmia pause.[25] However, the diseased sinus node, needless to say, requires an abnormally long recovery time until its automaticity as the primary pacemaker is reestablished. Thus there is a documented clear distinction between normal and abnormal responses.

It has been reported that the actual sinus node recovery time following the termination of atrial pacing is closely related to the resting sinus rate—the slower the resting sinus rate, the longer the maximum post-pacing pause.[4,68,69] When the resting sinus rate is between 75 and 85 beats per minute, the maximum post-pacing pause is estimated to be 115 and 128%, respectively, of the resting cycle length (the post-pacing pause is 800 to 900 msec).[4] In sinus bradycardia (45 to 60 beats per minute), the maximum post-pacing pause is expected to be much longer, and an abnormally long sinus node suppression can be easily recognized. In sinus rhythm with a rate of 60 beats per minute (the cycle length is 1000 msec), a post-pacing pause showing 125% of the resting value (1250 msec) strongly suggests the SSS; and the presence of the SSS is almost certain when the post-pacing pause is longer than 1250 msec.[4] When the resting sinus rate is 45 beats per minute (the cycle length is 1420 msec), the post-pacing pause of 1700 msec or greater is diagnostic of the SSS although the percentage increase is only 120%.[4] In severe SSS, the post-pacing pause may reach 2000 to 6000 msec.[67,68] Recently, I demonstrated extremely prolonged sinus node recovery times (13,680 msec following atrial pacing of 120 beats per minute and 19,400 msec following atrial pacing of 140 beats per minute) in a patient with far-advanced SSS due to cardiac amyloidosis.[84]

Narula and co-workers[67] proposed the concept of corrected sinus node recovery time (CSRT)—the difference between the post-pacing pause and the resting sinus P–P cycle. The normal maximum CSRT is calculated to be 525 msec or less, whereas the abnormal CSRT is calculated to be 1880 ± 1079 msec.

It should be noted that although the determination of the sinus node recovery time by atrial pacing is still the best indirect diagnostic approach for the SSS, the test may still have false negative results in some instances.

Determination of SA Conduction Time by the Atrial Extrastimulus Technique. In other kinds of electrophysiologic studies, the SA conduction times (SACTs) were measured indirectly by the atrial extrastimulus technique.[82,83] In one study, a prolonged (more than 152 msec) calculated SACT was associated with a high incidence of sinus node and/or atrial disease.[82] But in another study, the SACT in the control group was not significantly different from the SACT in the patients with the SSS.[83]

His Bundle Electrocardiography. Since the SSS is often associated with various abnormalities in the impulse formation and conduction elsewhere in the heart, His bundle electrocardiographic studies can provide useful information. For example, the presence of abnormal electrophysiologic properties in the AV junction may indirectly support the diagnosis of SSS. In addition, by recognizing the coexisting conduction disturbance, a specific type of artificial pacing may be selected for a given patient with the SSS.

THERAPEUTIC APPROACH[1-6,25,85]

The fact that antiarrhythmic drug therapy alone has been unsatisfactory in the treatment of the SSS has been repeatedly emphasized. At present, the use of a permanent artificial pacemaker is the treatment of choice for all patients with the SSS. Drug therapy alone for the SSS is unsuccessful because:

1. The drug used to treat the tachyarrhythmia component is harmful for or aggravates the bradyarrhythmia component and vice versa.

2. The drugs used to treat bradyarrhythmia (e.g., atropine sulfate and isoproterenol) are not effective enough.

3. Many patients experience significant and intolerable side effects from the drugs.

For those reasons it is generally agreed that artificial pacemaker therapy is mandatory in almost every case of advanced SSS even if the patient is asymptomatic. In fact, at present the most common indication for the artificial pacemaker is the SSS.

Artificial Pacemaker Therapy

Of the many types and modes of artificial pacemakers, the one most commonly used to treat the SSS is the demand asynchronous (ventricular) pacemaker (Fig. 9–14). The reason for that choice is that many patients with the SSS have a coexisting AV conduction disturbance and/or an intraventricular block. Use of the fixed-rate ventricular pacemaker is hazardous for a patient with the SSS because a competition between the patient's own rhythm and the pacemaker rhythm may lead to the development of ventricular fibrillation as a result of the R–on–T phenomenon. The demand pacemaker is very effective for marked sinus bradycardia as well as for sinus arrest, SA block, and AF or flutter with advanced AV block. As mentioned, the demand ventricular pacemaker is ideal for the patient with the SSS that coexists with advanced or complete AV block. In addition, the demand pacemaker is efficient enough for almost all people with the SSS because most people with the SSS are elderly and do not need the atrial contribution (kick) to increase the cardiac output; it is not essential for their daily activities. Thus for most people with the SSS the permanent demand ventricular pacemaker is the pacemaker of choice.

Coexisting AV conduction disturbances in the SSS can be identified

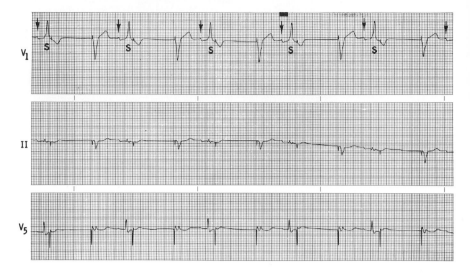

Figure 9–14.   The arrows indicate sinus P waves. The tracing shows marked sinus bradycardia (30 beats per minute) with demand ventricular pacemaker rhythm. Note that the patient's sinus beats and the pacing beats alternate throughout the tracing.

readily by the His bundle ECG. When the His bundle recording is not available, the atrial pacing can provide valuable information. Thus significant AV block is reasonably excluded when the P–R interval remains less than 0.22 sec during atrial pacing (120 to 140 beats per minute). But when AV block of any degree (commonly, the Wenckebach AV block) is produced by the atrial pacing, the presence of AV conduction disturbances is certain.

When the possibility of a coexisting AV block is reasonably excluded, atrial pacing may be considered. An important advantage of the atrial pacing (80 to 120 beats per minute) is that the atrial tachyarrhythmia component in the BTS can be suppressed (in up to 50% of cases) by pacing without the use of an antiarrhythmic drug. For that purpose, coronary sinus pacing is the preferred atrial pacemaker therapy. One of the disadvantages of coronary sinus pacing is that one cannot always be sure that the pacing will be stable and constant.

When the atrial kick is considered to be definitely needed in patients with coexisting AV block, the use of a bifocal demand pacemaker should be considered. The bifocal demand pacemaker, like the ventricular demand pacemaker, monitors ventricular electrical activity but it programs both atrial and ventricular stimulation. It consists of two demand pacemaker units—a conventional QRS-inhibited demand pacemaker and a QRS-inhibited atrial demand pacemaker.[25,85] The pacing escape interval of the atrial pacemaker is shorter than that of the ventricular pacemaker. The difference between those two escape intervals determines the AV sequential interval—the P–R interval. The ventricular electrodes have a dual function. They sense the ventricular signal and they stimulate the ventricles as required. The atrial electrode stimulates the atria but does not have a sensing function. Thus the signal detected by the ventricular electrode is responsible for both atrial and ventricular pacing. The bifocal demand pacemaker can stimulate both atria and ventricles in sequence, or it may stimulate the atria alone, or it may remain totally dormant. Thus the pacemaker functions automatically according to the individual patient's needs.

Recently, a programmable pacemaker has been introduced in clinical medicine, particularly for the treatment of the sick sinus syndrome. The programmable pacemaker is often ideal for many patients with sick sinus syndrome, particularly the brady-tachyarrhythmia syndrome, because the ideal pacing rate can be achieved non-invasively after implantation.[87] In many patients with the BTS, a slightly overdriving pacing rate (80 to 100 beats per minute) is required.

Antiarrhythmic Drug Therapy

As mentioned on page 179, antiarrhythmic drug therapy alone is unsatisfactory (and often hazardous) for the patient with the SSS. However, antiarrhythmic drug therapy can be instituted with relative safety following the implantation of a permanent pacemaker. Antiarrhythmic drugs are often required for the SSS because the tachyarrhythmia component is usually not suppressed by the pacing alone although atrial pacing may be capable of eliminating atrial tachyarrhythmias.

The indications for specific antiarrhythmic drugs are similar to those for various tachyarrhythmias[25] that are not associated with the SSS (Chapter 7). Digitalis is the drug of choice for AF, flutter, or tachycardia with rapid ventricular response (Figs. 9–3 and 9–7). Digitalis and diuretics may improve myocardial function and indirectly suppress the atrial tachyarrhythmias in patients with the SSS associated with congestive heart failure. At times, propranolol may be added when an atrial tachyarrhythmia with rapid ventricular response is not well controlled by digitalis alone. Quinidine is very useful for the prevention of atrial tachyarrhythmias. When a ventricular tachyarrhythmia is not controlled by artificial pacing, various drugs, such as procainamide, quinidine, diphenylhydantoin, or propranolol may be tried either one at a time or combined (Figs. 9–11 and 9–12). Every physician should be clearly aware of the fact that no patient is immune to any drug intoxication, particularly digitalis intoxication, even after artificial pacing (Chapter 16).

PROGNOSIS

The natural course of disease of the sinus node seems to be that it is chronic, progressive, and long-standing, but it is difficult to determine the long-term prognosis. At present, the diseased sinus node cannot be cured, and in most cases only symptomatic treatment with hemodynamic inprovement—artificial pacing to replace the natural pacemaker—can permit the patient with the SSS to lead a normal life. The exact length of time from the first manifestation of the SSS until death is unknown, but in most cases it seems to be from many months to 5 to 10 years. At present, it is more difficult to evaluate the natural course of the SSS because of the ready availability of artificial pacemakers to treat the SSS in the early stage. The danger of sudden death is always possible in people with untreated SSS.

The initial stage of the SSS is marked by chronic sinus bradycardia that is progressively followed by development of sinus arrest and/or SA block. Advanced SSS is manifested by chronic AF or flutter with slow ventricular rate due to advanced AV block and/or the BTS. Although chronic AF is considered to be the end stage of the SSS, it is difficult to predict when it will appear in a person with the SSS. In addition, it is also difficult to predict the life expectancy of people with the SSS who develop chronic AF. Careful clinical observations and more in-depth investigations may give more precise information about the long-term prognosis of the SSS.

In a recent study of 39 patients with the SSS, after pacemaker implantation, the long-term (6 to 59-month follow-up period) prognosis was reported to be poor.[86] In that study, 15 patients (42%) died during the follow-up period. Eleven of the 15 deaths (73%) were related to cardiac problems, but none were associated with either cardiac arrhythmias or pacemaker failure. Symptoms recurred or persisted after pacemaker implantation in 14 patients, and 9 of those 14 died. Twenty-two patients became asymptomatic after pacing, and 6 of those 22 died.

SUMMARY

1. The SSS may be manifested by a variety of ECG abnormalities, including marked and persistent sinus bradycardia (that is not due to drugs), sinus arrest, SA block, chronic AF or flutter with slow ventricular rate, AV junctional escape rhythm with or without unstable sinus activity, a hypersensitive response to carotid sinus stimulation or the Valsalva maneuver, a failure to restore sinus rhythm following cardioversion, and the BTS.

2. Sinus bradycardia is the earliest finding in the SSS.

3. Chronic AF is considered to be the end stage of the SSS.

4. The BTS is one of the common manifestations of advanced SSS.

5. Direct documentation of the typical ECG manifestations of the SSS by the 12-lead ECG or the Holter monitor ECG is the best diagnostic approach.

6. There are many provocative diagnostic tests available for the diagnosis of the SSS but none of them are perfect. The determination of the sinus node recovery time by atrial pacing is the best test, but it may have a false negative result.

7. The various clinical manifestations of the SSS are due to hypoperfusion of the vital organs, particularly the brain and the heart itself.

8. The most common clinical manifestations of the SSS are cerebral symptoms, including lightheadedness, near syncope, and syncope.

9. The next most common clinical manifestations of the SSS are cardiac symptoms, including palpitations, increased signs of congestive heart failure, and angina pectoris. Acute pulmonary edema may occur.

10. Antiarrhythmic drug therapy alone is unsatisfactory for the SSS, and all patients with significant SSS should be treated with permanent artificial pacemakers.

11. The demand ventricular pacemaker is the pacemaker of choice in most cases. Atrial pacing (coronary sinus pacing) or bifocal demand pacing is indicated in occasional cases, when an atrial contribution (kick) is desired. The programmable pacemaker has been introduced recently into clinical medicine, and it seems to be very popular among cardiologists.

12. After artificial pacing, some patients require one or more antiarrhythmic drugs (e.g., digitalis, propranolol, quinidine, procainamide) for the treatment of the tachyarrhythmia component of the BTS.

13. It is important to re-emphasize that no one is immune to any drug intoxication, particularly digitalis intoxication, even after artificial pacing.

14. The long-term prognosis in the SSS is uncertain, but it appears to take many months to 5 to 10 years after the onset of the first manifestations of the SSS to the patient's death. In one recent study, the long-term (6 to 59-month follow-up period) the prognosis following pacemaker implantation for 39 patients with the SSS was poor. Nevertheless, the immediate prognosis after pacing seems to be favorable in many cases of SSS.

15. The incidence of the SSS has been reported to reach a peak in people in their 60s and 70s, but a person of any age may have the SSS.

16. There is no sex preponderance.

17. The SSS is always a possibility in anyone, especially an elderly person who has marked and chronic sinus bradycardia (that is not due to drugs) with or without symptoms.

18. For a similar reason, the possibility of the SSS should always be considered in any person who experiences near-syncope or syncope.

19. Sudden death is always a possibility in anyone who has advanced, untreated SSS.

REFERENCES

1. Moss, A.J., and Davis, R.J.: Brady-tachy syndrome. Prog. Cardiovasc. Dis. 16:439, 1974.
2. Jordan, J.L., Yamaguchi, I., and Mandel, W.J.: The sick sinus syndrome. J.A.M.A. 237:682, 1977.
3. Ferrer, M.I.: The natural history of the sick sinus syndrome. J. Chronic Dis. 25:313, 1972.
4. Ferrer, M.I.: The sick sinus syndrome. Circulation 47:635, 1973.
5. Ferrer, M.I.: The sick sinus syndrome in atrial disease. J.A.M.A. 206:645, 1968.
6. Scarpa, W.J.: The sick sinus syndrome. Am. Heart J. 92:648, 1976.
7. Birchfield, R.I., Menefer, E.E., and Bryant, G.D.M.: Diseases of the sino-atrial node associated with bradycardia, asystole, syncope and paroxysmal atrial fibrillation. Circulation 16:20, 1957.
8. Fowler, N.O., Fenton, J.C., and Conway, G.F.: Syncope and cerebral dysfunction caused by bradycardia without atrioventricular block. Am. Heart J. 80:303, 1970.
9. Easley, R., and Goldstein, S.: Sino-atrial syncope. Am. J. Med. 50:166, 1971.
10. Rubinstein, J.J., Schulman, C.L., and Yurchak, P.M.: Clinical spectrum of the sick sinus syndrome. Circulation 46:5, 1972.
11. Arguss, N.S., Rosin, E.V., and Adolph, R.J.: Significance of chronic sinus bradycardia in elderly people. Circulation 46:924, 1972.
12. Kaplan, B., Langendorf, R., Lev, M., and Pick, A.: Tachycardia-bradycardia syndrome (so-called "sick sinus syndrome"). Am. J. Cardiol. 31:497, 1973.
13. Silverman, L.F., Mankis, H.T., and McGoon, D.C.: Surgical treatment of an inadequate sinus mechanism by implantation of a right atrial pacemaker electrode. J. Thorac. Cardiovasc. Surg. 55:264, 1968.
14. Tabatznik, B., Mower, M.M., Somson, E.B., and Prempree, A.: Syncope in the "sluggish sinus node syndrome." Circulation 40 (Suppl. III):200, 1969.
15. Bouvrain, Y., Slama, R., and Temkine, J.: Le bloc sino-auriculaire et les "maladies du sinus": Reflexions à propos de 63 observations. Arch. Mal. Coeur 60:753, 1967.
16. Lown, B.: Electrical reversion of cardiac arrhythmias. Br. Heart J. 29:469, 1967.
17. Short, D.S.: The syndrome of alternating bradycardia and tachycardia. Br. Heart J. 16:208, 1954.
18. Sandøe, E., and Flensted-Jensen, E.: Adams-Stokes seizures in patients with attacks of both tachy- and bradycardia: A therapeutic challenge. Acta Med. Scand. 186:111, 1969.
19. Keith, A., and Flack, M.: Form and nature of the muscular connections between the primary divisions of the vertebrate heart. J. Anat. Physiol. 41:172, 1907.
20. Wybouw, R.: Sur le point d'origine de la systole cardiaque dans l'oreilette droite. Arch. Int. Physiol. Biochim. 10:78, 1910.
21. Lewis, T., Oppenheimer, B.S., and Oppenheimer, A.: Site of origin of the mammalian heart beat: The pacemaker in the dog. Heart 2:147, 1910.
22. Patten, B.M.: Initiation and early changes in the character of the heart beat in vertebrate embryos. Physiol. Rev. 29:31, 1949.
23. James, T.N.: Anatomy of the human sinus node. Anat. Rec. 141:109, 1961.
24. Walmsley, T.: Comparative anatomy of the heart. In Quain's Elements of Anatomy, Part III. London, Longmans, Green and Co., 4:3, 1929.
25. Chung, E.K.: Principles of Cardiac Arrhythmias, 2nd ed. Baltimore, Williams & Wilkins Co., 1977.
26. James, T.N.: The specialized conducting tissue of the atria. In L.S. Dreifus and W. Likoff (eds.), Mechanisms and Therapy of Cardiac Arrhythmias. New York, Grune & Stratton, 1966. P. 97.

27. Lev, M.: The conduction system in the human heart. Military Med. 120:262, 1957.
28. James, T.N.: Pericarditis and the sinus node. Arch. Intern. Med. 110:305, 1962.
29. James, T.N.: Anatomy of the Coronary Arteries. New York, Hoeber, Medical Division of Harper & Row, 1961.
30. James, T.N., Sherf, L., and Fine, G.: Comparative ultrastructure of the sinus node in man and dog. Circulation 34:139, 1966.
31. West, T.C., Falk, G., and Cervoni, P.: Drug alteration of transmembrane potentials in atrial pacemaker cells. J. Pharmacol. Exp. Ther. 117:247, 1956.
32. Lu, H.H., Lange, G., and Brookes, C.M.: Factors controlling pacemaker action in cells of the sinoatrial node. Circ. Res. 17:460, 1965.
33. Brooks, C.M., and Lu, H.H.: The Sinoatrial Pacemaker of the Heart. Springfield, Ill., Charles C Thomas, 1972.
34. Stotler, W.A., and McMahon, R.A.: The innervation and structure of the conductive system of the human heart. J. Comp. Neurol. 87:57, 1947.
35. Woolard, H.H.: The innervation of the heart. J. Anat. 60:345, 1926.
36. Hoffman, B.F., and Cranefield, P.F.: Electrophysiology of the Heart. New York, McGraw-Hill, 1961.
37. Merideth, J., and Titus, J.L.: The anatomic atrial connections between sinus and AV node. Circulation 37:566, 1968.
38. Shaw, D.B.: The etiology of sino-atrial disorder (sick sinus syndrome). Am. Heart J. 92:539, 1976.
39. Parameswaran, R., Ohe, T., and Goldberg, H.: Sinus node dysfunction in acute myocardial infarction. Br. Heart J. 38:93, 1976.
40. Hatle, L., Bathen, J., and Rokseth, R.: Sinoatrial disease in acute myocardial infarction: Long-term prognosis. Br. Heart J. 38:410, 1976.
41. Jordan, J., Yamaguchi, I., and Mandel, W.J.: Characteristics of sinoatrial conduction in patients with coronary artery disease. Circulation 55:569, 1977.
42. Rokseth, R., and Hatle, L.: Sinus arrest in acute myocardial infarction. Br. Heart J. 33:639, 1971.
43. James, T.N.: The coronary circulation and conduction system in acute myocardial infarction. Prog. Cardiovasc. Dis. 10:410, 1968.
44. Thery, C., Gosselin, B., Lekieffre, J., and Warembourg, H.: Pathology of sinoatrial node. Correlations with electrocardiographic findings in 111 patients. Am. Heart J. 93:735, 1977.
45. Evans, R., and Shaw, D.B.: Pathological studies in sinoatrial disorder (sick sinus syndrome). Br. Heart J. 39:778, 1977.
46. Rasmussen, K.: Chronic sino-atrial heart block. Am. Heart J. 81:38, 1971.
47. Allensworth, D.C., Rice, G.J., and Lowe, G.W.: Persistent atrial standstill in a family with myocardial disease. Am. J. Med. 47:775, 1969.
48. Bloomfield, D.A., and Sinclair-Smith, B.C.: Persistent atrial standstill. Am. J. Med. 39:335, 1965.
49. Caponnetto, S., Pastorini, C., and Tirelli, G.: Persistent atrial standstill in a patient affected with facioscapulohumeral dystrophy. Cardiologia 53:341, 1968.
50. James, T.N., Rupe, C.E., and Monte, R.W.: Pathology of the cardiac conducting system in systemic lupus erythematosus. Ann. Intern. Med. 63:402, 1965.
51. Metzger, A.L., Goldberg, A.N., and Hunter, R.L.: Sick sinus node syndrome as the presenting manifestation of reticulum cell sarcoma. Chest 60:602, 1971.
52. Greenwood, R.D., Rosenthal, A., Sloss, L.J., et al.: Sick sinus syndrome after surgery for congenital heart disease. Circulation 52:208, 1975.
53. Spellberg, R.D.: Familial sinus node disease. Chest 60:246, 1971.
54. Caralis, D.G., and Varghese, P.J.: Familial sinoatrial node dysfunction. Increased vagal tone a possible aetiology. Br. Heart J. 38:951, 1976.
55. Nordenberg, A., Varghese, P.J., and Nugent, E.W.: Spectrum of sinus node dysfunction in two siblings. Am. Heart J. 91:507, 1976.
56. Vincent, G.M., Abildskov, J.A., and Burgess, M.J.: Q–T interval syndrome. Prog. Cardiovasc. Dis. 16:523, 1974.
57. Maron, B.J., Clark, C.E., Goldstein, R.E., and Epstein, S.E.: Potential role of QT interval prolongation in sudden infant death syndrome. Circulation 54:423, 1976.

58. Schwartz, P.J., Periti, M., and Malliani, A.: The long Q–T syndrome. Am. Heart J. 89:378, 1975.
59. Langslet, A., and Sørland, S.J.: Surdocardiac syndrome of Jervell and Lange-Nielsen, with prolonged QT interval present at birth, and severe anaemia and syncopal attacks in childhood. Br. Heart J. 37:830, 1975.
60. Guntheroth, W.G.: Sudden infant death syndrome (crib death). Am. Heart J. 93:784, 1977.
61. Fairfax, A.J., Lambert, C.D., and Leatham, A.: Systemic embolism in chronic sinoatrial disorder. N. Engl. J. Med. 295:190, 1976.
62. DeSilva, R.A., and Shubrooks, S.J.: Mitral valve prolapse with atrioventricular and sinoatrial node abnormalities of long duration. Am. Heart J. 93:772, 1977.
63. Leichtman, D., Nelson, R., Gobel, F.L., et al.: Bradycardia with mitral valve prolapse. A potential mechanism of sudden death. Ann. Intern. Med. 85:453, 1976.
64. Swartz, M.H., Teichholz, L.E., and Donoso, E.: Mitral valve prolapse. A review of associated arrhythmias. Am. J. Med. 62:377, 1977.
65. Hanne-Paparo, N., Drory, Y., Schoenfeld, Y., et al.: Common ECG changes in athletes. Cardiology 61:267, 1976.
66. Rosen, K.M., Loeb, H.S., Sinno, M.Z., Rahimtoola, S.H., and Gunnar, R.M.: Cardiac conduction in patients with symptomatic sinus node disease. Circulation 43:836, 1971.
67. Narula, O.S., Samet, P., Javier, R.P.: Significance of the sinus-node recovery time. Circulation 45:140, 1972.
68. Mandel, W., Hayakawa, H., Danzig, R., and Marcus, H.S.: Evaluation of sino-atrial node function in man by overdrive suppression. Circulation 44:59, 1971.
69. Mandel, W., Hayakawa, H., Allen, H.H., et al.: Assessment of sinus node function in patients with sick sinus syndrome. Circulation 46:761, 1972.
70. Chughtai, A.L., Yans, J., and Kwatra, M.: Carotid sinus syncope. Report of 2 cases. J.A.M.A. 237:2320, 1977.
71. Laslett, E.E.: Syncopal attacks associated with prolonged arrest of the whole heart. Q. J. Med. 2:347, 1909.
72. Ikeme, A.C., D'Arbela, P.G., and Somers, K.: The sick sinus syndrome in Africans. Am. Heart J. 89:295, 1975.
73. Reiffel, J.A., Bigger, J.T., Jr., Cramer, M., and Reid, D.S.: Ability of Holter electrocardiographic recording and atrial stimulation to detect sinus nodal dysfunction in symptomatic and asymptomatic patients with sinus bradycardia. Am. J. Cardiol. 40:189, 1977.
74. Dhingra, R.C., Amat-Y-Leon, F., Wyndham, C., et al.: Electrophysiologic effects of atropine on sinus node and atrium in patients with sinus nodal dysfunction. Am. J. Cardiol. 38:848, 1976.
75. Reiffel, J.A., Bigger, J.T., Jr., and Giardina, E.G.V.: "Paradoxical" prolongation of sinus nodal recovery time after atropine in the sick sinus syndrome. Am. J. Cardiol. 36:98, 1975.
76. Toyama, J., Ito, A., Sawada, K., et al.: Overdrive suppression in diagnosis of sick sinus syndrome. J. Electrocardiol. 8:209, 1975.
77. Kulbertus, H.E., De Leval-Rutten, F., Mary, L., and Casters, P.: Sinus node recovery time in the elderly. Br. Heart J. 37:420, 1975.
78. Steinbeck, G., and Lüderitz, B.: Comparative study of sinoatrial conduction time and sinus node recovery time. Br. Heart J. 37:956, 1975.
79. Gupta, P.K., Lichstein, E., Chadda, K.D., and Badui, E.: Appraisal of sinus nodal recovery time in patients with sick sinus syndrome. Am. J. Cardiol. 34:265, 1974.
80. Breithardt, G., Seipel, L., and Loogen, F.: Sinus node recovery time and calculated sinoatrial conduction time in normal subjects and patients with sinus node dysfunction. Circulation 56:43, 1977.
81. Benditt, D.G., Strauss, H.C., Scheinman, M.M., et al.: Analysis of secondary pauses following termination of rapid atrial pacing in man. Circulation 54:436, 1976.
82. Dhingra, R.C., Amat-Y-Leon, F., Wyndham, C., et al.: Clinical significance of prolonged sinoatrial conduction time. Circulation 55:8, 1977.

83. Crook, B., Kitson, D., McComish, M., and Jewitt, D.: Indirect measurement of sinoatrial conduction time in patients with sinoatrial disease and in controls. Br. Heart J. 39:771, 1977.
84. Gray, L.W., Duca, P., and Chung, E.K.: Sick sinus syndrome due to cardiac amyloidosis. Cardiology 63:212, 1978.
85. Lemberg, L., and Castellanos, A., Jr.: Artificial pacing. *In* E.K. Chung (ed.), Cardiac Emergency Care. Philadelphia, Lea & Febiger, 1974. Pp. 165–189.
86. Wohl, A.J., Laborde, J., Atkins, J.M., et al.: Prognosis of patients permanently paced for sick sinus syndrome. Arch. Intern. Med. 136:406, 1976.
87. Chung, E.K.: Artificial Cardiac Pacing: Practical Approach. Baltimore, Williams & Wilkins Co., 1979.

Chapter 10

DIRECT CURRENT SHOCK

LEON RESNEKOV

The drug management of cardiac arrhythmias continues to have serious limitations in clinical practice. Those limitations may be summarized as follows:

1. Success is by no means universal.

2. An unstandardized dose varying from patient to patient has to be given.

3. The margin between the therapeutic effects and the toxic effects may be small.

4. Current medical practice dictates that the dose be titrated against an observed effect, which requires keeping the patient under close observation, often for several days.

5. Many antiarrhythmic drugs (Chapter 7) are negatively inotropic. They may also be dromotropic.

6. Paradoxically, if toxic manifestations emerge following the use of a drug, they may be even more serious than the effects of the arrhythmia being treated.

7. A drug overdose may suppress the normal sinus mechanism, thereby actually inhibiting reversion to sinus rhythm.

An electrical shock causes momentary depolarization of the majority of heart fibers, thereby terminating an ectopic tachycardia and allowing the sinus node to be reestablished as the pacemaker of the heart. There is now abundant evidence that such therapy is both successful and safe provided certain procedures are carried out rigorously.

189

HISTORY

The rhythm disturbance now called ventricular fibrillation was first described in 1850 (by Hoffer). Some time thereafter, the first fatal electrical accident was reported in the medical literature, but several years passed before the idea that fatal electrocution often resulted from ventricular fibrillation gained general acceptance. In 1900 Prevost and Battelli[1] observed that a direct current shock across the heart would terminate ventricular fibrillation in dogs. Their important report, written as a postscript to an article on another subject, was generally unrecognized until the topic of electric defibrillation was restudied by Kouwenhoven and his co-workers[2] in a series of experiments over many years and by Ferris and his co-workers.[3] The latter group described a series of experiments undertaken between 1927 and 1935 on the effects of electricity on the heart from which they reached the following important conclusions:

1. Current, rather than voltage, is the proper criterion of shock intensity.

2. The passage of an electrical current across the heart may precipitate ventricular fibrillation, even in the absence of any recognizable myocardial damage.

3. Unless ventricular fibrillation is successfully treated by another shock within a few minutes, the animal will die.

Equally significant was the demonstration by King[4] that electrical shocks delivered in relation to the apex of the T wave of the ECG are more likely to cause ventricular fibrillation.

At about the same time, workers in Europe, particularly in the Soviet Union, had been doing pioneer work in the application of capacitor discharge (direct current) to clinical use. The studies of Gurvich and Yunyev[5] can be regarded as an important inspiration to later investigators, including Peleşka,[6] Tsukerman,[7] and Lown and his co-workers.[8]

ELECTRICAL DEFIBRILLATION

Whether direct current or alternating current is used, electrical defibrillation requires the passage of a high-energy impulse of short duration between two concave paddles closely applied to the surface of the heart (internal defibrillation) or between two flat paddles applied to the chest wall (external defibrillation). The total energy needed depends not only on the electrical current used but also on the resistance of the heart, the bony cage, and the skin. Hooker and his co-workers[9] reported that a minimal current of 1 amp is needed to bring all heart fibers instantaneously to the same refractory point. Delivery of that current requires about 100 volts and a power of 100 watts (voltage × current). Since the usual duration of an *alternating current* defibrillatory shock is 0.2 sec, the energy used for internal defibrillation is about 20 joules. For external defibrillation, however, the change in resistance may require a sixfold increase in current rating: 1800 watts of electrical power are usually used for 0.2 sec, which is equivalent to 360 joules of electrical energy. The waveform for alternating current defibrillation is, of course, standard, being produced at the electrical power station as a sinusoidal impulse and at a frequency of 60 Hz.

In contrast, *direct current* defibrillators discharge a single capacitor or a bank of capacitors that have been charged over a short period (2 to 10 sec) from line current and a step-up transformer. The duration of the impulse is 1.5 to 4 msec. An unmodified capacitor discharge has a characteristic waveform (Fig. 10–1), with an abrupt rise in voltage and current to a sharp peak, followed by an exponential decay to the baseline. The waveform may be shaped by adding varying amounts of inductance to the circuit, and an infinite variety of waveforms may thus be obtained. There is experimental evidence that suggests that defibrillation is not only more successful but also safer when inductance is introduced into the circuit.[10] When a capacitor of 16 microfarads charged to 7000 volts is used, the stored energy for a 3.5 msec direct current defibrillating waveform is 392 joules, but it must be stressed that the setting on the moving coil meter of the apparatus reflects only the energy delivered to the skin. The amount

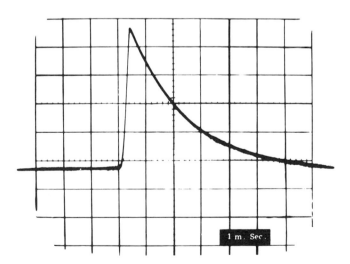

Figure 10–1.   Spike capacitor discharge. No additional inductance in circuit. Note the rapid rise time, sharp peak and exponential decay.

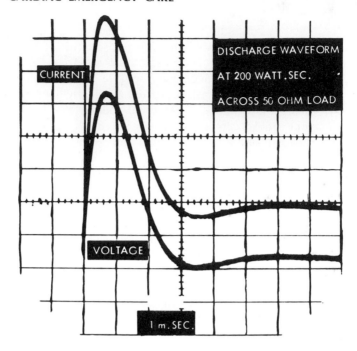

Figure 10–2.   Monophasic slightly underdamped current and voltage waveform. Capacitor 16 μf, inductance 100 mh, 5 kV (Lown circuit). (Reprinted with permission from Resnekov and McDonald.[23])

of true energy delivered to the heart is affected by the resistance of the skin, bones, and deeper tissues. Most commercially available direct current apparatus use capacitors in the range of 10 to 20 microfarads, and the inductance of the circuit is about 100 millihenrys. If a discharge of 400 joules lasting for 3 msec is assumed, the current delivered would be 19 amp and the power would be 133,000 watts. Its waveform is shown in Figure 10–2.

ALTERNATING CURRENT OR DIRECT CURRENT

Direct current develops many times the power of alternating current but requires less energy since the shock lasts only 3 to 4 msec. Several investigators have reported that alternating current shocks are more harmful than direct current shocks and produce greater deterioration of ventricular function.[11,12]

The first successful defibrillation in humans was performed by Beck and his co-workers (in 1947);[13] they used an alternating current discharge. For many years thereafter, the convenience of alternating defibrillation made it the standard method. It should be realized, however, that since the waveform and the duration of the current are so different in the two methods, any true comparison is extremely difficult. Two important clinical observations stimulated further investigation of the use of direct current in clinical practice:

1. Alternating current was frequently unsuccessful when ventricular fibrillation was caused by myocardial infarction.

2. There was a clinical need for the electrical conversion of rhythm disturbances other than ventricular fibrillation.

In regard to item No. 2, Lown and his co-workers[14] had reported that they had terminated an organized arrhythmia with alternating current, but the experience of others had already given clear warning of the risk of precipitating ventricular fibrillation and even death when alternating current was used for this purpose.[15] Although there are relatively few well-controlled defibrillation studies in which alternating and direct current have been compared, Nachlas and his co-workers[16] were able to show that direct current was unmistakably superior in terminating ventricular fibrillation.

From all the evidence then, the following conclusions can be drawn:

1. Alternating current can be used to treat ventricular fibrillation, but direct current is more effective.

2. Alternating current cannot be recommended for the elective treatment of atrial rhythm disturbances or ventricular tachycardia because of the risk that it will precipitate ventricular fibrillation.

DIRECT CURRENT SHOCK AND SYNCHRONIZED SHOCK

Although its waveforms are less likely to cause myocardial damage when appropriately shaped by an inductor in circuit, direct current shock has on occasion precipitated ventricular fibrillation. For many years, a vulnerable phase of ventricular excitability has been postulated,[17] and Wiggers and Wegria[18] were able to show that such a phase occurs 27 msec before the end of ventricular systole in dogs. It is due to non-uniform recovery from the refractory state allowing reentry of the depolarization wave and favoring self-sustained activity. That a similar phenomenon also occurs in the human heart has been shown by Castellanos and his co-workers.[19]

Those animal and human investigations, therefore, indicate that in the treatment of rhythm disturbances other than ventricular fibrillation, the direct current shock should be timed to avoid the apex of the T wave. Since it is almost impossible to avoid that vulnerable period when the longer-duration alternating current shocks are used (Fig. 10–3), direct

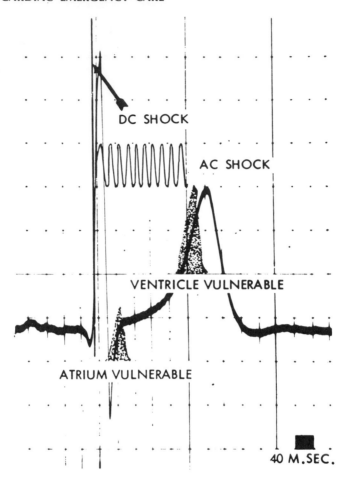

Figure 10–3.   Atrial and ventricular phases of vulnerability. Note that an AC shock of 0.2 sec may end at the T wave even if synchronized with the R wave of the ECG.

current defibrillators can incorporate a synchronizer to permit triggering of the shock by the R or the S wave of the ECG well away from the vulnerable phase. When ventricular fibrillation is being treated, the synchronizer has to be switched out of circuit.

The precipitation of ventricular fibrillation following randomized unsynchronized shock is 2%.[20] Some workers do not use a synchronizer in clinical practice, and they report no dire consequences.[21] If a synchronizer is not used, it is most important that sufficient energy be delivered so that a current of at least 1.5 to 2 amp passes across the heart;

lower energies may well be dangerous and precipitate ventricular fibrillation, particularly if temporally related to the T waves. Thus increased energy level settings are required when a synchronizer is not used.

CLINICAL USE OF SYNCHRONIZED DIRECT CURRENT SHOCK

Lown and his co-workers[8] were the first to use capacitor discharges with inductance in series for the treatment of ventricular tachycardia. Many thousands of patients suffering cardiac rhythm disturbances have now been successfully treated by that method and the total experience has completely justified the initial confidence in the technique. The overall success rate for the termination of atrial and ventricular rhythm disturbances approaches 90%.[22,23] In addition, it has been shown that a success rate of 86% occurs even after determined efforts at drug conversion have failed.[24] The correct choice of patients, meticulous attention to detail, including correction of any electrolyte imbalance, postponement of treatment when overdigitalization occurs, proper synchronization, and the correct choice of antiarrhythmic drugs (Chapter 7) immediately before and after treatment[25] insure immediate success and a low incidence of complications.

The important aspects of synchronized direct current shock are summarized in the following paragraphs.

Apparatus

1. Each month the electrical integrity of the equipment should be checked as follows:
   a. The waveform should be inspected when the paddles are discharged across a 50-ohm load in the laboratory.
   b. The delivered energy should be measured and compared with the setting of the apparatus.
2. Paddles. The paddles must be large enough to stimulate simultaneously most of the myocardial fibers. (Paddles that are too small permit a high current density in a localized pathway and produce myocardial damage.)
3. For external DC shock. Two anterior or, alternatively, an anterior and a posterior paddle should be used.

Note that anterior and posterior paddles are more convenient since the patient lies on the flat posterior paddle and only the anterior one needs to be held by the operator—an important safety measure, particularly with apparatus in which one paddle is grounded. Although it has been reported that the anteroposterior paddle position significantly lowers the amount of energy needed for electrical cardioversion,[26] others could not confirm that finding.[23] Indeed, experimental work[16] has shown that anterior positioning of the electrodes as originally suggested by Kouwenhoven and his co-workers[27] results in the delivery of approximately 2.5 times more current to the heart. The failure to note more striking clinical differences with variation in electrode placement is undoubtedly due to the excessive amounts of electrical energy that are consistently used in achieving electrical cardioversion. Thus the anteroposterior position is recommended because of the added safety offered by the flat posterior paddle held in place only by the weight of the patient.

Drugs

1. Digoxin and all other digitalis preparations should be withheld for 24 to 48 hours before electrical cardioversion.
2. If treatment cannot be postponed despite the presence of heavy digitalization, (a) the shock should be preceded by an intravenous injection of 50 mg of lidocaine, 50 to 100 mg of diphenylhydantoin, or 50 to 100 mg of procainamide, and (b) the energy level setting should be lowered to 5 to 10 joules.

At present there is little evidence that quinidine or other antiarrhythmic drugs (Chapter 7) given orally, intramuscularly, or intravenously as a routine before direct current shock produce the energy needed or help to maintain long-term sinus rhythm thereafter.[23] But those drugs may help to prevent premature beats following the shock that could precipitate a return to the arrhythmia after successful conversion (pp. 207–209).

Anesthesia

1. To prevent vomiting, food should be withheld for several hours before treatment.
2. Premedication is not needed.
3. Amnesia produced by 5 to 10 mg of diazepam intravenously, rather than general anesthesia, is recommended.[28,29,30] It significantly reduces the complication rate.[31]
4. Do not use muscle relaxants, especially halothane, which predisposes the patient to rhythm disturbances, particularly in the presence of carbon dioxide retention.
5. Do not use sympathomimetic drugs during attempts at electrical cardioversion.[32]

Note that the duration of action of diazepam is only three to four minutes, making it a safe, even ideal, drug for electrical cardioversion. Additional doses may be given within a few minutes of the initial injection if the first dose fails to induce drowsiness. But it should be remembered that patients with congestive heart failure should be given diazepam cautiously and that it is very unusual for more than 20 mg to be needed in any patient.[33] An added point in favor of diazepam is that its safety and speed of action mean that the skilled help of an anesthesiologist is not mandatory and that elaborate anesthetic equipment is not needed.

The Treatment Room

The treatment room should:
1. Be fully equipped for cardiac monitoring
2. Have full cardiac resuscitation facilities
3. Permit emergency pacemaking (Chapter 11)
4. Permit the display of the heart rate on a tachometer
5. Permit the monitoring of the ECG on an oscilloscope throughout the procedure
6. Permit the recording of specific ECG leads as needed before, during, and after electrical cardioversion.

Routine Preparation

1. A short strip of lead V_1 should be recorded—to confirm the presence of an arrhythmia before the shock and to confirm that sinus rhythm has returned after the shock.
2. ECG paste should be applied liberally to the patient and rubbed well into his skin to reduce electrical resistance.
3. It should be ascertained that no part of the patient's skin is in direct contact with the metal of the trolley or the bed on which he is lying.
4. No one should touch the patient, his bed, or any apparatus to which he is attached at the moment of shock.

When the electrical resistance of the skin is reduced by the use of ECG paste or saline-soaked pads, the substance used should not be allowed to run between the two paddles. Current takes the path of least resistance, and unless strict attention is paid to that detail, most of the electrical energy could be diverted from the heart muscle, resulting in failure of the attempt at electrical cardioversion.

Levels of Electrical Energy

As mentioned, the shock may be administered across two anterior paddles or, preferably, with paddles in the anterior and posterior positions. Low energy levels should be used first. If the low levels are unsuccessful, the shock may be repeated at an increased energy level (Table 10–1). It is important to use a low initial energy level if the patient is heavily

Table 10–1.   *Energy Level Settings for the Emergency or Elective Electrical Cardioversion of Cardiac Arrhythmias in Adults*

	Atrial Arrhythmia or Ventricular Tachycardia				Ventricular Fibrillation
	Acute: Emergency Electrical Cardioversion		Chronic: Elective Electrical Cardioversion		
	Digitalized 1, 2	Not Digitalized 2	Digitalized 1, 2, 3	Not Digitalized 2, 3	
Synchronizer Used?	Yes	Yes	Yes	Yes	No
Shock No. 1	5 joules	25 joules	5 joules	25 joules	200 joules
Shock No. 2	10 joules	50 joules	10 joules	50 joules	300 joules
Shock No. 3	25 joules	100 joules	25 joules	100 joules	400 joules
Shock No. 4	50 joules	150 joules	50 joules	150 joules	
Shock No. 5, etc.	Thereafter by 50-joule increments to 400 joules if needed		Thereafter by 50-joule increments to 300 joules if needed		

1. Precede the initial shock with the intravenous administration of 50 to 100 mg of lidocaine, 50 to 100 mg of procainamide, or 100 mg of diphenylhydantoin.
2. If any shock is followed by premature beats, give drugs as indicated in No. 1 before giving any incremental shock.
3. Precede the initial shock with the intravenous administration of 1 mg of atropine if atrial arrhythmia has been present for three years or more and if the ventricular rate is less than 70 beats per minute.

digitalized and to use intravenous lidocaine (1) if extrasystoles follow the first shock and (2) routinely before treating a patient who is heavily digitalized. Initial energy settings for children delivered across appropriately-sized pediatric paddles is also indicated.

There should be great reluctance to use more than 300 joules in an adult being treated for chronic rhythm disturbances, but when an acute arrhythmia has serious hemodynamic effects, the maximum energy (400 joules) can be used.

The initial setting for ventricular fibrillation (no synchronizing circuit) is 200 joules increasing by 100-joule increments to a maximum of 400. An appropriate range for internal defibrillation (with special spoon-shaped paddles) is 20 to 100 joules in 20-joule increments.

Following the Shock

With the reinstitution of sinus rhythm (or if sinus rhythm should fail to occur), after optimal amounts of energy have been delivered:
1. The amnesic drug should be discontinued

2. The 12-lead ECG should be recorded

3. The ECG should be monitored for the next 24 hours or longer if premature beats or other arrhythmias occur

4. The blood pressure should be determined every half hour until it reaches the control value before the shock

5. A chest roentgenogram should be taken again within 24 hours to exclude pulmonary edema, which sometimes follows a high-energy-level shock (p. 202).

TREATMENT OF INDIVIDUAL RHYTHM DISTURBANCES

Atrial Fibrillation

Atrial fibrillation is the most common rhythm disturbance that is to be treated. Lone or idiopathic atrial fibrillation deserves special mention since the success rate of electrical cardioversion is low, the incidence of complications is high, and the length of time during which sinus rhythm persists is disappointingly short.[34] For atrial fibrillation due to rheumatic heart disease, the initial success rate is 87 to 90%,[23] but for idiopathic atrial fibrillation, it is less than 75%.[34] The rate of initial success is not related to the age or sex of the patient, the type of heart disease (except for lone atrial fibrillation), nor even to overall body size. The success rate does depend on:

1. The duration of the rhythm disturbance (Fig. 10–4). The rate of success is 50% or less when atrial fibrillation has been present five years or longer.

2. The overall increase in size of heart. The larger the heart, the less likely is the chance of success.

3. Enlargement of the left atrium. Enlargement of the left atrium significantly reduces the chance of success.

It is clear therefore, that every patient with chronic atrial fibrillation requires individual assessment to determine whether treatment is worthwhile. There is no doubt, however, that hemodynamic benefit may be achieved by conversion to sinus rhythm,[35] particularly during exercise. Certain groups of patients can be kept free of cardiac failure only by repeated electrical termination of atrial fibrillation.

Open Chest Electrical Cardioversion. Although cardioversion is easy to achieve at the time of surgery, reversion to atrial fibrillation in the postoperative phase is almost universal. Atrial fibrillation with a ventricular rate controlled by digoxin is preferred to rapidly changing cardiac rhythms postoperatively, and it is recommended, therefore, that the electrical cardioversion of the patient be postponed until he is convalescent following open or closed valvular surgery.[25,36]

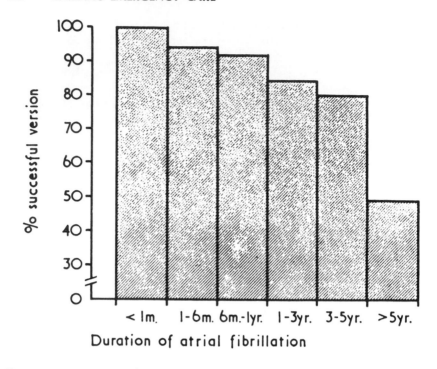

Figure 10–4.   Percentage of successful electrical cardioversion and duration of atrial fibrilla-tion before treatment (idiopathic atrial fibrillation excluded). (Reprinted with permission from Resnekov and McDonald.[23])

Relative Contraindications. Electrical cardioversion for atrial fibrillation should be attempted only under exceptional circumstances in the following groups of patients:

1. Those with idiopathic or lone atrial fibrillation

2. Those with coronary heart disease and atrial fibrillation with a slow ventricular response in the absence of digoxin

3. Those unable to maintain sinus rhythm for more than a very brief period of time, even when they are given quinidine or other antiarrhythmic drugs (Chapter 7) in adequate doses

4. Those displaying varying atrial rhythm disturbances in rapid succession.

5. Those in the tachycardia phase of the brady-tachyarrhythmia syndrome (unless emergency pacemaking is at hand) since dangerous asystole may follow a transmyocardial shock in that phase

6. Those with longstanding atrial fibrillation (more than five years) with considerable enlargement of the heart (a cardiothoracic ratio of more than

2:1) unless they are to undergo cardiac surgery for an associated valvular heart disease

7. Those whose atrial fibrillation is associated with conduction disturbances.

Atrial Flutter

A 90 to 95% success rate for electrical cardioversion of atrial flutter is common. The electrical energy setting needed is usually much lower than that for atrial fibrillation, averaging 50 joules. Unlike idiopathic atrial fibrillation, atrial flutter not associated with detectable heart disease may still be successfully reverted by direct current shock at relatively low energy settings, and sinus rhythm may be maintained for significantly long periods.[34]

Paroxysmal Atrial Tachycardia

The success rate for electrical cardioversion in paroxysmal atrial tachycardia varies from 75 to 80%, depending on the underlying cause. Even so, electrical cardioversion is preferred to drug therapy. It should not be used, however, for digitalis-induced arrhythmias, such as atrial tachycardia with AV block of varying degrees and nonparoxysmal AV junctional tachycardia (Chapter 16), except under the most unusual circumstances, because the risk of precipitating ventricular fibrillation is very high.[37]

Paroxysmal AV Junctional Tachycardia

The success rate for electrical cardioversion in AV junctional tachycardia is similar to that in paroxysmal atrial tachycardia, and the same caution must be exercised if a digitalis preparation is also being used.

Ventricular Tachycardia

The initial success rate of electrical cardioversion exceeds 97%. The energies needed are low. Again, great caution must be exercised when ventricular tachycardia is digitalis-induced (Chapter 16). In such a case, electrical cardioversion is contraindicated, except in rare instances, and it is always preceded by the intravenous administration of a drug such as lidocaine to protect against the emergence of ventricular fibrillation, with full resuscitative equipment at hand in case of need.

Ventricular Fibrillation

Controlled clinical comparisons of unsynchronized direct current shock and alternating current shock are difficult to design, but experimental animal studies have shown direct current shock to be superior.[16] In clinical practice, successful resuscitation, as judged by the patients being able to leave the hospital, can be achieved in more than 60% of cases with direct current shock and proper applications of the principles of resuscitation.[38]

COMPLICATIONS

Initially, complications were thought to be rare following synchronized DC shock, but an incidence of 14.5% among 220 patients has been reported.[39] That incidence does not include minor complications, such as superficial burns due to poor preparation of the skin or transient rhythm disturbances immediately after the shock. It does include the following complications:

1. Raised levels of serum enzymes (in 10% of the cases). The cause of the increases is still debated. Many consider damage to skeletal muscle to be the cause.[40] Nevertheless, other signs of myocardial damage are frequently seen,[39] including positive technetium pyrophosphate myocardial scintiscan results.

2. Hypertension (in 3% of the cases). The hypertension is not due to the kind of anesthesia used, and it is more common when higher levels of electrical energy are used. The hypertension may persist for several hours, but it usually requires no particular treatment.

3. ECG evidence of myocardial damage (in 3% of the cases). Patterns of myocardial infarction recorded even in the absence of obvious symptoms may persist for many months. They are most common following electrical cardioversion at high energy settings (Fig. 10–5).

4. Pulmonary and systemic embolism (in 1.4% of the cases). Embolism does occasionally follow electrical cardioversion, indicating the need for anticoagulation therapy.

5. Ventricular arrhythmias. Serious ventricular rhythm disturbances are common, even at low energy settings, when the patient is heavily digitalized and at higher settings whether or not digoxin has been given. Their emergence requires the use of an intravenous antiarrhythmic drug (Chapter 7) before the energy level setting is increased.

6. An increase in heart size and in pulmonary edema (in 3% of the cases) occurs within one to three hours after treatment and can be confirmed by chest roentgenogram.[39] Unlike any of the other complications of electroversion, it seems to occur only in patients actually brought

into sinus rhythm.[41] While Lown considered pulmonary embolism to be a cause,[22] others believe that there is considerable depression in the mechanical function of the heart following electrical cardioversion.[42] Despite the fact that sinus rhythm is recorded on the ECG, mechanical left atrial systole may be depressed or absent. Any additional obstruction to flow across the mitral valve or any left ventricular dysfunction will

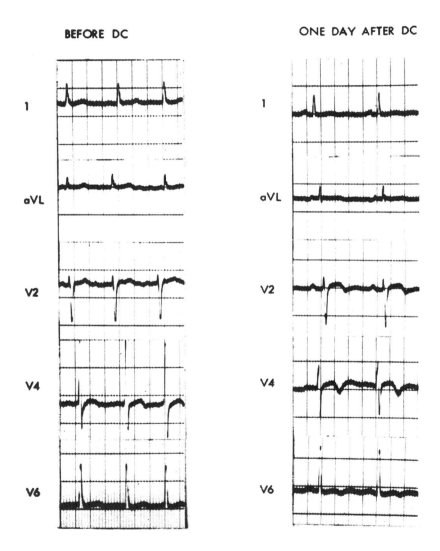

Figure 10–5.   Idiopathic atrial fibrillation. ECG one day before and after electroversion. Note the deep T-wave inversion following the direct current shock. It was associated with elevation of serum enzymes. (Reprinted with permission from Resnekov and McDonald.[39])

aggravate the situation and result in pulmonary edema. As with other complications, its incidence is greatest following high energy level settings.

In the series already mentioned,[39] the incidence of complications was 6% when an electrical energy level setting of up to 150 joules was used, but it increased to more than 30% at 400 joules (Fig. 10–6). High energy level settings are often needed for treating longstanding atrial fibrillation, and complications are likely in patients:

1. Who have been in atrial fibrillation for three years or more
2. Who have cardiomyopathy or coronary heart disease as the cause
3. In whom idiopathic atrial fibrillation is present.

From all the foregoing evidence one may conclude the following:

1. There rarely is an indication for exceeding an energy level setting of 300 joules in patients who present with longstanding atrial fibrillation.

2. Particular caution must be exercised in (a) those who are heavily digitalized, (b) those whose arrhythmia is due to cardiomyopathy or coronary heart disease, and (c) those with lone atrial fibrillation.

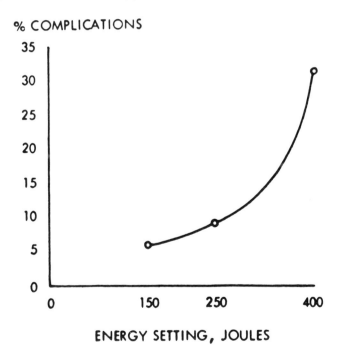

Figure 10–6.   Percentage of complications in 220 patients treated by electrical cardioversion related to the maximal energy setting used. (108 patients were treated at an energy setting of <150 joules, 55 at <250 joules, and 37 at <400 joules.) (Reprinted with permission from Resnekov and McDonald.[39])

FOLLOW-UP STUDIES

While electrical cardioversion is highly successful, the number of patients who remain in sinus rhythm is disappointingly small, particularly when atrial fibrillation is treated.[25] A 36-month follow-up study involving 183 patients successfully converted to sinus rhythm showed that less than 30% remained in sinus rhythm.[23] The majority who revert to their original rhythm disturbance do so by the end of the first month of treatment (Fig. 10–7), but the highest incidence of reversion is actually in the first 24 hours (Fig. 10–8).

The following groups of patients are particularly prone to revert to their original rhythm disturbance:

1. Those in whom significant heart disease is associated with radiographic evidence of cardiac enlargement

2. Those who have atrial fibrillation of long duration. If they have had atrial fibrillation more than three years, they have a 70% chance of reverting to atrial fibrillation following successful electrical cardioversion (Fig. 10–9)

3. Those who have significant enlargment of the left atrium

4. Those whose sinus node function is inadequate (Chapter 9)

5. Those in whom electrical cardioversion is followed by atrial ectopic beats, particularly in association with poor sinus node function and sinus bradycardia (Chapter 9).

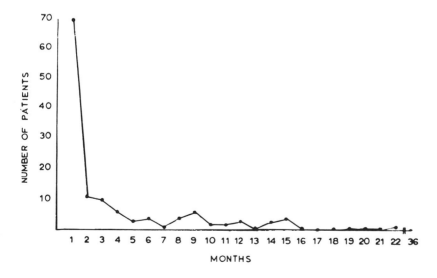

Figure 10–7. Thirty-six-month follow-up of 183 patients in whom electrical cardioversion succeeded: 131 (72%) reverted to their original arrhythmia, 70 (53%) within the first month (see also Fig. 10 8). (Reprinted with permission from Resnekov and McDonald.[11])

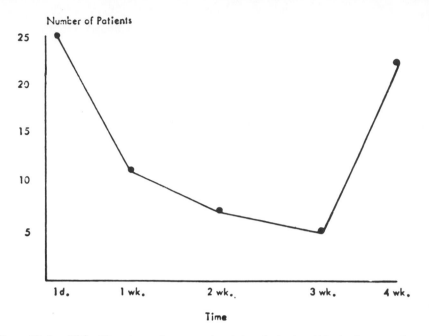

Figure 10–8. Of the 70 patients who reverted to their arrhythmia within the first 4 weeks, 25 (35%) did so within the first day of electrical cardioversion (see also Fig. 10–7). (Reprinted with permission from Resnekov and McDonald.[23])

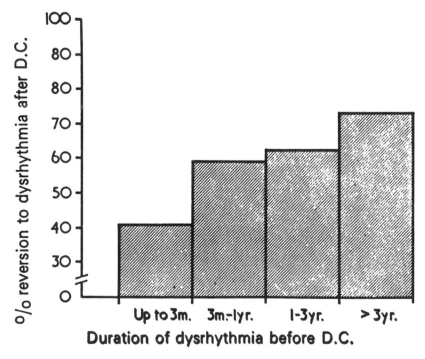

Figure 10–9. Percentage of patients who reverted to atrial fibrillation related to the duration of the arrhythmia before electrical cardioversion. (Reprinted with permission from Resnekov and McDonald.[23])

DRUGS AND DIRECT CURRENT SHOCK

Anticoagulants

As mentioned, the incidence of embolism following electrical car-dioversion is 1.4 to 2.4%,[39,43] a rate similar to the reported incidence of embolism following quinidine cardioversion.[44] The need for anticoagulant protection was the subject of much debate when well-controlled studies were lacking, but such a study has now been reported,[45] and the results indicate that there is a statistical benefit in patients who had electrical cardioversion while undergoing anticoagulation therapy.

The following groups of patients with clear risk for embolism should have electrical cardioversion while they are undergoing anticoagulation therapy control:

1. Those with recent myocardial infarction
2. Those with chronic coronary heart disease, particularly with left ventricular dyskinetic segments or aneurysm
3. Those suffering cardiomyopathy
4. Those with prosthetic heart valves
5. Those with a history of embolism.

Anticoagulation therapy using a coumarin derivative should be given long enough before electrical cardioversion to insure a protective effect; heparin should be used when the need for direct current shock is urgent.

Since the risk of the patient's reverting to the arrhythmia is highest within the first month of treatment (Fig. 10–8), anticoagulation therapy should be maintained for at least four weeks, even after successful direct current shock; thereafter it may be discontinued unless the underlying heart disease requires its continuance.

Digitalis

In a study involving heavily digitalized dogs, the direct current threshold for ventricular tachycardia fell by some 2000% to 0.2 joules.[46] The clinical importance of that phenomenon is that digitalis effects not clinically apparent may be unmasked by an electrical shock, and any associated intramyocardial cell potassium deficit could enhance the digitalis effects. Conversely, administering potassium to raise the serum potassium level to normal may reverse the undesirable effect. The higher the level of electrical energy, the greater the risk of serious ventricular arrhythmia; and death has been reported to result.[37] Thus electrical cardioversion should rarely be used in the management of a rhythm disturbance known to be digitalis induced (Chapter 16), since despite the occasional report of success,[47] fatal ventricular fibrillation may follow, even when the shock is properly synchronized.

If electrical cardioversion is needed when the patient is heavily digitalized:

1. The direct current shock should be preceded by an intravenous injection of an antiarrhythmic drug, such as lidocaine, diphenylhydantoin, and procainamide, as previously indicated.

2. The initial energy setting (in an adult) should be 5 to 10 joules.

3. Any incremental energy settings should be at 5 to 10 joules.

Propranolol may also be helpful in reducing the dangerous myocardial sensitivity to high-energy electrical currents, but it should be combined with intravenous atropine[48] to protect the patient against cardiac arrest, which may follow direct current shock in patients primed with propranolol.[49] It is essential that a normal serum potassium level be achieved before electrical cardioversion, particularly in patients being given digoxin and diuretic therapy, since hypokalemia may well precipitate serious ventricular disturbances, even when only small amounts of digoxin are used[50] (Chapter 16).

Antiarrhythmic Drugs

For electrical cardioversion to succeed:

1. An energy setting sufficient to instantly depolarize the majority of heart fibers is needed.

2. Adequate functioning of the sinus node is essential for the maintenance of sinus rhythm.

3. Ectopic beats should be kept to a minimum immediately after a shock.[51]

Abnormalities of the sinus node, including fibrosis, are commonly associated with atrial rhythm disturbances, particularly atrial fibrillation (Chapter 9).

As mentioned, excess electrical energy may be harmful. Any interruption of the rhythm disturbance by the direct current shock is good evidence that depolarization of the heart occurred, indicating that the level of electrical energy was adequate. If sinus rhythm fails to emerge or if it is only short lived despite the delivery of adequate electrical energy to the myocardium, the likely explanations are:

1. The sinus node is no longer capable of functioning as the pacemaker of the heart because of structural change or disease (Chapter 9).

2. Ectopic rhythms were precipitated by the sudden catecholamine release that followed the electrical discharge.

Improved Pacemaker Functioning Following Direct Current Shock

Improved pacemaker functioning can best be achieved by the routine intravenous injection of 1 to 2 mg of atropine for patients who have had atrial fibrillation for five years or more. But it should be realized that the chance that those patients will convert to sinus rhythm easily or will maintain sinus rhythm for a significant length of time after conversion is small.[23] It should also be realized that any tendency to bradycardia following direct current shock will enhance the likelihood that atrial or ventricular premature beats will escape.[23] It should be recalled that although the antiarrhythmic drugs are successful in suppressing ectopic beats, quinidine, procainamide, lidocaine, and propranolol all depress pacemaker functioning. Furthermore, since there is already a likelihood of intense parasympathetic stimulation immediately after direct current shock,[52] the *routine* use of those drugs is not advised because they may precipitate dangerous asystole.

Isolated ventricular premature beats or ventricular tachycardia immediately after direct current shock often results from a combination of:

1. Overdigitalization (Chapter 16)
2. The effects of the shock itself on the heart
3. A lowered myocardial potassium content.

As mentioned, patients with those conditions should be protected by:

1. Postponing treatment if at all possible
2. Insuring an adequate serum potassium level and intramyocardial cellular potassium content
3. Administering antiarrhythmic drugs immediately before the shock.

Although there is good evidence in the literature that no antiarrhythmic drug now available, alone or in combination, can maintain sinus rhythm (1) when SA function is faulty, (2) when serious underlying myocardial valvular heart disease is present, or (3) when atrial fibrillation has existed for five years or longer, particularly when the heart is considerably enlarged, the maintenance of sinus rhythm may be hemodynamically important and can keep such patients free of cardiac failure. In such circumstances, quinidine or procainamide may be used in an attempt to maintain sinus rhythm over the long term.

If cardiac failure is not too severe, it may be possible to prolong sinus rhythm by combining quinidine and propranolol;[53] the combination allows reduction of the dose of quinidine, thus lessening the incidence of intoxication.

SUMMARY

1. Electrical cardioversion of cardiac arrhythmias should be undertaken only by those who understand the apparatus, the indications, the technique, and the potential risks of the technique.

2. Electrical cardioversion should be undertaken in an area equipped for full cardiac monitoring, resuscitation, and emergency pacemaking.

3. A monthly check of the electrical safety of the apparatus should be

made routinely. The waveform should be inspected following discharge across a 50-ohm load, and the amount of energy delivered should be measured and compared with the manufacturer's specifications.

4. The shock should always be synchronized with the R or the S wave to avoid the vulnerable phase of the ventricles, except when ventricular fibrillation is being treated, in which case the synchronizer has to be switched out of circuit.

5. The minimal amounts of energy needed to instantly depolarize the majority of the myocardial fibers should be delivered rather than the maximal amounts of energies.

6. The electrical resistance of the skin should be reduced as much as possible by the localized application of ECG paste or saline-soaked pads to insure that the substance used does not run between the paddles.

7. Anticoagulation therapy should precede the shock in most instances. Oral coumadin administered to therapeutic levels should be given, or in urgent cases intravenous heparin.

8. Anticoagulation therapy should be maintained for at least one month in those who have been treated successfully. Reversion to the original rhythm disturbance is most likely to occur within the first month of treatment.

9. If possible, digitalis preparations should be stopped 24 to 48 hours before treatment.

10. Treatment should be postponed in any patient with evidence of a digitalis overdose.

11. If it is not possible to delay treatment in those heavily digitalized, serious ventricular rhythm disturbances should be protected against as follows: (a) Any electrolyte imbalance, especially a potassium imbalance should be corrected. (b) The shock should be preceded by an intravenous injection of lidocaine, 50 to 100 mg, or diphenylhydantoin, 50 to 100 mg, or procainamide, 50 to 100 mg. (c) The initial energy level setting should be 5 to 10 joules. (d) If the first shock is followed by ventricular premature beats, the injection of lidocaine, diphenylhydantoin, or procainamide should be repeated before the energy level setting is increased.

12. The pacemaker activity of the SA node should be enhanced following direct current shock by injecting 1 to 2 mg of atropine intravenously just before electrical cardioversion in (a) patients who have had artrial fibrillation for three or more years, (b) patients whose ventricular response to atrial fibrillation is 70 beats per minute or less, and (c) patients taking beta-adrenergic blocking drugs (e.g., propranolol). Postshock sinus bradycardia and/or asystole may thus be prevented.

13. The initial energy settings for adults who are not heavily digitalized should be 25 to 50 joules, and the levels should increase in 25 to 50 joule steps to 300 joules.

14. Energy levels higher than 300 joules should be used cautiously in people with chronic rhythm disturbances since the complication rates are proportional to the amounts of energy delivered.

15. People with an acute rhythm disturbance producing severe cardiac dysfunction should be given incremental amounts of energy to a maximum setting (400 joules) if needed.

16. At the end of treatment, the rhythm should be confirmed by comparing the post–direct current shock lead V_1 with that pretreatment lead.

17. Patients should be observed for any complications over a 24-hour period, ideally by monitoring the ECG, insuring the stability of the blood pressure, and obtaining a chest roentgenogram within the first 24 hours.

18. Complications are frequent, and often they are multiple: raised levels of serum enzymes, hypotension, ECG changes characteristic of myocardial infarction, positive technetium pyrophosphate scintiscan results, pulmonary edema, and increases in the size of the heart, in sinus rhythm, and in the incidence of pulmonary and/or systemic embolism. Less serious complications include transient rhythm disturbances and superficial skin burns.

19. The complications are related to the energy levels and they increase dramatically when the energy levels are more than 300 joules.

20. The success rate of electrical cardioversion is 90%, even when antiarrhythmic drugs have failed.

21. Definite indications for electrical cardioversion are all *acute rhythm disturbances*—(supraventricular or ventricular), particularly if the disturbances cause circulatory depression.

22. Relative indications for electrical cardioversion are chronic arrhythmias, especially in patients with atrial fibrillation, who require careful assessment before treatment is decided on.

23. The patients with chronic atrial fibrillation most likely to benefit from electrical cardioversion are (1) those in whom the arrhythmia has been present for three years or less, (2) those who have only mild enlargement of the heart and left atrium, and (3) those who do not have a hemodynamically important valvular heart disease, coronary heart disease, or cardiomyopathy.

24. Patients in chronic atrial fibrillation without the favorable signs mentioned in No. 23 convert only with difficulty, require high energy settings, have high complication rates, and usually revert to atrial fibrillation within one month of electrical cardioversion.

25. Rhythm disturbances thought to be due to an overdose of digitalis should be treated by electrical cardioversion, even when synchronized, only when every other treatment has failed since the risk of precipitating ventricular fibrillation and death is high.

26. In patients undergoing open heart surgery, electrical cardioversion is best postponed until convalescence since reversion during the immediate postoperative phase in those brought into sinus rhythm at the time of surgery is usual.

27. Patients with idiopathic atrial fibrillation are unsuitable for electrical cardioversion, except under unusual circumstances.

28. The following groups of patients are also unsuitable for synchronized electrical cardioversion, except under unusual circumstances: (a) Those with slow ventricular rates, even in the absence of digitalis. (b) Those who do not maintain sinus rhythm despite antiarrhythmic drugs. (c) Those who have varying atrial rhythm disturbances in rapid succession. (d) Those who have had atrial fibrillation for more than five years, particularly if the fibrillation is associated with considerable enlargement of the heart. (e) Those in the tachycardia phase of the brady-tachyarrhythmia syndrome (Chapter 9). (f) Those whose atrial rhythm disturbance is associated with conduction defects.

29. The drug regimen immediately before, during, and after electrical cardioversion should be defined for every patient according to the following principles: (a) The pacemaker activity of the sinus node should be enhanced by preceding the shock with intravenous atropine. (b) The incidence of atrial or ventricular premature beats should be reduced by intravenous lidocaine, diphenylhydantoin, or procainamide before the shock. (c) The long-term antiarrhythmia management should be tailored to the needs of the patient; the choice of regimen is based on its potential for preserving sinus rhythm.

30. Electrical defibrillation of the heart is an exciting advance that is now known to be safe and effective, particularly if the principles for its use are strictly adhered to. Great efforts must be expended on uncovering the basic mechanisms of rhythm disturbances and thus encouraging the development of more physiologic approaches to their treatment and, especially, to the long-term maintenance of sinus rhythm.

REFERENCES

1. Prevost, J.L., and Battelli, F.: Quelques effets des décharges electriques sur le coeur des mammifères. J. Physiol. Path. Gen. 2:40, 1900.
2. Kouwenhoven, W.B., Hooker, D.R., and Langworthy, O.R.: The current flowing through the heart under conditions of electric shock. Am. J. Physiol. 100:344, 1932.
3. Ferris, L.P., King, B.G., Spence, P.W., and Williams, H.B.: Effects of electrical shock on the heart. Elec. Eng. 55:498, 1936.
4. King, B.G.: The Effect of Electric Shock on Heart Action with Special Reference to Varying Susceptibility in Different Parts of the Cardiac Cycle. Aberdeen, Scotland, The Aberdeen University Press, 1934.
5. Gurvich, N.L., and Yunyev, G.S.: O vosstanovlenii normalnoi deyatel'nosti gibril-liroyuschego sevdtsa teplokrovaikh possedstrom kondensatornogo vazvyada. Byul. Eksp. Biol. Med. 8:55, 1939.

6. Peleşka, B.: Transthorákalni přimá defibrilace. Rozhl. Chir. 36:731, 1957.
7. Tsukerman, B.M.: Opit electricheskoi defibrillyatsii predserdii u 20 bol'nikh s mitralmini porokami sevdsta. Vestn. Akad. Med. Nauk SSSR 8:32, 1961.
8. Lown, B., Amarasingham, R., and Neuman, J.: New method for terminating cardiac arrhythmias. Use of synchronized capacitor discharge. JAMA 182:548, 1962.
9. Hooker, D.R., Kouwenhoven, W.B., and Langworthy, O.R.: The effect of alternating electrical currents on the heart. Am. J. Physiol. 103:444, 1933.
10. Kouwenhoven, W.B., and Milnor, W.R.: Treatment of ventricular fibrillation using a capacitor discharge. J. Appl. Physiol. 7:253, 1954.
11. Main, F.B., Aberdeen, E., and Gerbode, F.L.A.: Comparison of ventricular function subsequent to multiple defibrillations using the alternating current and the direct current defibrillators. Surg. Forum 14:258, 1963.
12. Yarbrough, R., Ussrey, G., and Whitley, J.: A comparison of the effects of AC and DC countershock on ventricular function in thoracotomized dogs. Am. J. Cardiol. 14:504, 1964.
13. Beck, E.S., Pritchard, W.H., and Feil, H.S.: Ventricular fibrillation of long duration abolished by electric shock. JAMA 135:985, 1947.
14. Alexander, S., Kleiger, R., and Lown, B.: Use of external electric countershock in the treatment of ventricular tachycardia. JAMA 177:916, 1961.
15. Zoll, P.M., and Linenthal, A.J.: Termination of refractory tachycardia by external countershock. Circulation 25:596, 1962.
16. Nachlas, M.M., Bix, H.H., Mower, M.M., and Siebano, M.P.: Observations on defibrillation and synchronized countershock. Prog. Cardiovasc. Dis. 9:64, 1966.
17. DeBoer, S.: On the fibrillation of the heart. J. Physiol. 54:400, 1921.
18. Wiggers, C.J., and Wegria, R.: Ventricular fibrillation due to single, localized induction and condensed shocks applied during vulnerable phase of ventricular systole. Am. J. Physiol. 128:500, 1940.
19. Castellanos, A., Jr., Lemberg, L., and Berkovits, B.V.: Repetitive firing during synchronized ventricular stimulation. Am. J. Cardiol. 17:119, 1966 (Abst.).
20. Peleşka, B.: Cardiac arrhythmias following condensed discharges and their dependence upon strength of current and phase of the cardiac cycle. Circ. Res. 13:21, 1963.
21. Kreus, K.E., Salokannel, S.J., and Waris, E.K.: Non-synchronized and synchronized direct-current countershock in cardiac arrhythmias. Lancet ii:405, 1966.
22. Lown, B.: Electrical reversion of cardiac arrhythmias. Br. Heart J. 29:469, 1967.
23. Resnekov, L., and McDonald, L.: Appraisal of electroversion in treatment of cardiac dysrhythmias. Br. Heart J. 30:786, 1968.
24. McDonald, L., Resnekov, L., and O'Brien, K.: Direct current shock in treatment of drug resistant arrhythmias. Br. Med. J. i:1468, 1964.
25. Resnekov, L.: Synchronized capacitor discharge in the management of cardiac arrhythmias with particular reference to the haemodynamic significance of atrial systole. M.D. Thesis, University of Cape Town, 1965.
26. Lown, B., Kleiger, R., and Wolff, G.: The technique of cardioversion. Am. Heart J., 67:282, 1964.
27. Kouwenhoven, W.B., Jude, J.R., Knickerbocker, G.G., and Chestnut, W.R.: Closed chest defibrillation of the heart. Surgery 42:550, 1957.
28. Stock, R.J.: Cardioversion without anesthesia. N. Engl. J. Med. 269:534, 1963.
29. Lown, B.: Cardioversion without anesthesia. N. Engl. J. Med. 269:535, 1963.
30. Kahler, R.I., Burrow, G.N., and Felig, P.: Diazepam induced amnesia for cardioversion. JAMA 200:997, 1967.
31. Shephard, D.A.E., and Vandam, L.D.: Anesthesia for cardioversion. Am. J. Cardiol. 15:55, 1965.
32. Johnstone, M., and Nisbet, H.I.A.: Ventricular arrhythmia during halothane anaesthesia. Br. J. Anaesth. 33:9, 1961.
33. Nutter, D.O., and Massumi, R.A.: Diazepam in cardioversion. N. Engl. J. Med. 273:650, 1965.
34. Resnekov, L., and McDonald, L.: Electroversion of lone atrial fibrillation and flutter, including haemodynamic studies at rest and on exercise. Br. Heart J. 33:339, 1971.

35. Resnekov, L.: Haemodynamic studies before and after electrical conversion of atrial flutter and fibrillation to sinus rhythm. Br. Heart J. 29:100, 1967.
36. Yang, S.S., Maranhao, V., Monheit, R., Ablaza, S.G.G., and Goldberg, H.: Cardioversion following open-chest valvular surgery. Br. Heart J. 28:309, 1966.
37. Rabbino, M.D., Likoff, W., and Dreifus, L.: Complications and limitations of direct-current countershock. JAMA 190:417, 1964.
38. Gilston, A.: Clinical and biochemical aspects of cardiac resuscitation. Lancet ii:1039, 1965.
39. Resnekov, L., and McDonald, L.: Complications in 220 patients with cardiac dys-rhythmias treated by phased direct-current shock and indications for electroversion. Br. Heart J. 29:926, 1967.
40. Mandecki, T., Biec, L., and Kargul, W.: Serum enzyme activities after cardioversion. Br. Heart J. 32:600, 1970.
41. Resnekov, L., and McDonald, L.: Pulmonary oedema following treatment of ar-rhythmias by direct current shock. Lancet i:506, 1965.
42. Logan, W.F.W.E., Rowlands, D.J., Howitt, G., and Holmes, A.M.: Left atrial activity following cardioversion. Lancet ii:471, 1965.
43. Sjorstein, D.: DC Cardioversion Session 18, p. 418. In E. Sandøe, E. Flensten-Jensen, and K.H. Olesen. (eds.), Symposium on Cardiac Arrhythmias. Sodertalje, Sweden, A.B. Astra, 1970.
44. Goldman, J.: The management of chronic atrial fibrillation: indications for and method of conversion to sinus rhythm. Progr. Cardiovasc. Dis. 2:465, 1959–1960.
45. Bjerkelund, C.J., and Orning, O.M.: The efficacy of anticoagulant therapy in preventing embolism following DC electrical conversion of atrial fibrillation. Am. J. Cardiol. 23:208, 1969.
46. Lown, B., Kleiger, R., and Williams, J.: Cardioversion and digitalis drugs: Changed threshold to electric shock in digitalized animals. Circ. Res. 17:519, 1965.
47. Corwin, N.D., Klein, M.J., and Friedberg, C.K.: Countershock conversion of digitalis associated paroxysmal tachycardia with block. Am. Heart J. 66:804, 1963.
48. Sloman, G., Robinson, J.S., and McClean, K.: Propranolol in persistent ventricular fibrillation. Br. Med. J. i:895, 1965.
49. Lown, B.: Discussion, p. 127. In D.G., Julian and M.F. Oliver (eds.), Acute Myocardial Infarction: Proceedings of a Symposium. Edinburgh, Livingstone, 1968.
50. Lown, B., and Wittenberg, S.: Cardioversion and digitalis. III. Effect of change in potassium concentration. Am. J. Cardiol. 21:513, 1968.
51. Resnekov, L.: Drug therapy before and after the electroversion of cardiac dys-rhythmias. Prog. Cardiovasc. Dis. 16:531, 1974.
52. Childers, R.W., Rothbaum, D., and Arnsdorf, M.: The effects of DC shock on the electrical properties of the heart. Circulation 36:II-85, 1967 (Abstr.).
53. Byrne-Quinn, E., and Wing, A.J.: Maintenance of sinus rhythm after DC reversion of atrial fibrillation. Br. Heart J. 32:370, 1970.

Chapter 11

ARTIFICIAL PACING

LOUIS LEMBERG
AGUSTIN CASTELLANOS

GENERAL CONSIDERATIONS

The fundamental principles for the utilization of an artificial pacemaker were established in 1932 by Hyman[1] and promulgated by Callaghan and Bigelow in 1951.[2] External cardiac pacing was introduced into clinical medicine in 1952 by Zoll.[3] In 1957 Weirich and his co-workers introduced temporary direct myocardial stimulation for the treatment of complete AV block,[4] and in 1960 Chardack and his co-workers introduced a transistorized, self-contained implantable pacemaker for long-term correction of complete AV block.[5] Artificial pacemakers are now indispensable, and they are the most reliable method of treating the Adams-Stokes syndrome.

At first, fixed-rate pacemakers were used, but they have been gradually replaced by demand pacemakers, which have several advantages over the earlier type.

Artificial pacemakers are used primarily for the treatment of various bradyarrhythmias, particularly complete AV block. However, they also provide a life-saving measure in the treatment of drug-resistant and refractory tachyarrhythmias, especially those of ventricular origin.

INDICATIONS FOR PACING

Artificial pacing is performed primarily for symptomatic arrhythmias.[6] Asymptomatic patients may be candidates for pacing when there are specific ECG changes that are considered to be harbingers of symptomatic arrhythmias. The indications for pacing are discussed in this chapter from the clinical viewpoint because it is symptoms and the clinical setting that determine the need for cardiac pacing.

Pacing in Symptomatic Patients

Patients with Adams-Stokes Syndrome. The Adams-Stokes syndrome is an attack of syncope, with or without a convulsive seizure, resulting from a sudden marked bradycardia, ventricular standstill, or transient ventricular repetitive beats associated with complete AV block. Brief episodes of faintness, dizziness, or weakness are variants of the syndrome.

Complete AV block in the Adams-Stokes syndrome occurs in the elderly patient. There are no known predisposing diseases; however, the pathologic entities are known as Lev's disease and Lenegre's disease.[7] Lev described fibrosis or calcification of the connective tissue skeleton of the heart that envelops the conduction pathways, and Lenegre reported sclerodegenerative changes in the conduction pathways.

The first appearance of the Adams-Stokes syndrome, corroborated by the presence of AV block, is an indication for immediate permanent pacemaker implantation.

Patients with Heart Failure. When congestive heart failure associated with a bradyarrhythmia is unresponsive to medical management, permanent cardiac pacing is indicated. Pacing at physiologic rates usually results in diuresis and compensation.

Patients with Altered Mentation. Altered mentation due to reduced cerebral blood flow may result from bradyarrhythmias. Pacing at physiologic rates augments the minute volume and cardiac output and thus improves cerebral perfusion.

Patients with the Sick Sinus Syndrome. The term sick sinus syndrome (SSS) refers to a constellation of signs, symptoms, and arrhythmias with ECG manifestations of sinus node dysfunction and without any relation to the administration of cardiac drugs or to electrolyte imbalance.

The SSS may occur at any age but it occurs more commonly in the elderly patient. The SSS is characterized by one or more of the following: near syncope, syncope, vertigo, or any manifestation of cerebral dysfunction associated with specific ECG abnormalities. Since congestive heart failure may either be initiated or augmented by slow ventricular rates, it is included in the SSS.

The ECG manifestations of the SSS include:

1. Persistent and severe sinus bradycardia
2. SA block or sinus arrest
3. Chronic atrial fibrillation or flutter with slow ventricular response
4. Alternating tachycardia and bradycardia (the brady-tachyarrhythmia syndrome)
5. Carotid sinus hypersensitivity
6. AV junctional escape rhythm with or without slow, unstable sinus activity
7. Inability to resume sinus rhythm following cardioversion of atrial fibrillation or atrial flutter

Coronary artery atherosclerosis is the most common disease responsible for the SSS. Sclerodegenerative disease, fibrosis, or amyloid infiltration may also involve the SA and AV nodes and be responsible for the SSS.[8-12]

The elements in the diagnosis of the SSS are shown in Table 11–1.

Extended ECG recordings (Holter monitor ECGs) often uncover the presence of the SSS when the arrhythmia occurs infrequently.

The provocative tests described in the following paragraphs may be used to help establish a diagnosis.

1. Atropine sulfate administered intravenously in 1 to 2 mg doses results in an increase in sinus rate of approximately 65% in the normal heart. In contrast, in the SSS the sinus node fails to make an appropriate increase in rate in response to atropine sulfate.

2. Isoproterenol administered intravenously in 1 to 2 mg doses in a 500-ml 5% solution of dextrose in water is titrated to increase the heart rate to 90 to 100 beats per minute. In the SSS the sinus node fails to increase its rate in response to isoproterenol. Careful attention is necessary to avoid ectopic beats when isoproterenol is used. However, those adverse effects are very transient after discontinuing the drug.

Table 11–1. *The Sick Sinus Syndrome: Diagnostic Approach*

Clinical manifestations
12-lead ECG
Extended ECG recording (Holter monitor ECG)
Carotid sinus stimulation and Valsalva maneuver
Cardioversion
Exercise (stress) ECG test
Drugs (e.g., atropine, isoproterenol)
Electrophysiologic studies
Determination of sinus node recovery time by atrial pacing
Determination of SA conduction time by extrastimulus technique
His bundle electrocardiography

3. Measuring the sinus node recovery time by atrial pacing at rates of 120 to 180 beats per minute for two to five minutes at each level and then stopping abruptly. The time of appearance of the first sinus P wave should be 1400 msec or less following the termination of pacing. A pause greater than 1400 msec is consistent with a diagnosis of the SSS.

4. Measuring SA conduction time indirectly by the atrial extrastimulus technique.

The SSS is often associated with AV nodal disease that is not manifested in the surface ECG. His bundle electrograms may show abnormalities in AV nodal or His-Purkinje conduction. Demand or standby pacing is indicated in the management of the SSS. It is accomplished by pacing the ventricles or the atria provided AV transmission is intact. Pacemaking prevents the development of bradycardia, but it has little effect in preventing supraventricular tachycardia. However, suppressive doses of antiarrhythmic drugs can be used safely and effectively after pacemaker implantation in patients with supraventricular tachycardia. Both atrial and ventricular sequential pacing may also be employed by using a bifocal sequential demand pacemaker when significant AV conduction disturbance coexists and when the atrial contribution is desired. That type of demand pacemaker, which was developed recently, can pace the atria only or the atria and ventricles in sequence; or it can remain dormant when normal sinus rhythm prevails.[13]

The sick sinus syndrome is discussed in detail on pp. 157–187.

Patients with Bradycardia. Patients with bradycardia-induced ventricular ectopic beats or ventricular tachycardia can benefit from suppression of the ventricular arrhythmias at an overdriving pacing rate. The successful use of permanently implanted pacemakers for the control of recurrent ventricular tachycardia or ventricular fibrillation refractory to drug therapy has been reported extensively.[14] Demand or standby pacing has been effective in those cases. Pacemakers have also been used for patients with atrial fibrillation or atrial flutter and slow ventricular response accompanied by congestive heart failure who were otherwise difficult to manage. Bradycardia resulting from a hypersensitive carotid sinus reflex has at times required pacing.

After pacemaker implantation for symptomatic bradycardia, cardioactive drugs can be employed in therapeutic ranges without the danger of added suppression of SA nodal discharge or AV nodal conduction.

Pacing in Asymptomatic Patients

The indications for electrical stimulation in the absence of any symptoms are less clear than when symptoms are present. The presence of Mobitz type II AV block is a definite indication for pacing. Correct ECG identification of that conduction disturbance is imperative. A diagnosis of Mobitz type II AV block is made when a nonconducted sinus P wave suddenly occurs and is preceded by conducted beats that have constant P–R intervals. Some patients may be symptomatic when the number of successively blocked P waves is significant. However, if the block is temporarily stabilized as a 2:1 or 3:1 AV block, the symptoms may be absent or mild.

There are several processes that can simulate 2:1 AV block in the presence of fairly regular P–R intervals. Foremost among the processes are the recording of the end of a long run of Mobitz type I (Wenckebach) AV blocks in which the increase in the P–R interval is very slight before the blocked P wave. If a Mobitz type II AV block emerges after a normal P–R interval, the possibility is less likely.

Concealed His bundle or fascicular extrasystoles can produce a similar phenomenon.[15,16] Mobitz type II AV block should be diagnosed with caution in patients having manifest AV junctional (His bundle) and fascicular beats.

The asymptomatic patient with right bundle branch block (RBBB) and left anterior hemiblock (LAHB) or left posterior hemiblock (LPHB) poses difficult problems in regard to prophylactic therapy. According to Rosenbaum and his co-workers,[17] prophylactic pacemaker implantation is indicated whenever RBBB coexists with an abnormal right axis deviation due to LPHB (other causes of right axis deviation have to be excluded).

Pacemaker therapy in patients who have RBBB and LAHB due to chronic conducting system disease has also been a subject of debate and speculation.[9] Because the time of onset of symptomatic complete AV block in those patients is unpredictable, definite guidelines for prophylactic pacing have not been established.

Recent His bundle studies suggest that a prolonged H–V interval does not adversely affect the short-term prognosis in patients with RBBB and LAHB. The implications are that His bundle electrograms may not be indicated for the evaluation of those patients. However, longer follow-up periods are required to prove that assumption. Some of those patients are prone to develop tachycardia-dependent or bradycardia-dependent AV block. Bradycardia-dependent AV block is precipitated by sinus slowing, which delays the subsequent P wave long enough that it falls during phase 4 depolarization.[18] In other cases, the AV block is triggered by a premature beat when the post-extrasystolic P wave falls sufficiently late.[18] Continuous 24-hour ECG monitoring in patients with chronic RBBB and LAHB can be used to reveal bradycardia-dependent AV block.

Atrioventricular Block in Acute Myocardial Infarction

Site of Infarction. There are specific features and specific therapeutic problems associated with AV block complicating acute myocardial infarction. Although AV block is an infrequent complication (it occurs 7 to 10% of cases), it has generated more controversy than any of the other arrhythmias that occur in the coronary care unit. The differences of opinion are related to the indications for the use of pacemakers and to their beneficial effects.[19]

Knowledge of the site of the infarction is a critical factor in determining the prognosis as well as the management of AV block complicating acute myocardial infarction.[19] As Table 11–2 indicates, it is apparent that although AV block complicates diaphragmatic (inferior wall) infarctions more than twice as often as it does anterior wall infarctions, the mortality of AV block is three times greater in anterior wall infarctions than in diaphragmatic infarctions.

The pathogenesis of acute AV conduction disturbances helps to explain those differences. AV block in acute infarction of the inferior wall is located high in the AV node (above the His bundle) and consists pathologically of edema or inflammation due to transient injury of the node or infarction of the contiguous myocardium rather than involvement of the conduction tissue proper. The block is usually transient, and there is seldom a residual conduction defect. In anterior wall infarctions, AV block is secondary to destruction and necrosis of the bundle branches and distal parts of the conducting tissues, so that permanent damage results, with residual block of one or both bundles. Analysis of His bundle electrograms of patients with AV block following acute myocardial infarction has localized the conduction disturbance to an area above the His bundle in diaphragmatic infarction and below the bundle of His in anterior wall infarction. Table 11–3 shows the other differences that characterize those two forms of AV block.

In general, first-degree AV block alone, regardless of the site of infarction, requires no treatment. In the presence of high degrees of block complicating diaphragmatic infarctions, initial drug therapy is indicated if

Table 11–2.   *Incidence of and Mortality in Complete Atrioventricular Block Complicating Acute Myocardial Infarction*

Site of Infarction	Incidence of AV Block (%)	Mortality (%)
Inferior wall	7	30
Anterior wall	3	80

Table 11–3. *Atrioventricular Block Complicating Acute Myocardial Infarction*

	AV Block Complicating Inferior Wall Infarction	AV Block Complicating Anterior Wall Infarction
Pathogenesis	Edema or inflammation due to transient ischemia of AV node and contiguous myocardium	Destruction due to infarction of the bundle branches
Location of block	Above the His bundle	Below the His bundle
Premonitory signs	Sinus bradycardia often. First-degree AV block or second-degree block. Wenckebach type often precedes complete AV block	RBBB plus LAH—often RBBB plus LPH—infrequent Alternating BBB or sudden asystole
Adams-Stokes attacks	Rare (7 to 10%)	Almost always present
QRS complexes	Usually narrow, maintaining a supraventricular pattern	Usually wide (idioventricular)
Subsidiary pacemaker	Probably junctional	Ventricular
Mobitz II	Rare	Usual
Residual block	Very rare	BBB and/or fascicular block
Treatment	Drugs usually effective	Pacemaker
Prognosis	Good	Poor

the existing ventricular rate is inadequate and symptoms of bradyarrhythmia develop. In that clinical setting, therefore, the critical factor is the heart rate and not the degree of block.[19,20]

In diaphragmatic infarctions, early acute AV block of any degree may result from excessive vagal discharge, and in that clinical setting, sinus bradycardia is also present. Atropine sulfate improves AV conduction in more than 50% of these cases (Fig. 11–1). Intravenous infusion of isoproterenol may improve AV conduction when atropine is ineffective. Excessive sinus rates and ventricular rates should be avoided when isoproterenol is used.

Diaphragmatic Infarction. The clinical course and prognosis of AV block in diaphragmatic infarction are not significantly altered by endocardial pacing. Pacing in AV block due to acute diaphragmatic infarction is indicated in the following situations:

1. When the ventricular rate cannot be effectively maintained at optimal levels by drug therapy

2. In Mobitz type II AV block

3. In symptomatic complete AV block (usually a ventricular rate slower than 50 beats per minute)

Anterior Wall Infarction. Early experiences in coronary care units showed that the prognosis for most patients who develop acute AV block following anterior wall infarctions is poor, even with artificial pacing. The

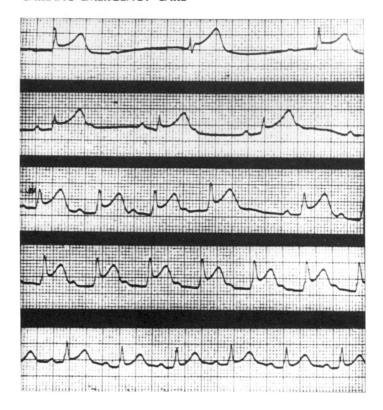

Figure 11–1.   Regression of third-degree AV block to sinus rhythm with a normal P–R interval following the intravenous administration of 0.6 mg of atropine sulfate in a patient with an acute inferior wall myocardial infarction. Wenckebach periods followed by first-degree A–V block precede the return to normal sinus rhythm.

poor prognosis was attributed to the extensive myocardial damage, which was frequently complicated by cardiogenic shock, heart failure, or myocardial rupture.

With recent advances in electrophysiology and after retrospective reviews of particular clinical situations, it has been noted that AV block with anterior wall infarctions is frequently ushered in by the appearance of block in any of the bundle branches. Specific ECG patterns are produced by interruption of the right bundle or of the two fascicles (anterosuperior and posteroinferior) of the left bundle, or of any combination of those elements. With this knowledge, prophylactic insertion of a pacing catheter may improve the prognosis when any two of those branches are blocked.

Therapy for AV block complicating anterior myocardial infarction is quite different. Atropine is ineffective, but isoproterenol may be transiently helpful if advanced AV block or asystole occurs before a pacing catheter can be introduced. Therefore, in the following conditions, a pacemaker catheter should be inserted prophylactically for demand or standby pacing:

1. Complete RBBB and LAHB
2. Complete RBBB and LPHB
3. Complete RBBB and first-degree AV block
4. Complete LBBB and first-degree AV block
5. Complete LBBB alternating with complete RBBB

Indications for Pacing. AV conduction disturbances that follow diaphragmatic infarctions are transient and seldom require permanent pacing. Because regular sinus rhythm may return at any time during the course of an acute myocardial infarction, the pacemaker of choice is the ventricular-inhibited, or demand, pacemaker. That type of pacemaker reduces the risk of repetitive ventricular beats or ventricular fibrillation. Figure 11–2 shows an episode of repetitive ventricular beating initiated by a stimulus from a continuous asynchronous pacemaker in a patient with an acute myocardial infarction.

Permanent demand pacemaker implantation is indicated in a few patients who survive transient AV block due to acute anterior myocardial infarction. Atkins and his co-workers[21] reported that of 13 patients with RBBB and LAHB who had transient AV block during the acute phase of myocardial infarction and survived, 11 died within six months of discharge. The posthospital mortality in that group is much higher than that of patients with otherwise uncomplicated myocardial infarction. The report continues with information about eight similarly ill patients in whom pacemakers were implanted before discharge. There were no deaths in that group during the 8- to 18-month follow-up.

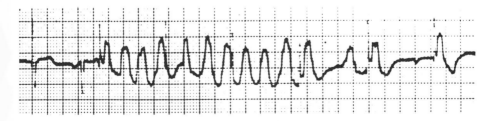

Figure 11–2.   A continuous asynchronous (fixed-rate) pacemaker stimulus artifact falling in the vulnerable period of a natural beat initiates repetitive ventricular beats.

Reciprocating Tachycardia

An increasing number of patients with reciprocating tachycardia are being treated by artificial pacing. The type of pacemaker therapy for reciprocating tachycardias is determined by the particular mechanism of the tachycardia. Knowledge of the tachycardia mechanisms permits the physician to choose the optimal therapy and to avoid conceptual errors that may threaten the life of the patient. The widespread modern use of pacemakers dictates the need for a discussion of the reciprocating tachycardias.

A classification of the reciprocating tachycardias is shown in Tables 11–4 and 11–5. It is important to stress that the newer methods of intracardiac recording and stimulation have shown that multiple circuits can be involved in the origin and perpetuation of those arrhythmias.[21] The mechanisms of reciprocating tachycardias in patients with preexcitation Wolff-Parkinson-White (WPW) syndrome are discussed first.

Preexcitation is said to be present when a sinus (or atrial) impulse is conducted through pathways other than the normal AV route and activates a portion or all of the ventricles earlier than the impulse that is conducted through the normal AV pathways at the usual speed. From the

Table 11–4.   *Types of Reciprocating Atrial and Ventricular Tachycardias*

Sinus node-atrial reciprocation

Intra-atrial or interatrial reciprocation
    Reciprocating atrial flutter
    Rare cases of reciprocating atrial tachycardia

Intraventricular or interventricular reciprocation
    Reciprocation around the stimulating electrodes, as in classic "vulnerability"
    Reciprocation involving the bundle branches
    Reciprocation involving an area of acute myocardial infarction
    Reciprocation involving a scarred area
    Combinations of the above

Table 11–5.   *Types of Reciprocating Atrioventricular Tachycardias*

Functional longitudinal dissociation of the AV node
Reciprocation involving the AV node and the Kent bundle
Reciprocation involving the AV node and the James bundle
Combinations of the above
When ventricular stimulation is performed at short coupling intervals, any of the reciprocating
    intraventricular or interventricular tachycardias described in Table 11–4 can be associated
    with any of the above reciprocating tachycardias.

---

clinical standpoint, any patient with recurrent, repetitive, supraventricular tachyarrhythmias can be considered to have a form (or a variant) of the preexcitation syndrome.[22] The resting ECG obtained during sinus rhythm may be deceptive because of the coexistence of congenital, atherosclerotic, or primary conduction system disease.

The short P–R interval with the wide QRS complex in the WPW syndrome is presumably due to a Kent bundle, but AV conduction time may be normal in the presence of atrial enlargement or intra-atrial conduction defects. A short P–R interval, narrow QRS complexes, and repetitive tachyarrhythmias suggest the Lown-Ganong-Levine (LGL) syndrome, perhaps due to total bypass of the area where the major AV nodal delay occurs. The P–R interval can be normal in the presence of atrial or bundle branch disease, but the ventricular complexes are wide and the A–H interval is short.

Some patients with recurrent tachyarrhythmias and normal P–R and A–H intervals but a narrow QRS complex may have a partial AV nodal bypass. Those patients, as well as patients with the LGL syndrome, are characterized by a dynamic response to atrial pacing at increasing rates and not by the measurement of conduction intervals at natural rates.[22] The A–H interval does not show the increase that is normally seen. At times, 1:1 AV conduction occurs at rates as high as 240 beats per minute. Adults with atrial flutter and 1:1 AV conduction are likely to have an AV nodal bypass.

A premature atrial beat with prolonged AV conduction time usually triggers the reciprocating tachycardia. However, the initiating event need not be an atrial extrasystole in the true sense since retrograde atrial activation of ventricular extrasystoles or marked sinus arrhythmia may produce the same effect.

In the WPW syndrome, the reciprocating arrhythmias appear when the premature atrial impulse is conducted to the ventricles through the AV node while being blocked at the Kent bundle. It can, nevertheless, return to the atria through the accessory pathway. Yet there is no reason a reciprocating tachycardia involving a single functionally dissociated anatomical pathway (AV node) cannot occur in patients with the WPW syndrome. Similar considerations apply to patients with the LGL syndrome and its variants.

Various types of pacemakers have been implanted for the treatment of symptomatic patients with drug-resistant recurrent supraventricular tachycardias. There is no single mode of pacing that is appropriate for all forms of reciprocating tachycardias. Electrophysiologic evaluation is essential before selection of the best mode of stimulation.[22]

Specialized studies are needed to distinguish among the types of reciprocating mechanisms that may be present (Table 11–4). Those studies can establish the presence or absence of preexcitation and can evaluate the type of preexcitation, as well as the functional properties of the normal and accessory pathways. Finally, those studies can help to reach an understanding of the effects of electrical stimuli and the response to intravenously administered drugs.

The WPW syndrome is discussed in detail on pp. 101–142.

Rapid Atrial Stimulation. Rapid atrial stimulation can transform an AV reciprocating tachycardia into atrial fibrillation or flutter, which, in the absence of atrial disease, is self limited. Since the arrhythmia subsides promptly, sinus rhythm is generally reestablished. However, in some patients with preexcitation (usually those with the WPW syndrome and, rarely, those with the LGL syndrome or its variants), the effective refractory period of the accessory pathway is very short. In those patients (especially if they have organic disease), atrial fibrillation may be persistent and associated with clinically significant rapid ventricular rates. Cardioversion may be needed to terminate the arrhythmia.

Stimulation of the Atria at Varying Coupling Intervals. Properly timed single or double atrial stimuli can break a reciprocating circuit, thus stopping the tachycardia. That type of pacing may at times induce vulnerability-related atrial fibrillation with the same potential hazards just mentioned. Such atrial fibrillation is generally triggered by stimuli delivered at short coupling intervals, immediately after the end of the atrial effective refractory period.

Ventricular Pacing. Stimulation of the ventricles can abolish a reciprocating tachycardia if the impulses are conducted retrograde to the atria provided that the P wave falls in the moment of the cycle when it can break the tachycardia. At times, concealed retrograde conduction into the AV tissues collides with the oncoming supraventricular impulse, thus stopping the tachycardia.

However, premature ventricular stimuli delivered at short coupling intervals can produce additional reciprocating circuits (Table 11–5). The latter can be short lived or persistent, at times interrupting (permanently or transiently) the original AV tachycardia.

As mentioned, several types of permanent pacemakers have been used in the treatment of reciprocating AV tachycardias.[19] Undesirable sinus bradycardia is prevented by QRS-inhibited ventricular demand pacemakers in patients receiving high doses of beta-blocking drugs. Sequential AV bifocal units can abolish certain reciprocating circuits. Several authors have reported the use of an implanted pacemaker that can be activated externally by magnets or radiofrequency signals during bouts of tachycardia; conventional QRS-inhibited ventricular demand units, rapid atrial stimulators, and atrial- or ventricular-triggered pacemakers with preselected (fixed or varying) coupling (or triggering) intervals have also been used in the treatment of reciprocating tachycardia.[22]

MODALITIES OF PACING

Since the advent of electronic cardiac pacemakers, a variety of pacing modalities have been developed. The physician who uses pacemakers must understand the various types of pacing available so that he can select the type best suited to the particular patient.

The following is a basic classification of the modalities of pacing.[24]

1. Stimulation of the ventricles only
   a. Continuous asynchronous ventricular pacing
   b. QRS-inhibited ventricular (demand) pacing
   c. QRS-triggered ventricular (standby) pacing
   d. P wave–triggered ventricular pacing
2. Stimulation of the atria only
   a. Continuous asynchronous atrial pacing
   b. P wave–inhibited atrial pacing
   c. P wave–triggered atrial pacing
   d. QRS-inhibited atrial pacing
3. Stimulation of both atria and ventricles
   a. Continuous sequential atrial and ventricular pacing
   b. QRS-inhibited sequential atrial and ventricular (bifocal demand) pacing

Stimulation of the Ventricles Only

The Continuous Asynchronous Pacemaker. The continuous asynchronous pacemaker delivers stimuli to the ventricles continuously at rates of 60 to 80 beats per minute. The rate can be altered manually in some units, and since the output of the pacemaker is neither inhibited nor synchronized, the term continuous asynchronous (Fig. 11–3) is more suitable than the term fixed rate. During normal functioning, the interval between pacemaker stimuli does not change, even in the presence of natural beats (either sinus or ectopic). All stimulus artifacts, except those appearing during the absolute refractory period of the ventricles, result in propagated responses.

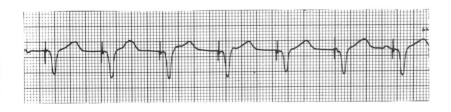

Figure 11–3.   A continuous asynchronous (fixed-rate) pacemaker that is functioning normally.

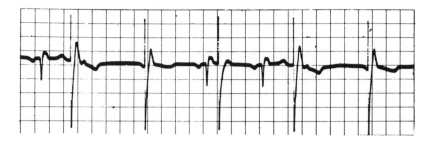

Figure 11–4.   Summated heartbeats due to the coaction of natural beats and pacemaker beats (continuous asynchronous pacemaker).

Table 11–6.   Pacemaker Characteristics

Pacemaker	Type	Mode of Action	Stimulates	Senses	General Indications
Continuous asynchronous ventricular	Ventricular	Continuous asynchronous	Ventricles	—	SA arrest; AV block
QRS-inhibited ventricular	Ventricular	QRS-inhibited (demand)	Ventricles	QRS	SA arrest; AV block electrical overdrive
QRS-triggered ventricular	Ventricular	QRS-triggered (standby)	Ventricles	QRS	SA arrest; AV block
P wave–triggered ventricular	Ventricular	P wave–triggered	Ventricles	P waves	AV block in children
Continuous sequential atrial and ventricular	Atrial and ventricular	Continuous sequential	Atria and ventricles	—	AV block; Sinus bradycardia; AV synchrony when needed to enhance cardiac output
QRS-inhibited sequential atrial and ventricular	Atrial and ventricular	QRS-inhibited sequential (bifocal demand)	Atria and ventricles	QRS	Sick sinus syndrome; AV block overdrive; reciprocating tachycardia; AV synchrony when needed to enhance cardiac output

The transient appearance of natural beats occurs commonly in patients with pacemakers. Potential hazards due to competition are created as a result of the coaction of natural and artificial pacemaker rhythm (Fig. 11–4). Summated heart rates are seen, and repetitive ventricular beats may occur when pacemaker stimuli fall during the vulnerable period of the cardiac cycle (Fig. 11–2). Those problems led to the development and widespread use of noncompetitive (QRS-inhibited, QRS-triggered, and P wave–triggered) pacemakers.[25] Because of the risks of competition, the continuous asynchronous pacemaker is not widely used today. The characteristics of that pacemaker are summarized in Table 11–6.

The QRS-Inhibited Ventricular (Demand) Pacemaker. The QRS-inhibited pacemaker is the most widely used pacemaker. It has both stimulating and sensing mechanisms. When natural ventricular activity is sensed, the output of the pacemaker is suppressed. A stimulus is emitted only after a preset interval following a natural ventricular beat has been exceeded. Pacing automatically ceases when the natural rate exceeds that of the pacemaker (Fig. 11–5). The significant characteristics of the safe and useful QRS-inhibited pacemaker are outlined in Table 11–6.[23]

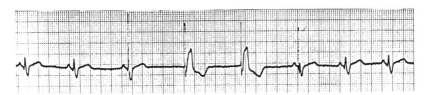

Figure 11–5.   QRS-inhibited (demand) pacemaker pacing when the natural rate is below that of the pacemaker. With an increase in the natural rate (shown at the right end of the trace), pacing stimulus artifacts are no longer seen.

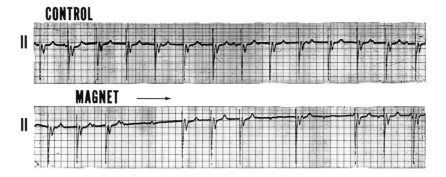

Figure 11–6.   Erratic firing of a normally functioning QRS-inhibited ventricular pacemaker due to improper application of a magnet over the neck of the pulse generator. (Reprinted by permission of the American Heart Association.[24])

Because of the difficulties of evaluating the stimulating properties of the QRS-inhibited pacemaker during periods of pacemaker inhibition, a magnetic reed switch was added to the pulse generator. Application of a magnet to the skin overlying the pulse generator activates the switch and causes a change to a continuous mode of operation at a fixed rate, which is not necessarily the same as its automatic rate. However, that feature introduced new problems. For instance, improper application of the magnet over the neck of pulse generators can lead to erratic firing in some normally functioning units (Fig. 11–6). In other units with component failure manifested by significant rate variations, the magnet can produce complete pacemaker inhibition.

Ventricular fusion beats result if portions of the ventricles are activated by the natural impulse and other portions by the pacemaker.[25] A true fusion beat appears when the pacemaker escape interval ends after the onset of ventricular depolarization but before the moment (within the QRS complex) at which inhibition would have occurred. That occurs if the perielectrode tissues have not been rendered absolutely refractory by the activation front propagating from the area first depolarized by the natural impulse.

Pseudo-fusion beats are due to the ECG superimposition of an ineffective stimulus artifact on a natural ventricular complex.[26] Pseudo-fusion beats appear when the pacemaker escape interval ends after the beginning of ventricular depolarization but before the moment (within the QRS complex) at which inhibition would have occurred.[24] However, the perielectrode tissues have been rendered absolutely refractory by the impulse propagating from the area first activated by the natural impulse. (Figure 11–7 is a diagrammatic representation of the mechanisms of true fusion beats and pseudo-fusion beats.)

The escape interval following a sensed ventricular beat is shorter or longer than (but rarely equal to) the interval between two consecutive stimulus artifacts (the automatic interval). That is so because the moment within the QRS complex at which inhibition starts cannot be determined from the surface ECG.[25,26] Moreover, the escape interval also changes in accordance with the structure and origin of the ventricular beats.[23] Some manufacturers have preset the duration of the escape intervals in demand pacemakers, thus adding the function of rate hysteresis. In rate hysteresis,[28] the escape intervals are intentionally longer than the automatic interval (Fig. 11–8). The clinical significance of rate hysteresis is that it can lead to an otherwise paradoxical situation in which a slower natural rhythm inhibits a faster artificial pacemaker. That phenomenon reflects a malfunction when it occurs in pacemakers that do not have rate hysteresis.

The QRS complexes appearing after the end of the pacemaker refractory period may be sensed by normally functioning QRS-inhibited pace-

ONSET OF ARP   PART OF QRS INHIBITING

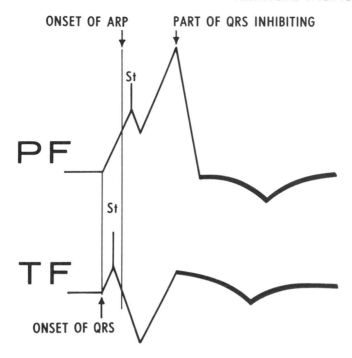

Figure 11–7.   Diagrammatic representation of the mechanisms of true fusion (TF) beats and pseudo-fusion (PF) beats. (See text for explanation.) Onset of QRS = the beginning of ventricular depolarization (in an area distant from the electrodes). Onset of ARP = the moment at which the muscle surrounding the electrodes is rendered refractory by the impulse propagating from its site of origin. Part of QRS inhibiting = the moment within the ventricular complex at which pacemaker inhibition would occur. St = pacemaker spike. For those events to occur, a built-in lag between the onset of ARP and the part of QRS inhibiting must be present. (Reprinted by permission of the American Heart Association.[24])

St - St = 840   R - R = 960

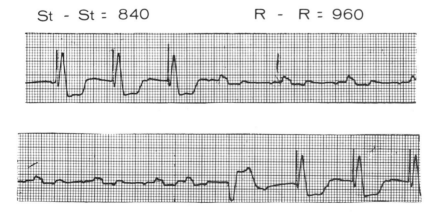

Figure 11–8.   QRS-inhibited ventricular pacemaker with rate hysteresis. A slower natural rhythm (R–R cycle length of 960 msec) inhibits a faster automatic rate (St–St interval of 840 msec). St = stimulus artifact. (Reprinted by permission of the American Heart Association.[24])

makers. Since intracavity ventricular electrograms of 1 mv or less have been observed in the presence of myocardial infarction, nonsensing might occur in the absence of pacing system failure if the catheter electrodes are improperly positioned.[24] At times, unipolarization of a bipolar system is required. It should be emphasized that a good threshold for stimulation does not necessarily imply that sensing is adequate. If voltages greater than 2.5 mv are not found, transvenous QRS-inhibited pacing should not be attempted. Contrary to commonly held assumptions, sensing is not an all-or-none phenomenon. It has been shown that borderline intracavity signals can produce an incomplete recycling of the sensing mechanism that is characterized by escape intervals of longer duration than if the beat had not been detected at all. However, the escape interval is significantly shorter than that seen when normal sensing occurs.[29-32]

Partial sensing (Fig. 11–9) may occur in patients with normally functioning pacing systems if the intracardiac signals are from 1.5 to 5 mv. The most frequent cause of partial sensing, however, is improper electrode placement. Thus repositioning of the electrodes or unipolarization of the pacing system (and not replacement of the pulse generator) prevents partial sensing. As with any problem involving sensing, the presence of partial sensing can be confirmed by magnet conversion to continuous asynchronous pacing, which will differentiate the stimulating and the sensing functions of the pacing system.

The QRS-Triggered Ventricular Pacemaker. The QRS-triggered ventricular pacemaker is similar to the QRS-inhibited type, and it has both stimulating and sensing mechanisms (Table 11–5). Unlike the ventricular-inhibited type, the QRS-triggered pacemaker delivers an electrical stimulus during the formation of the patient's QRS complex when the natural rate exceeds that of the pacemaker (Fig. 11–10). In addition, the pacemaker fires automatically after a preset escape interval, the duration of which is determined by the rate of the pacemaker. Triggered pacemaker stimuli falling within the QRS complexes are generally considered to be safe and ineffective.

A stimulus artifact seen in the middle of the QRS complex indicates that the sensing mechanism is functioning normally. However, it distorts the QRS structure thus interfering with the evaluation of the ventricular complex. The interference is a problem in the interpretation of certain acute conditions. At rates greater than 100 beats per minute, firing occurs only after the second or third ventricular complex. During atrial fibrillation, a chaotic arrhythmia results from the interplay of normal or aberrantly conducted supraventricular beats, pure pacemaker beats, and true fusion and pseudo-fusion beats. In the presence of sinus rhythm, the function of capture can be tested by conversion to a continuous asynchronous mode of operation by the use of an external magnet. Improper

S

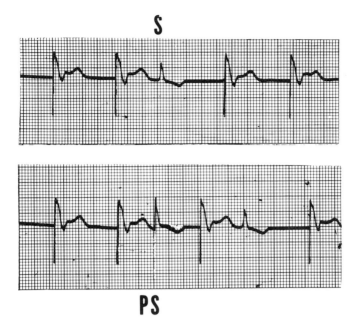

PS

Figure 11–9.   Differences between "normal" and "partial" sensing. The escape intervals of "normally" sensed (S) beats are slightly longer (880 msec) and those of "partially" sensed (PS) QRS complexes are significantly shorter (610 msec) than the automatic intervals (840 msec) (Reprinted by permission of the American Heart Association.[24])

V-S ESCAPE

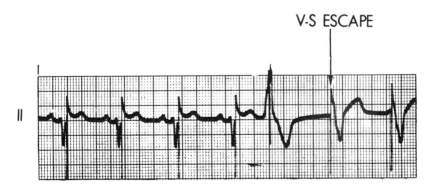

Figure 11–10.   Pacemaker stimulus artifacts appear during the formation of the QRS complex as seen with the sinus conducted beats as well as with the ventricular premature beat. When a natural beat fails to appear, the pacemaker takes over ventricular-stimulus (V–S) escape and paces the ventricles.

II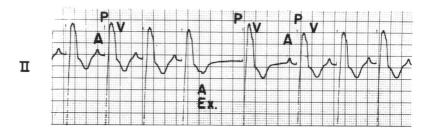

Figure 11-11. Wave-triggered ventricular pacemaker. An atrial extrasystole occurs during the refractory period of the pacemaker. In the absence of a P wave, the pacemaker captures the ventricles after preset interval. A = P waves; P = pacemaker artifact; V = QRS complex; AEx = atrial extrasystoles.

application of the magnet over the neck of the pulse generator produces intermittent activation of the magnetic switch that is perceived by the corresponding circuit as an ectopic beat; as a result, a pacemaker stimulus is delivered. That causes irregular pacemaker firing not due to malfunctioning. The fact that the QRS-triggered pacemaker makes the ECG interpretation more difficult has resulted in a general decline in its use.

The P Wave–Triggered Ventricular Pacemaker. The P wave–triggered pacemaker also has both stimulating and sensing mechanisms. The P wave–triggered ventricular pacemaker functions as an artificial AV node. A sensing electrode in the atrium detects the P waves, and after a delay corresponding to the normal P–R interval, the ventricle is stimulated by a ventricular electrode (Fig. 11-11). If a P wave does not appear, the pacemaker stimulates after a preset escape interval and it maintains the ventricular output at a preset rate. It has been found useful in the management of chronic AV block in children.

The features of the P wave–triggered pacemaker are summarized in Table 11-6.

Stimulation of the Atria Only

The various modalities of atrial pacing are presented diagrammatically in Figure 11-12.[24,33–40]

Stimulation of Both Atria and Ventricles

The Continuous Sequential Atrial and Ventricular Pacemaker. Diagrams illustrating the ECG features of continuous sequential atrial and ventricular pacing and of QRS-inhibited sequential atrial and ventricular pacing (bifocal demand stimulation) are presented in Figure 11-13.[24]

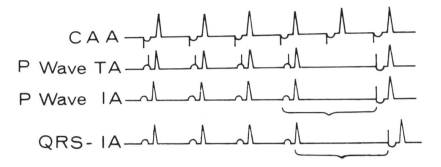

Figure 11–12.   Diagrammatic illustration of the modalities of pacing used for atrial stimulation. During continuous asynchronous atrial pacing (CAA), the stimulus artifacts precede and capture the atria; AV transmission is intact. With P wave–triggered atrial pacing (P Wave TA), the stimulus artifacts appear during the formation of the sinus P wave. When SA block occurs, the stimulus artifact appears at the end of the escape interval and precedes the P wave. In P wave–inhibited atrial pacemakers (P Wave IA), the faster atrial rates suppress or inhibit the output of the atrial pacemaker. Pacemaker atrial escapes occur when a P wave fails to appear before a preset interval. With QRS-inhibited atrial pacemakers (QRS–IA), faster ventricular rates suppress the output of the pacemaker. A pacemaker atrial escape occurs when a QRS complex fails to appear before a preset interval. (Reprinted by permission of the American Heart Association.[24])

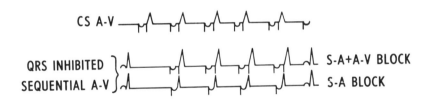

Figure 11–13.   ECG features of implantable transvenous pacemakers that have been used for both atrial and ventricular stimulation. Continuous sequential A–V pacemakers (CS A–V) stimulate the atria and, after a preset delay, the ventricles. They are neither inhibited nor triggered by P waves or ventricular complexes. On the other hand, QRS-inhibited sequential AV (bifocal demand) pacemakers are inhibited by faster natural rates. Only the atria will be paced if intermittent pure sinoatrial (S–A) block occurs. However, both atria and ventricles will be stimulated when intermittently coexisting SA and AV blocks appear. (Reprinted by permission of the American Heart Association.[24])

In the continuous sequential atrial and ventricular mode of pacing, electrodes in the atrium and in the ventricle stimulate at a continuous rate but with a sequential delay between the stimuli equal to that of the normally functioning AV node (Fig. 11–14). The competitive rhythms that often occur with continuous asynchronous pacemakers are potential problems in continuous sequential atrial and ventricular pacing. The characteristics of the continuous sequential atrial and ventricular pacemaker are listed in Table 11–6.

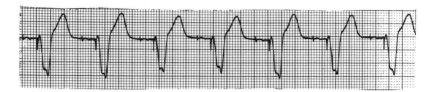

Figure 11–14. Continuous sequential atrial and ventricular pacing. Stimulus artifacts capture the atria and the ventricles with a delay equal to the normal P–R interval.

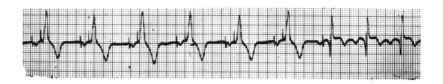

Figure 11–15. QRS-inhibited AV sequential pacing (bifocal demand). At the right end of the trace, when normal sinus rhythm returns, the ventricular pacemaker stimulus artifact is inhibited first, and then both atrial and ventricular pacemaker stimuli are inhibited.

The QRS-Inhibited Sequential Atrial and Ventricular (Bifocal Demand) Pacemaker. Like the ventricular demand pacemaker, the QRS-inhibited sequential atrial and ventricular pacemaker monitors ventricular electrical activity but programs both atrial and ventricular stimulation (Table 11–6). It consists of two demand units, a conventional QRS-inhibited demand pacemaker and a QRS-inhibited atrial demand pacemaker.[13,40] The escape interval of the atrial pacemaker is shorter than the escape interval of the ventricular pacemaker. The difference between the two escape intervals defines the AV sequential interval: that is, the P–R interval. Both pacemakers acting in synchrony provide QRS-inhibited AV sequential stimulation (Fig. 11–15).

The ventricular electrodes have a dual function. They sense the ventricular signal and they stimulate the ventricles when required. The atrial electrode stimulates the atrium, but it does not have a sensing function. Therefore the signal detected by the ventricular electrode is responsible for both atrial and ventricular pacing.

COMPLICATIONS OF PACEMAKERS

Pacemaker Arrhythmias

Pacemaker arrhythmias were included in the discussion of the different modes of pacing (pp. 227–236) because the different modes of pacing have their characteristic rhythm problems. The discussion was confined to the arrhythmias related to the most commonly used pacemakers.

Malpositioning of the Transvenous Pacemaker Catheters

Proper positioning of the electrode catheter in the apex of the right ventricle is not always achieved. Misplacement of the catheter tip can be avoided by (1) radiographic localization using both posteroanterior (P–A) and lateral views and (2) recording at least two ECG leads. Exclusive reliance on the posteroanterior view is to be discouraged since the catheter tip may appear to be located in the right ventricular apex on the P–A film when it actually lies in the middle cardiac vein, as can be seen in a lateral view (Fig. 11–16). To have arrived at that location, the electrode catheter had to have been passed through the coronary sinus.

The position of the pacing catheter can be determined by the QRS pattern produced by the stimulus artifacts (Fig. 11–17). Right chest lead V_1 is the best single lead to determine whether the impulse is produced by an electrode located within the right ventricular cavity or in the coronary sinus or great and middle cardiac vein.[41] The superior or inferior location of the stimulating electrode is determined by the inferior or superior

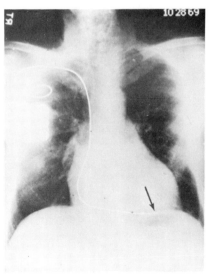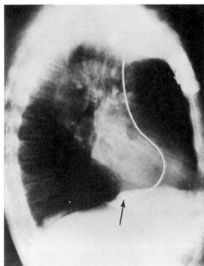

Figure 11–16.   The posteroanterior view on the left shows the catheter tip position to be in the area of the right ventricular apex. However, the lateral view on the right indicates the true position of the catheter tip, in the inferior and posterior region of the cardiac shadow—probably in the middle cardiac vein

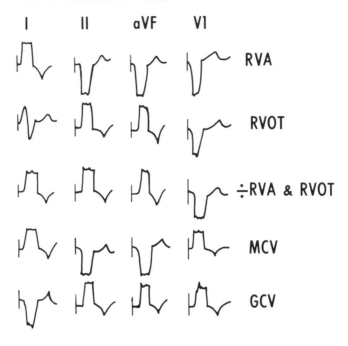

Figure 11–17.   QRS patterns produced by pacing from different ventricular sites. RVA = right ventricular apex; RVOT = right ventricular outflow tract; ÷ = between; GCV = great cardiac vein; MCV = middle cardiac vein. Right chest lead V₁ is the best single lead to determine whether the catheter electrodes induce beats arising in the right ventricular cavity (top three rows) or at the epicardial left posterior wall (bottom two rows) stimulated through the corresponding veins (GCV and MCV) entering the coronary sinus. On the other hand, the direction of the electrical axis as deterrmined from leads I, II, and aVF is a function of the caudal (first and fourth rows), cephalic (second and fifth rows) or intermediate (third row) location of the catheters.

orientation of the frontal plane electrical axis of QRS as determined from leads I, II, and aVF.[42]

Displacement of the Electrode Tip and Perforation of the Electrode Catheter Tip into the Pericardial Space.

Those complications of permanent transvenous pacing are infrequent. Loss of pacemaker capture, either intermittent or permanent, during the normal life of the pacemaker battery should alert the physican to those possible complications. Pericardial irritation or diaphragmatic stimulation may occur because of perforation of the catheter tip into the pericardial space.

SUMMARY

1. Pacemaker implantation was initially used for the treatment of complete AV block resulting from chronic conduction system disease, but at present the most common indication for pacing is the sick sinus syndrome.

2. Since experience has been gained in coronary care units, basic principles have been established that serve as guidelines for the treatment of AV block following acute myocardial infarction. Since very few patients develop chronic AV block as a result of acute myocardial infarction, the need for permanent pacing in that condition is not too common.

3. Permanent pacing is indicated primarily for complete AV block associated with anterior wall myocardial infarction, *not* with diaphragmatic myocardial infarction.

4. Artificial pacing has been established as useful for the management of reciprocating tachycardias, which may be initiated and perpetuated by a variety of mechanisms. Effective pacemaker therapy must be based on an understanding of the electrophysiologic aspects of reciprocating tachycardia. Those aspects were discussed in detail in this chapter.

5. The sophisticated use of pacemakers must be based on the knowledge of the various types of pacing modes. Such knowledge permits the physician to select the mode of pacing best suited to each patient. Various types of artificial pacemakers were described in detail in this chapter.

6. Familiarity with the complications of pacemakers is vital for those who treat patients with artificial pacemakers. ECG criteria have been established that allow precise location of the tip of the pacemaker electrode catheter; malposition of transvenous pacemaker catheters can be responsible for pacemaker failures. Radiographic localization requires two views, the posteroanterior and the lateral. Reliance on the posteroanterior view alone is unacceptable.

REFERENCES

1. Hyman, A.S.: Resuscitation of the stopped heart by intracardiac therapy: Further use of the artificial pacemaker. J.A.M.A. 99:1888, 1932.
2. Callaghan, J.C., and Bigelow, W.G.: An electrical artificial pacemaker for standstill of the heart. Ann. Surg. 134:8, 1951.
3. Zoll, P.M.: Resuscitation of the heart in ventricular standstill by external electric stimulation. N. Engl. J. Med. 247:768, 1952.
4. Weirich, W.L., Gott, V.L., and Lillehei, C.W.: Treatment of complete heart block by combined use of myocardial electrode and an artificial pacemaker. Surg. Forum 8:360, 1957.
5. Chardack, W.M., Gage, A.A., and Greatbatch, W.: A transistorized self-contained, implantable pacemaker for the long-term correction of complete heart block. Surgery 48:643, 1960.

6. Zoll, P.M.: Development of electrical control of cardiac rhythm. J.A.M.A. 266:881, 1973.
7. Rosenbaum, M.B., Elizari, M.V., and Lazzari, J.O.: The Hemiblocks. Oldsmar, Fla., Tampa Tracings, 1970. P. 107.
8. DeSanctis, R.W.: Sick sinus syndrome. ACCEL 6 (No. 1): 1974.
9. Narula, O.S.: Advances in clinical electrophysiology: Contribution of His bundle recordings. In P. Samet (ed.), Cardiac Pacing. New York, Grune & Stratton, 1973.
10. Jordan, J.L., Yamaguchi, I., and Mandel, W.J.: The sick sinus syndrome: Pathophysiology, significance, and treatment. Cardiol. Digest 12:11, 1977.
11. Narula, O.S.: Sick sinus syndrome. Part I. Primary Cardiol. 4 (No. 1): 27, 1978.
12. Narula, O.S.: Sick sinus syndrome. Part II. Primary Cardiol. 4 (No. 2): 12, 1978.
13. Castellanos, A., Jr., Berkovits, B.V., Castillo, C.A., and Befeler, B.: Sextapolar catheter electrode for temporary sequential atrioventricular pacing. Cardiovasc. Res. 8:712, 1974.
14. Haft, J.I.: Treatment of arrhythmias by intracardiac electrical stimulation. Prog. Cardiovasc. Dis. 16:539, 1974.
15. Langendorf, R., and Mehlman, J.S.: Blocked (non-conducted) A–V nodal premature systoles imitating first and second degree A–V block. Am. Heart J. 34:500, 1947.
16. Castellanos, A., Befeler, B., and Myerburg, R.J.: Pseudo A–V block produced by concealed extrasystoles arising below the bifurcation of the His bundle. Br. Heart J. 36:457, 1974.
17. Rosenbaum, M.B., Elizari, M.V., and Lazzari, J.O.: Los Hemibloqueos. Buenos Aires, Paidos, 1968. P. 19.
18. Corrado, G., Levi, R.J., Nau, G.J., and Rosenbaum, M.B.: Paroxysmal atrioventricular block related to phase 4 bilateral bundle branch block. Am. J. Cardiol. 33:553, 1974.
19. Lemberg, L., Castellanos, A., Jr., and Arcebal, A.G.: The treatment of arrhythmias following acute myocardial infarction. Med. Clin. North Am. 55:273, 1971.
20. Lemberg, L., Arcebal, A.G., Castellanos, A., Jr., and Claxton, B.W.: Cardiac drugs in the coronary care unit. Chest 59:289, 1971.
21. Atkins, J.M., Leshin, S.J., Blomquist, G., and Mullins, C.B.: Ventricular conduction blocks and sudden death in acute myocardial infarction. N. Engl. J. Med. 288:281, 1973.
22. Castellanos, A., Jr., and Myerburg, R.J.: Repetitive supraventricular tachycardias in context. Am. Heart J. 90:131, 1975.
23. Lemberg, L., Castellanos, A., Jr., and Berkovits, B.V.: Pacemaking on demand in A–V block. J.A.M.A. 191:12, 1965.
24. Castellanos, A., Jr., and Lemberg, L.: Pacemaker arrhythmias and electrocardiographic recognition of pacemakers. Circulation 47:1382, 1973.
25. Castellanos, A., Jr., and Lemberg, L.: Electrophysiology of Pacing and Cardioversion. New York, Appleton-Century-Crofts, 1969.
26. Spitzer, R.C., Donoso, E., Gadboys, H.L., and Friedberg, C.K.: Arrhythmias induced by pacing on demand. Am. Heart J. 77:619, 1969.
27. Kastor, J.A., Berkovits, B.V., and DeSanctis, R.: Variations in discharge rate of demand pacemakers not due to malfunction. Am. J. Cardiol. 25:344, 1970.
28. Medtronic, Chardac: Model 5943 implantable unipolar demand pulse generator. Minneapolis, Medtronic, Inc., 1971.
29. Barold, S.S., and Gaidula, J.J.: Evaluation of normal and abnormal sensing functions of demand pacemakers. Am. J. Cardiol. 28:201, 1971.
30. Barold, S.S., and Gaidula, J.J.: Failure of demand pacemaker from low voltage bipolar electrogram. J.A.M.A. 215:923, 1971.
31. Barold, S.S., Gaidula, J.J., Lyon, J.L., and Carbol, M.: Irregular recycling of demand pacemaker from borderline electrographic signals. Am. Heart J. 87:477, 1971.
32. Barold, S.S., Pupillo, G.A., Gaidula, J.J., and Linhart, J.W.: Chest wall stimulation in evaluation of patients with inplantable ventricular-inhibited pacemakers. Br. Heart J. 32:783, 1970.
33. Silverman, L.F., Mankin, H.T., and McGoon, D.C.: Surgical treatment of an inadequate sinus mechanism by implantation of a right atrial pacemaker electrode. J. Thorac. Cardiovasc. Surg. 55:264, 1968.

34. Harris, P.D., Malm, J.R., Bowman, F.O., et al.: Epicardial pacing to control arrhythmias following cardiac surgery. Circulation 37 (Suppl. II): 178, 1968.
35. Kastor, J.A., DeSanctis, R.W., Leinbach, R.L., et al.: Long-term pervenous atrial pacing. Circulation 40:535, 1969.
36. Lister, J.W., Cohen, L.S., Hildner, F.J., et al.: Electrical stimulation of the atria in patients with an intact conduction system. Ann. N.Y. Acad. Sci. 167:785, 1969.
37. DeSanctis, R.W.: Diagnostic and therapeutic uses of atrial pacing. Circulation 43:748, 1971.
38. Kramer, D.H., and Moss, A.J.: Permanent pervenous atrial pacing from the coronary vein. Circulation 42:427, 1970.
39. Nathan, D.A., Lister, J.W., Castillo, R., et al.: Current status of atrial pacing. Ann. Cardiol. Angeiol. 20:451, 1971.
40. Siddons, H.: Long-term sequential and atrial ventricular pacing. Ann. Cardiol. Angeiol. 40:431, 1971.
41. Castillo, C.A., Berkovits, B.V., Castellanos, A., Jr., et al.: Bifocal demand pacing. Chest 59:360, 1971.
42. Castellanos, A., Jr., and Lemberg, L.: A Programmed Introduction to the Electrical Axis and Action Potential. Oldsmar, Fla., Tampa Tracings, 1974.

Chapter 12

CARDIOPULMONARY RESUSCITATION

PAUL WALINSKY
EDWARD K. CHUNG

GENERAL CONSIDERATIONS

Sudden and unexpected cessation of effective cardiopulmonary performance is a cardiac emergency that requires immediate recognition and proper management. Rapid and effective institution of measures to maintain the delivery of oxygen to vital organs and to reverse the initiating pathophysiologic derangements is essential. Although the techniques for sustaining critical tissues and returning cardiac performance to a level adequate to sustain life are now universally practiced, they have been generally accepted and practiced only within the past 20 years.[1] Before that time, cardiac resuscitation was performed, if at all, primarily by thoracotomy with open-chest cardiac massage. The demonstration by Kouwenhoven and his co-workers in 1960 of the effectiveness of closed-chest cardiac massage freed cardiac resuscitation from the requirement of proximity to trained surgical hands and made it possible for all appropriately trained physicians and paramedical personnel to successfully perform cardiac resuscitation.[2] Even before the demonstration of the efficacy of closed-chest cardiac massage, the development of an external alternating current cardiac defibrillator capable of reverting ventricular fibrillation to a normal sinus rhythm was reported by Zoll and his co-workers.[3] Since then, the direct current defibrillator has been demonstrated to be the preferred mode of cardiac defibrillation[4] (Chapter 10).

Appropriate use of those modalities has saved countless lives. Perhaps the most important factor (aside from those related to the underlying cause) in determining the outcome of a sudden cardiac catastrophe is the presence of personnel skilled in cardiac resuscitation. Every physician, regardless of his subspecialty or interest, should make the acquisition and maintenance of cardiac resuscitation skills an essential part of his training and practice. Were all medical and paramedical personnel so trained in cardiac resuscitation, even more people could be successfully resuscitated.

ETIOLOGY OF THE CESSATION OF CARDIAC PERFORMANCE

The primary causes of sudden and unexpected cessation of effective cardiac performance and cessation of spontaneous respiratory activity may be neurologic, pulmonary, or cardiovascular disorders. Table 12–1 lists the findings of Johnson and his co-workers,[5] who evaluated the causes of cardiovascular collapse in a review of 552 patients for whom cardiopulmonary resuscitation (CPR) was attempted. Similar distributions of causes have been reported by others.

The likelihood of recovery is determined by the underlying primary pathophysiologic derangements and by how rapidly effective CPR is instituted. Although cardiovascular stability may be achieved following anatomic damage, the phenomena most likely to be reversible are those associated with abnormal cardiac electrical events (cardiac arrhythmias). When it can be determined, the nature of the cardiac arrhythmia causing cardiopulmonary collapse is found to be either a tachyarrhythmia (usually

Table 12–1. *Etiology of Cardiovascular Collapse*

Causative Factor	Number of Patients
Coronary artery disease	239
Respiratory failure	55
Pulmonary embolism	18
Stokes-Adams syndrome	11
Cardiomyopathy	7
Uremia	32
Reaction to angiography	6
Miscellaneous	184
Total	552

Source: Johnson et al.[5]

ectopic) or a bradyarrhythmia, ventricular tachycardia or fibrillation being the most common tachyarrhythmia and ventricular standstill the most common bradyarrhythmia. It is possible, but less common, for a rapid supraventricular tachyarrhythmia to cause cardiovascular collapse; likewise, a severe degree of bradyarrhythmia of various potential mechanisms may result in cardiovascular collapse.

The inciting cardiac arrhythmia may have disparate causes. Recent experience with cardiac care units has demonstrated a high incidence of such arrhythmia related to acute myocardial infarction or ischemia[6] (Chapter 5). However, catastrophic arrhythmia may develop de novo or in the presence of chronic but self-limited arrhythmia. Thus chronic ventricular ectopic beats may be observed before the development of ventricular tachycardia or fibrillation and may be related to myocardial fibrosis, cardiomyopathy, mitral valve prolapse syndrome, electrolyte disturbance, or drug intoxication, particularly digitalis intoxication (Chapter 16).

INDICATIONS

CPR should be instituted immediately on recognition of the sudden cessation of effective cardiopulmonary performance. The following will be manifested on loss of cardiopulmonary performance:

1. Loss of consciousness
2. Loss of carotid and femoral pulses
3. Loss of respiration
4. Loss of heart tones
5. Loss of blood pressure

Unless cardiac monitoring is continuous, there may be delays in recognizing the arrest of cardiopulmonary function. Thus in a cardiac or intensive care unit (Chapters 5 and 6), where continuous monitoring is available, the need for CPR should be immediately recognized. In a general hospital ward, the recognition of cardiovascular collapse depends on the presence of medical personnel, who may be alerted by hospital personnel or visitors. In that setting, the recognition of cardiovascular catastrophe may be delayed because there was no observer. Outside the hospital even more critical delays are likely to be encountered before adequate resuscitative measures are initiated (Chapter 4).

ORGANIZATION

Cardiopulmonary resuscitation can be performed by one person, but it is best performed by a team. In the hospital, where a team is likely to be present, there must be a plan so that the people needed for CPR can be immediately summoned to the scene. The members of the team should be assigned clearly defined duties. The following is a suggested plan of organization.

1. Senior physician. Assumes overall responsibility for the resuscitative efforts and directs all necessary procedures and drug therapy.

2. Junior physician or nurse. Performs closed-chest cardiac resuscitation and artificial ventilation.

3. Junior physician. Starts the intravenous line.

4. Nurse. Has access to and prepares the required drugs, administers intravenous medications, and monitors cardiac rhythm and blood pressure.

5. Laboratory technician. Is available for performing required laboratory procedures.

CANDIDATES

For whom should CPR be performed? The question can be a difficult one—and one not readily answered by strict categorization because different philosophical views can be involved. For patients with an incurable or a terminal disease, such as terminal cancer, and for patients with severe neurologic disturbances, particularly those involving loss of higher cortical function, CPR would seem to be inappropriate. CPR should be aimed primarily at the patient in whom restoration of cardiopulmonary stability will result in a potential for continued productive life and not in a perpetuation of preterminal agony or a vegetative existence. In the hospital setting, if there is sufficient reason not to resuscitate a patient, that fact should be clearly indicated as part of the orders in the patient's chart in order to prevent possible medicolegal problems and to avoid unnecessary CPR. It is also important to discuss the nature of the disease with the patient's family in detail so that there will be no misunderstanding about the indication (or non-indication for CPR) for the patient. However, if the medical status of a patient is not known before cardiopulmonary collapse, it is mandatory to proceed with CPR without hesitation.

INITIAL MEASURES AND TECHNIQUES

The goals of initial emergency measures for CPR are to maintain ventilation of the lungs and to deliver adequate amounts of oxygenated blood to tissues. The initial measures have been described as the ABCs of therapy:[7] A = Clearing the airway, B = Instituting breathing, C = Restoring circulation.

It has been reported that a direct blow to the sternum can revert ventricular fibrillation, ventricular tachycardia, and asystole to normal sinus rhythm. It is thus appropriate to attempt that maneuver first; it should take only 1 to 2 seconds.[8-10] A forceful blow should be delivered to the sternum with the heel of the hand. It may be repeated once or twice if there is no response. If the maneuver is not successful, one should immediately proceed to measures required to support life, as follows.

A = Clear the Airway

Place the patient in a supine position (Fig. 12–1). Place one hand behind the neck and the other on the forehead. Tilt the head back; that maneuver lifts the tongue from the back of the throat and results in an intrinsically unobstructed airway. At the same time, remove any obvious foreign body or obstructions in the mouth or nasal passages. Those maneuvers alone may lead to a restoration of breathing and to recovery.

B = Institute Ventilation

Mouth-to-Mouth Technique. Maintain the backward tilt of the head with one hand (Fig. 12–2). Pinch the nostrils closed with the other hand. Place the mouth over the patient's mouth, completely sealing the patient's mouth, so that there is no leak of air. At the end of inspiration, exhale a larger than normal breath into the patient's mouth. If the procedure is performed correctly, a rise should be noted in the patient's chest as the intrathoracic volume is increased. There should be no loss of air through

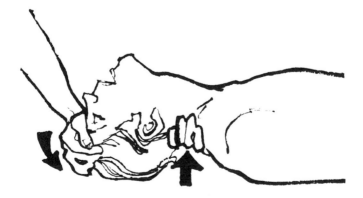

Figure 12–1.   Head-tilt method of opening the airway. (Reprinted with permission from the *Journal of the American Medical Association*.)

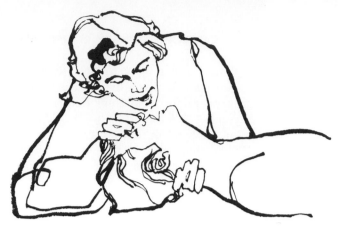

Figure 12–2. Mouth-to-mouth resuscitation. (Reprinted with permission from the *Journal of the American Medical Association*.)

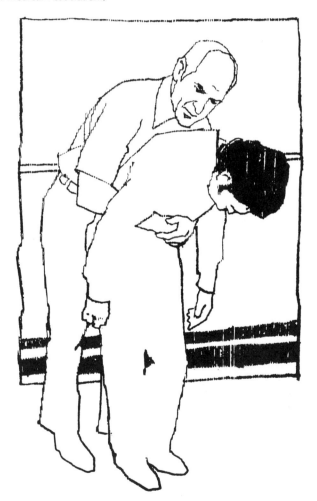

Figure 12–3. Application of the Heimlich maneuver with the patient upright. (Reprinted with permission from the *Journal of the American Medical Association*.)

the nose or mouth as the lungs are inflated. After inflation of the lungs, remove your mouth from the patient's mouth, allowing his lungs to deflate. Air should be heard escaping from the lungs during that period.

Mouth-to-Nose Technique. Maintain the backward head tilt with one hand. Close the patient's jaw and seal his mouth with your hand. Place your mouth over the patient's nose, and after inhaling deeply, again exhale through the patient's nose. The indications for a successful maneuver are the same as those described for mouth-to-mouth techniques. Perform ventilation at a rate of 12 per minute whichever technique of ventilation is used.

Problems with Ventilation. If there is resistance to inflation of the lungs, suspect a foreign body in the airway. Roll the patient onto his side and deliver a firm blow between the shoulder blades in an attempt to dislodge the foreign body. The patient's mouth and oropharynx should then be explored for a foreign body. Another maneuver that has recently been popularized for the removal of a foreign body is the Heimlich maneuver.[11] The patient can be either upright or supine (Figs. 12–3 and 12–4). If the

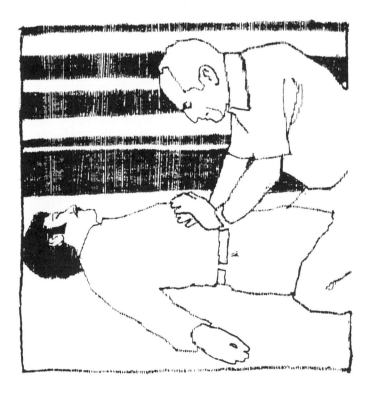

Figure 12–4.   Application of the Heimlich maneuver with the patient supine. (Reprinted with permission from the *Journal of the American Medical Association*.)

patient is upright, grasp him from behind, below the rib cage, with your fist against his abdomen. If the patient is supine, place your hands one on top of the other on the patient's abdomen, between the rib cage and the navel. In both cases the hand is thrust quickly into the patient's abdomen. The thrust increases the pressure within the large airway, and thus "pops" out the foreign body.

Vomiting may occur during CPR. Adequately functioning suction equipment should be readily available for that emergency. Gastric distention is best managed by inserting an indwelling nasogastric tube. If such a tube is not available, gastric distention may be corrected by pressing over the epigastrium. Recurrence of gastric distention may be prevented by intermittent epigastric pressure. Caution should be exercised with that maneuver since reflux of gastric contents may be induced.

The first two steps of CPR aim to institute ventilation. The procedures may be performed in any setting, even by a single person. In the hospital setting, where more help and more facilities may be available, there may be some modifications, but the basic approach is the same. In the hospital, a bag-and-mask technique may be used instead of either of the expired-air techniques. The prime advantages of that technique are that oxygen may be added to the intake and that some physicians find it is esthetically less distressing.

C = Restore Circulation

The final step of the initial resuscitative measures is the institution of cardiac massage. Except when the patient is already in the operating room or when chest wounds preclude open-chest massage, there is virtually no situation in which one would not perform closed-chest cardiac massage rather than open-chest massage.

Closed-Chest Cardiac Massage. 1. Position. The patient's back must be on a firm surface. Place hard board under the patient's back if he is on a soft surface, such as a bed. Position yourself alongside the patient. Place the heel of one hand over the lower third of the patient's sternum (but not on the xyphoid process). Your hand should not be in touch with the patient's chest, except for the heel of the hand. The other hand may rest on the first hand (Fig. 12–5).

2. Compression. Depress the patient's chest 1.5 to 2 inches (approximately one-fifth of the anterior-posterior thickness). The pressure should be smooth and uninterrupted. Following compression, release the sternum and ready the hand for the next compression. The duration of chest compression should approximate the duration of relaxation.

3. Rate. Compress the chest approximately 60 times per minute. Cardiac compression should be coordinated with ventilation. If only one

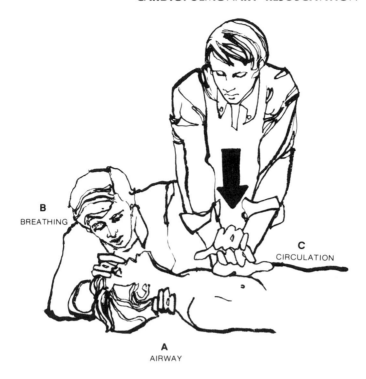

B
BREATHING

C
CIRCULATION

A
AIRWAY

Figure 12–5. Two-rescuer cardiopulmonary resuscitation. (Reprinted with permission from the *Journal of the American Medical Association.*)

resuscitator is present, it is recommended that 15 chest compressions be performed followed by two quick lung ventilations. If two or more resuscitators are present, every fifth chest compression should be followed by a lung inflation.

4. Pulse. Although it is not an ideal way to measure the efficiency of closed-chest cardiac massage, palpation of peripheral pulses during chest compression may provide a rough guideline. If an indwelling arterial line is present, the contour of the pressure pulse obtained may be of value in assessing the efficiency of cardiac compression.

Complications of Cardiac Massage. Although cardiac massage is a safe procedure, one must not be overly vigorous in sternal compression, particularly in children (Chapter 17). Reported complications, primarily those caused by inappropriate application of cardiac massage techniques, include fractures of the ribs and sternum, hemothorax, hemopericardium, pneumothorax, bone marrow emboli, gastric rupture, lacerations of the spleen and liver, and rupture of the aorta.[12]

Mechanical Devices. A number of mechanical devices, some manual and some automatic, are available for closed-chest cardiac massage. In the hands of trained persons, they may make cardiac massage easier and facilitate resuscitative efforts. But they should never be used by inexperienced personnel. Misapplication of those devices may result in not only ineffective resuscitation but also further injury to the patient.

EVALUATION OF SUCCESS

During the emergency measures, one must check for the presence or absence of several signs that indicate the success or failure of your efforts. Those signs are essentially those that were initially affected in cardiovascular collapse:

1. Pulses in the femoral or carotid arteries
2. Heart tones
3. Spontaneous respiratory efforts
4. Palpable or recordable blood pressure

One should also be alert to any change in the patient's neurologic status.

If there is evidence that the resuscitative efforts have been successful, one may stop and observe the patient for several seconds. If a reversal of cardiovascular collapse has been achieved, the patient should continue to be observed closely, and the cause of the collapse should be determined. If, however, there is no change in the patient's status, artificial ventilation and cardiac massage must be continued while further, more sophisticated, diagnostic and therapeutic approaches are sought. During that period, cardiac massage and ventilation must be continuous, and they should not be halted for longer than five seconds.

SECONDARY MEASURES

If there is no response to the initial resuscitative measures, perform the following measures while artificial support is continued:

1. Quickly review the chart (if you are not familiar with the patient's condition) to extract any relevant information.

2. Obtain an ECG to assess cardiac rhythm and to evaluate the possibility of abnormalities, including acute myocardial infarction, pulmonary embolism, electrolyte imbalance, and digitalis intoxication (Chapters 2, 3, 5, and 16).

3. Obtain an arterial blood gas analysis to assess the acid-base balance and the adequacy of ventilation.

4. Obtain a venous or arterial blood sample for the determination of serum electrolytes.

5. If an intravenous infusion site is not already available, one should be established.

When those steps have been taken, further therapeutic intervention may be instituted. Determination of cardiac rhythm is based on either a conventional 12-lead ECG or an oscilloscopic monitored ECG tracing. The treatment of the various cardiac arrhythmias is described in the following paragraphs (see also Chapters 7 and 8).

Treatment of Ventricular Fibrillation

Ventricular fibrillation should be treated as follows:

1. Attempt electrical cardioversion with a direct current defibrillator at 400 Wsec. If successful in restoring sinus rhythm, institute intravenous lidocaine (Xylocaine; Table 12–2). If a cardiac rhythm other than sinus rhythm ensues, institute appropriate therapy.

2. If direct current cardioversion is unsuccessful initially, repeat the procedure.

If coarse ventricular fibrillatory waves are present, administer lidocaine, 1 mg/kg in an intravenous bolus, and start an infusion of 4 mg/min. Repeat direct current cardioversion at 400 Wsec.

If fine ventricular fibrillatory waves are present, attempt to induce coarser, higher-amplitude waves by administering epinephrine (0.2 to 1 cc of a 1:1000 dilution, i.e., 200 to 1000 μg) intravenously or by intracardiac injection. Calcium chloride, 10 cc administered intravenously or by intracardiac injection, may have a similar effect on the fibrillatory waves.

Table 12–2. *Drugs Commonly Used in Cardiopulmonary Resuscitation*

Indication	Drug	Dosage
Asystole	Isoproterenol	200 mg–1000 mg IV or IC infusion of 2–12 mg/min
	Epinephrine	200 mg–1000 mg IV or IC infusion of 2–12 mg/min
	Calcium chloride	10 ml (10% solution) IV to a total of 30 ml
Bradycardia	Atropine	0.3–1.2 mg IV bolus
	Isoproterenol	IV infusion of 2–6 mg/min
Ventricular tachycardia/fibrillation	Lidocaine	50–100 mg bolus to a total of less than or equal to 300 mg IV infusion 2–4 mg/min
	Pronestyl	100-mg bolus to a total of less than 1000 mg IV infusion of 2–4 mg/min
	Dilantin	100 mg over 5 minutes Repeated to a total of less than 500 mg
	Propranolol	1 mg IV q 5–10 min to a total of 5–10 mg

Following the development of high-amplitude fibrillatory waves, electrical cardioversion should be repeated.

If ventricular fibrillation cannot be terminated, assess metabolic factors, such as acidosis or hypoxia. Those factors may make cardioversion difficult.

Treatment of Ventricular Tachycardia

1. Quickly assess the patient's stability. If ventricular tachycardia results in significant hypotension or congestive heart failure (Chapters 1 and 3), immediate direct current cardioversion should be performed as just described. Following the restoration of sinus rhythm, intravenous lidocaine should be administered as just described.

2. If the patient is hemodynamically stable, initiate pharmacologic cardioversion.

a. The drug of choice is lidocaine. It should be given as just described for ventricular fibrillation. If ventricular tachycardia persists or recurs, give repeated boluses of 100 mg, up to a total of 300 to 400 mg.

b. If ventricular tachycardia is refractory to lidocaine, administer procainamide (Pronestyl) in intravenous boluses of 100 mg given slowly. Boluses of 100 mg may be administered every five minutes, up to a total of 1000 mg or until hypotension or successful cardioversion occurs. A procainamide drip of 2 to 4 mg/min may likewise be instituted if ventricular irritability persists.

c. Other drugs that may be effective for persistent ventricular tachycardia include quinidine and propranolol (Inderal). Diphenylhydantoin (Dilantin) is the drug of choice for digitalis-induced ventricular tachycardia (Chapter 16).

3. If pharmacologic conversion is unsuccessful or if recurrent bouts of ventricular tachycardia occur, artificial pacing with an overdriving rate and in an atrial or a ventricular mode should be considered (Chapter 11).

Treatment of Supraventricular Tachyarrhythmias

In elderly patients with an underlying impairment of cardiovascular performance, rapid supraventricular tachyarrhythmias may cause profound hypotension and cardiovascular collapse. If a profound degree of cardiovascular decompensation is caused by a supraventricular tachyarrhythmia, direct current cardioversion is appropriate. But if in the presence of such an arrhythmia the patient has no evidence of a lack of organ perfusion, no significant neurologic change, and an adequate blood pressure, one may use appropriate drugs that may require a modest period of time to take effect.

Treatment of Bradyarrhythmias

Mild-to-Moderate Sinus Bradycardia (More than 40 Beats per Minute). As an isolated phenomenon, mild-to-moderate sinus bradycardia unaccompanied by other cardiovascular abnormalities may not require treatment. On the other hand if there is associated hypotension, atropine, 0.3 to 1 mg, may be administered intravenously. Administration of a volume load may be of value if hypotension persists.

Severe Sinus Bradycardia (Less than 40 Beats per Minute) or Second-Degree or Advanced AV Block. The clinical setting dictates the therapeutic approach. If increased vagal tone seems to play a role in the genesis of the bradyarrhythmias—as it does in patients with acute diaphragmatic (inferior wall) myocardial infarction—the administration of atropine would be of value in increasing the heart rate. Administer atropine as a bolus of 0.4 mg intravenously. If the heart rate does not increase within three minutes, administer additional boluses of 0.3 mg every 3 minutes to a total of 1 mg. If there is no response to atropine, proceed as with complete AV block.

When marked and persisting sinus bradycardia is refractory to atropine and/or isoproterenol (Isuprel), the presence of the sick sinus syndrome should be strongly considered (Chapter 9).

The use of an artificial pacemaker is mandatory in Mobitz type II AV block.

Intraventricular Block. Prophylactic artificial pacing is recommended for all patients who develop acute left bundle branch block, left posterior hemiblock, or bifascicular block (a combination of right bundle branch block and left anterior or posterior hemiblock) with or without coexisting AV block as a result of acute anterior wall myocardial infarction (Chapter 11).

Complete AV Block. Start an intravenous infusion of isoproterenol of 2 to 4 μg/min. If the ventricular rate is slow, a 100-μg bolus of isoproterenol may be given intravenously while the infusion is continued.

If there is no response to isoproterenol, an epinephrine 100-μg bolus and an infusion of 2 to 4 μg/min may be effective.

If despite the measures just described the bradycardia is not reversed, insertion of a transvenous pacemaker is indicated (Chapter 11).

When complete AV block is found to be chronic, especially when the block is considered to be in the infranodal region (complete trifascicular block), permanent implantation of an artificial pacemaker is indicated (Chapter 11).

Asystole. Administer epinephrine (Adrenalin) or isoproterenol as a 200 to 1000-μg bolus intravenously or by intracardiac injection. Calcium chloride may have a synergistic chronotropic effect. Calcium chloride should likewise be administered intravenously or by intracardiac injection. If the patient has been treated with propranolol and is likely to have continuing beta-blockade, intravenous injection of 10 mg of glucagon may also be effective. If it is technically and logistically feasible to insert an artificial pacemaker, that also should be done.

Hemodynamic Status

When a stable cardiac rhythm is restored, attention must be directed toward the adequacy of perfusion. Significant depression of cardiac performance may occur during the period of resuscitation as well as from the underlying cause of the cardiovascular collapse. A long-term approach to insuring adequacy of cardiac performance must be formulated, based on the underlying primary problems. The short-term approach to maintaining cardiac performance may include the use of a variety of inotropic drugs, including isoproterenol, epinephrine, norepinephrine, dopamine, metaraminol, calcium chloride, and glucagon.

OTHER MEASURES

Ventilation

If continued resuscitative efforts are required following the institution of artificial ventilation, consideration should be given to the insertion of an endotracheal or nasotracheal tube. Such a tube permits more effective pulmonary expansion, the administration of oxygen in high concentration, and the removal of secretions or vomitus from the bronchi by suction. Although such an airway is desirable, it should be inserted only by someone who can do so quickly and adequately. It should not be inserted by a novice, whose fumbling efforts may stop resuscitation for a prolonged period. Following the insertion of a tracheal airway, the cuff should be inflated to prevent any further aspiration of vomitus. Manual control of ventilation coordinated with cardiac massage should continue. Self-triggering ventilators should not be used unless they are fully coordinated with cardiac massage. The adequacy of ventilation should be determined by serial assessments of the arterial blood gases.

Treatment of Acidosis

Metabolic acidosis is a result of inadequate tissue perfusion and oxygenation. Respiratory acidosis occurs if there is significant underlying pulmonary disease, airway obstruction, or inadequate artificial ventilation. If resuscitative efforts are initiated without delay, there may be only minimal metabolic acidosis. The best way to assess the need for bicarbonate replacement is to sample arterial blood to determine the pH, HCO_3^-, PCO_2, and PO_2. Acidosis with an elevated PCO_2 and a normal or slightly decreased HCO_3^- indicates respiratory acidosis. In such a case, bicarbonate replacement will not be of major value, and more effective ventilation is required.[13] But if acidosis is accompanied by a normal PCO_2 and a decrease in bicarbonate metabolic acidosis is present, bicarbonate should be administered with serial assessments of the arterial blood gases to evaluate the efficacy of the treatment and continuing needs. If arterial blood gas values cannot be determined, it is difficult to assess the need for bicarbonate. Several regimens are prescribed in the literature as guides to bicarbonate therapy.[14,15] Sodium bicarbonate should be given if the arrest is longer than one minute. The initial amount is 100 cc (89.2 mEq) of $NaHCO_3$ followed by 50 cc of $NaHCO_3$ every 10 minutes. It is important to correct acidosis because it decreases cardiac and peripheral responses to catecholamines, lowers the threshold of ventricular fibrillation, and may induce cardiac asystole.

Treatment of Electrolyte Imbalance

Significant derangements of serum electrolytes may lead to various cardiac arrhythmias. Either hyperkalemia or hypokalemia may cause various cardiac arrhythmias, including ventricular irritability. In particular, hypokalemia frequently predisposes to digitalis-induced cardiac arrhythmias (Chapter 16). Serum electrolyte values should be determined, and appropriate replacement therapy is essential.

TERMINATION OF CARDIOPULMONARY RESUSCITATION

There are two major reasons to terminate CPR. The first reason is failure to restore an appropriate cardiac rhythm and adequate pump performance. The second reason is evidence of severe and irreversible cerebral damage. CPR should be continued until all the methods of restoring cardiopulmonary stability have been tried. If at that point the heart appears to be unable to maintain an adequate cardiac rhythm and mechanical performance, CPR should be terminated.

Determination of the severity of the neurologic damage is often difficult (and it can have medicolegal ramifications). Severe neurologic damage is suggested by unconsciousness, lack of spontaneous movement, lack of spontaneous respiration, pupillary dilatation without response to light, and "boxcarring" of the retinal vessels. Although those are not absolute signs of permanent neurologic impairment, they suggest severe, potentially irreversible, damage and they point toward termination of CPR.

CARE AFTER CARDIOPULMONARY RESUSCITATION

Following successful CPR, assessment of the initial cause and recognition of any persistent risk factors are essential. If any premonitory abnormalities of cardiac rhythm are present, they should be treated prophylactically (Chapters 7 and 8). If there is evidence of acute myocardial infarction, assessment of the patient's hemodynamic status and cardiac rhythm should be continued in a cardiac care unit (Chapter 5). If there is evidence of pulmonary insufficiency, careful attention should be directed to assuring adequacy of ventilation by monitoring the blood gases. If pulmonary embolism is suspected, the patient must be given anticoagulation therapy with heparin (Chapter 2).

A complete assessment of the degree of recovery should be part of post–CPR care. Particular attention should be directed to the patient's neurologic status. If cerebral edema is suspected, intravenous dexamethasone should be given, 10 mg initially and 4 mg every 12 hours for 3 to 6 days.

All patients who have been revived with CPR should be observed for several weeks to insure their stability. During that time, emergency resuscitative facilities should be immediately available.

RESULTS OF CARDIOPULMONARY RESUSCITATION

Many factors determine the success of CPR. The speed with which CPR is instituted and the underlying cause of the cardiopulmonary collapse are of major importance in determining ultimate recovery. The best survival rates seem to occur in coronary artery disease, cardiomyopathy, pulmonary embolism, and respiratory insufficiency. Although one would expect the best results to be noted in an intensive or coronary care unit (because of the constant attention given the patients), that has actually not been the case. Because only the sickest patients are in the intensive care unit, survival has been found to be as good (if not better) in a well-staffed medical ward, where patients are generally less acutely ill.

There is no universal agreement as to what cardiac rhythm disturbances are most amenable to CPR. However, most reviews of CPR results indicate that ventricular fibrillation is more amenable than asystole to reversion. Age and sex have not been found to be major determinants of success in CPR.

Survival figures vary from series to series, and they are difficult to compare because of different criteria of inclusion and different criteria of success.[16-19] However, a majority of studies have demonstrated that 4 to 15% of patients who undergo CPR are discharged from the hospital.

However, there are few long-term studies of CPR survivors once they have been discharged; also lacking is some assessment of the quality of the survivors' lives.

SUMMARY

1. Unexpected cardiopulmonary collapse is a medical emergency that requires immediate institution of artificial measures to support life and to reverse the initiating pathophysiologic event. To approach the problem efficiently, one must have a plan that can be implemented at a moment's notice.

2. The initial goals of CPR are to establish an airway, to institute artificial breathing, and to restore circulation. If those measures do not result in immediate recovery, assessment of cardiac rhythm, cardiac pump performance, ventilatory adequacy, acid-base balance, and serum electrolytes is required.

3. The primary therapeutic modalities are direct current defibrillation, intervention to restore normal sinus rhythm and normal blood pressure, and procedures to restore normal oxygenation and acid-base balance.

4. If CPR is successful, continued surveillance of the patient is required for complete assessment and for immediate intervention if cardiopulmonary collapse recurs.

5. Successful resuscitation, as defined by hospital discharge, has been reported in various series to occur in 4 to 15% of the patients who undergo CPR.

6. Every physician, nurse, and paramedical person should be capable of delivering CPR, regardless of his or her specialty.

7. Detailed descriptions of antiarrhythmic therapy, direct current shock, and artificial pacemakers are found in Chapters 7 to 11.

REFERENCES

1. Kouwenhoven, W.B.: The development of the defibrillator. Ann. Intern. Med. 71:449, 1969.
2. Kouwenhoven, W.B., Ing, J.J.R., and Knickerbocker, G.G.: Closed-chest cardiac massage. J.A.M.A. 173:94, 1960.
3. Zoll, P.M., Paul, M.H., Linenthal, A.J., et al.: The effects of external electrical currents on the heart. Circulation 14:745, 1956.
4. Lown, B., Neuman, J., Amarasingham, R., and Berkovits, B.V.: Comparison of alternating current with direct current electroshock across the closed chest. Am. J. Cardiol. 10:223, 1962.
5. Johnson, A.L., Tanser, P.H., Ulan, R.A., and Wood, T.E.: Results of cardiac resuscitation in 552 patients. Am. J. Cardiol. 20:831, 1967.
6. Pantridge, J.F., and Geddes, J.S.: A mobile intensive-care unit in the management of myocardial infarction. Lancet ii:271, 1967.
7. Standards for cardiopulmonary resuscitation (CPR) and emergency cardiac care (ECC). J.A.M.A. 227 (Suppl.).833, 1974.

8. Harwood-Nash, D.C.F.: Thumping of the precordium in ventricular fibrillation. S. Afr. Med. J. 36:280, 1962.
9. Pennington, J.E., Taylor, J., and Lown, B.: Chest thump for reverting ventricular tachycardia. N. Engl. J. Med. 283:1192, 1970.
10. Scharf, D., and Bonnemann, C.: Thumping of the precordium in ventricular standstill. Am. J. Cardiol. 5:30, 1960.
11. Heimlich, H.J.: A life-saving maneuver to prevent food-choking. J.A.M.A. 234:398, 1975.
12. Nelson, D., and Ashley, P.F.: Rupture of the aorta during closed-chest cardiac massage. J.A.M.A. 193:115, 1965.
13. Chazan, J.A., Stenson, R., and Kurland, G.S.: The acidosis of cardiac arrest. N. Engl. J. Med. 278:360, 1968.
14. Gilston, A., and Leeds, M.B.: Clinical and biochemical aspects of cardiac resuscitation. Lancet ii:1039, 1965.
15. Goldberg, A.H.: Cardiopulmonary arrest. N. Engl. J. Med. 290:381, 1974.
16. Hollingsworth, J.H.: The results of cardiopulmonary resuscitation. A 3-year university hospital experience. Ann. Intern. Med. 71:459, 1969.
17. Saphir, R.: External cardiac massage. Prospective analysis of 123 cases and review of the literature. Medicine 47:73, 1968.
18. Linko, E., Koskinen, P.J., Siitonen, L., and Ruosteenoja, R.: Resuscitation in cardiac arrest. An analysis of 100 successful medical cases. Acta Med. Scand. 182:611, 1967.
19. Wildsmith, J.A.W., Dennyson, W.G., and Myers, K.W.: Results of resuscitation following cardiac arrest. Br. J. Anaesthesiol. 44:716, 1972.

Chapter *13*

INFECTIOUS HEART DISEASE

ALBERT S. KLAINER

Infectious diseases involving the three basic anatomic compartments of the heart—the pericardium, the myocardium, and the endocardium—uncommonly present as acute emergencies that necessitate the immediate institution of therapy without affording the physician time to obtain the information required for an adequate presumptive or definitive diagnosis. Some of those diseases, such as acute bacterial endocarditis, demand urgent attention in that they need to be treated before the culture results are available. In contrast, more slowly progressive infections, such as subacute bacterial endocarditis, usually allow time to obtain specific bacteriologic information to aid the physician in making the correct diagnosis and choosing the proper therapy. Still others, such as viral infections, should not be treated because there are no effective drugs available. In other words, there is no parallel in infectious heart disease to the immediate urgency precipitated by such entities as the acute, potentially fatal arrhythmias (e.g., ventricular tachycardia or fibrillation). It is imperative, therefore, that any discussion of infectious heart disease be preceded by the admonition that the diagnostic and therapeutic approaches to infections involving the heart be taken in an orderly, rational manner based on clinical judgment and that therapy be instituted only when there is evidence to suggest that a treatable disease is present.

Infectious diseases involve the heart in two basic ways:

1. The pericardium, myocardium, and endocardium, together or separately, may be the site of primary infection or of infection resulting from bacteremia or contiguous spread from surrounding structures.

2. The heart may be affected by hemodynamic abnormalities resulting from extracardiac infection, especially septic shock.

In this chapter an attempt is made to provide the physician with a practical, orderly approach to the diagnosis and treatment of infections involving the heart, as well as of noncardiac infections that ultimately affect the heart through a variety of pathophysiologic events.

PERICARDITIS (See also Chapter 14)

Pericarditis is an inflammatory state involving the parietal and/or visceral pericardium, including the pericardial space. Diseases of the pericardium usually do not affect heart function unless tamponade or constriction develops to cause restriction of ventricular filling or unless cardiac arrhythmias occur.

Almost any infectious agent may cause pericarditis (Table 13–1); however, since a myriad of non-infectious diseases also may affect the pericardium, an accurate differential diagnosis is necessary if proper therapy is to be instituted.

In infectious pericarditis, involvement of the heart may occur via the blood or by contiguous spread of infection from neighboring structures, such as occurs in pneumonia or mediastinitis.

Signs and Symptoms

The signs and symptoms of pericarditis (Table 13–2) can be arbitrarily divided into those due to inflammation or infection, effusion, tamponade (if it occurs), and constriction.

Signs and Symptoms due to Inflammation and Infection per Se. Fever, a nonspecific response to infection or inflammation of non-infectious cause, is usually present, but it may be absent because (1) the process affecting

Table 13–1.   *Etiology of Pericarditis*

Infectious
  Bacterial
    Staphylococcus aureus
    Streptococcus pneumoniae
    Streptococcus pyogenes
    Neisseria meningitidis, Neisseria gonorrhoeae
    Hemophilus influenzae
    Salmonella species
    Coliforms
    Mycobacterium tuberculosis, atypical mycobacteria

Viral
  Coxsackie A, B
  ECHO
  Adenoviruses
  Influenza
  Infectious mononucleosis
  Varicella
  Mumps
  Rubeola
Fungal
  Histoplasma
  Coccidioides
  Blastomyces
  Aspergillus
Rickettsial
  Typhus
  Q fever
Other
  Actinomyces
  Nocardia
  Chlamydia (psittacosis–lymphogranuloma venereum group)
  Echinococci
  Amoebae
  Toxoplasma
  Trypanosomes
Non-infectious
  Acute rheumatic fever
  Collagen–vascular diseases
    Systemic lupus erythematosus
    Rheumatoid arthritis
    Scleroderma
    Polyarteritis nodosa
  Hypersensitivity reactions
    Postbacterial infections
    Drugs (e.g., hydralazine, procainamide)
    Serum sickness
    Allergic vasculitis
  Neoplastic
    Primary
      Benign (lipoma, fibroma, angioma)
      Malignant (mesothelioma, sarcoma)
    Metastatic
      Lymphoma, leukemia
      Carcinoma (esp. breast, lung, pancreas, ovary, esophagus)
      Thymoma
      Undifferentiated carcinomas
  Other
    Uremia
    Myxedema
    Myocardial infarction (post-myocardial infarction syndrome)
    Trauma
    Postcardiotomy syndrome
    Radiation
    Rupture of aortic aneurysm into pericardium
    Chylopericardium
  Acute idiopathic or nonspecific pericarditis

Table 13–2.   *Clinical Features of Acute Pericarditis*

Signs of infection, inflammation
  Fever
  Shaking chills
  Sweats
  Headache
  Malaise, myalgia, arthralgia
Chest pain
  Precordial
  Increased by lying flat
  Decreased by sitting up and bending forward
  May be referred to neck, shoulders, upper arms
Pericardial friction rub
Ewart's sign if pericardial effusion is present
Low pulse pressure, pulsus paradoxus if large effusion or tamponade is present
Cardiac arrhythmias may be present (paroxysmal supraventricular tachycardia, premature
  contractions, atrial flutter or fibrillation, especially if myocarditis is present)
Heart sounds distant or muffled if effusion is present
Chest roentgenogram showing normal-sized heart (heart is enlarged if effusion is present)

---

the pericardium does not evoke fever, (2) the patient is being treated with antipyretic, anti-inflammatory, or specific chemotherapeutic drugs (e.g., aspirin, corticosteroids, or antibiotics), or (3) the patient is unable to elicit a febrile response (e.g., the immunosuppressed host).

The presence of shaking chills and sweats is simply a reflection of rapid rises and falls in body temperature respectively and does not imply septicemia. Similarly, fatigue, malaise, myalgia, arthralgia, and nonspecific headaches are usually no more than nonspecific manifestations of infection.

Signs and Symptoms due to Specific Pericardial Involvement: Effusion, Tamponade or Constriction. Chest pain is usually sudden in onset. But although it is the most common symptom, it may be absent. It is usually severe, and it may mimic myocardial infarction. It is precordial. It is made worse by lying flat, relieved by sitting up and leaning forward; and it may be referred to the neck, shoulders, and upper arms. If pleuropericarditis is present, the pain may be pleuritic and aggravated by deep inspiration.

The signs and symptoms of congestive heart failure are usually absent unless tamponade or constriction is present. Right upper quadrant, epigastric, or diffuse abdominal pain may result from congestion if tamponade or constriction occurs.

Ewart's sign is not diagnostic, but it is common in patients with large pericardial effusions. It consists of an area of dullness, bronchial breathing, whispered pectoriloquy, and egophony in the region of the inferior angle of the left scapula. Those findings are due to compression of the lungs and bronchi by the accumulating fluid, which forces the heart and great vessels backward.

Cardiac arrhythmias, especially paroxysmal supraventricular tachycardias, premature contractions, or atrial flutter or fibrillation may occur, especially if myocarditis accompanies pericarditis.

The pulse pressure may be low in the presence of tamponade or constriction; pulsus paradoxus may be elicited.

Jugular venous pressure is elevated when tamponade or constriction alters ventricular filling.

Heart sounds are distant and muffled in the presence of significant effusion. In constrictive pericarditis, a "pericardial knock," an early diastolic sound, may be heard.

The pericardial friction rub is diagnostic of pericarditis. It may be diffuse or localized and persistent or transitory, and it may persist or disappear with the development of a significant pericardial effusion. Classically, the rub consists of three components: (1) the component caused by ventricular systole (it may sound like a click, and it occurs in early, middle, or late systole—or it may occupy all of systole), (2) the component that coincides with ventricular diastole and that occurs during early or mid-diastole, and (3) the presystolic component, which is due to atrial contraction. Characteristically, all three components blend to cause the usual to-and-fro sound.

Diagnosis

The clinical evaluation of the patient with pericarditis is outlined in Table 13–3. The basic responsibility of the physician is to decide, using all available data, whether an infectious cause exists, and if it does, whether it is treatable. Since viral pericarditis is most common, the large majority of patients with acute pericarditis need not be given specific therapy. But every effort must be made to determine whether treatable infection, especially one that is bacterial in origin, exists; if it does, the appropriate antimicrobial drug should be administered. Therefore any approach to the diagnosis of pericarditis must include:

History Taking. 1. Obtain an accurate chronologic story of symptoms characteristic of pericarditis.

2. Obtain epidemiologic data that may suggest a specific infectious cause; information about exposure, diet, travel, vaccinations, or recent antimicrobial therapy is of particular importance.

3. Evaluate the presence or absence of related or associated symptoms and signs suggestive of non-infectious diseases.

Physical Examination. 1. Fever may or may not be present.

2. A rash may suggest the causative agent (e.g., the scarlatiniform rash

Table 13–3.   *Clinical Evaluation of the Patient with Acute Pericarditis*

History and physical examination
Echocardiography to determine the presence of pericardial effusion
ECG to:
   Document the changes of acute pericarditis
     Elevation of S-T segments
     T-wave inversion
     S-T segment vector pointing toward apex
     T-vector tending to point upward and to the right shoulder
     S-T and T changes that may vary from day to day. S-T segment changes usually disappear
       with clinical improvement; T-wave inversion may persist
   Examine for presence of Q waves and reciprocal changes suggestive of acute myocardial
     infarction or AV block suggestive of acute rheumatic fever
Chest roentgenogram for heart size and silhouette and for evidence of bacterial pneumonia,
   tuberculosis, fungous disease, neoplasm
Hemoglobin and hematocrit determinations, WBC and differential counts to evaluate the
   possibility of leukemia, lymphoma, or other blood dyscrasia
Urinalysis
Test for antinuclear antibody, rheumatoid factor; appropriate serologic studies for the common
   infectious agents (acute sera and convalescent sera—obtained 2 to 4 weeks later—should be
   examined)
PPD test
ASLO titer
Serum creatinine test to exclude uremia
Thyroid function tests to exclude myxedema
Blood, throat, sputum, urine, stool cultures to evaluate for the presence of possible causative
   infectious agents
Pericardiocentesis to obtain material for cell count, differential count, tests for protein and sugar
   (to be compared to a simultaneous blood sugar test), Gram stain, acid-fast stain, cultures (for
   aerobes, anaerobes, fungi, mycobacteria), viral studies, cytologic studies
Open pericardial biopsy should be considered to obtain material for culture and histologic
   studies.

of a *Streptococcus pyogenes* infection or the central petechial rash of meningococcemia). Other rashes (e.g., the butterfly rash of systemic lupus erythematosus) may suggest that the cause of pericarditis is not an infectious agent.

3. Pericardial friction rub

4. Abnormal findings on examination of the lungs, especially those of pneumonia, may indicate contiguous spread of infection of the pericardium and thus suggest the pathogenesis.

5. Lymphadenopathy and splenomegaly may accompany viral infection, such as infectious mononucleosis on the one hand or tumor on the other.

6. Arthritis may be a part of a systematic infectious process or a manifestation of a non-infectious disease.

Ancillary Procedures. 1. Echocardiography is valuable in determining the presence of a pericardial effusion.

2. An ECG that manifests (1) elevation of S–T segments, (2) T-wave inversion, (3) an S–T vector pointing toward the apex, (4) a T-vector tending to point upward to the right shoulder, and (5) S–T and T-wave abnormalities that change from day to day and return to a normal pattern as the patient's condition improves is helpful in the diagnosis of acute pericarditis. T-wave inversion may persist. The ECG should be examined carefully for the presence of Q waves, reciprocal changes suggestive of acute myocardial infarction, or AV block suggestive of acute rheumatic fever.

3. The chest roentgenogram is usually normal unless congestive heart failure or pericardial effusion is present; in addition, the presence of pneumonitis, tuberculosis, or fungal disease of the lung or neoplasm may help to pinpoint the cause of pericarditis.

4. With the exception of changes that suggest leukemia, lymphoma, or other blood dyscrasias, the hemoglobin and hematocrit levels and the white blood cell and the differential cell counts are usually not helpful. It should be emphasized that leukocytosis may be seen in viral pericarditis and that leukopenia may be seen in significant bacterial infection.

5. Doing antinuclear antibody and rheumatoid factor tests and appropriate serologic studies for the common infectious agents may be useful in both the acute and retrospective diagnosis of pericarditis; the value of most serologic studies lies in the comparison of an acute serum sample with a convalescent serum sample obtained two to four weeks later.

6. The tuberculin skin test may be of value in the diagnosis of tuberculosis, but it should be remembered that the tuberculin test, which reflects delayed hypersensitivity, merely represents previous exposure to the agent. In the presence of overwhelming disease or very early disease, the skin tests may be negative; older people may also manifest decreased reactivity.

7. Information about the antistreptolysin O titer (ASLO) is helpful in the retrospective diagnosis of acute streptococcal disease; a strongly positive titer may suggest rheumatic fever.

8. A urinalysis, serum creatinine, creatinine clearance, and other appropriate tests of renal function are necessary to document uremia as a cause of pericarditis.

9. Thyroid function tests are needed to exclude the presence of myxedema.

10. Appropriate Gram stains of the throat, nasopharynx, sputum, urine, stool, and any skin lesions are helpful in documenting possible infectious causes; acid-fast smears are needed to diagnose tuberculosis; appropriately obtained cultures of the blood, throat, nasopharynx, sputum, urine, stool, and any pericardial fluid are extremely valuable in documenting the causative agent of pericarditis.

Table 13–4. Characteristics of Pericardial Fluids

	Suppurative	Viral	Tuberculous	Rheumatic	Neoplastic
Cells	Many (polymorphonuclear leukocytes, RBC)	Moderate number (lymphocytes, RBC)	Moderate number (lymphocytes, RBC)	Moderate number (polymorphonuclear leukocytes, RBC)	Moderate number (mixed cells, RBC)
Specific gravity	>1.016	Usually <1.016	>1.016	>1.016	>1.016
Protein	>3 g	Usually <3 g	>3 g	Usually >3 g	Usually >3 g
Stains for microorganisms	Causative agent may or may not be seen	Negative	Occasionally seen by acid-fast stain	Negative	Negative
Routine culture	May or may not be positive	Negative (virus isolation possible)	Cultures for mycobacteria may be positive	Negative	Negative
Cytology	Negative	Negative	Negative	Negative	Positive

11. Pericardiocentesis (Table 13–4; Chapter 14) to obtain material for a complete blood count, a differential cell count, protein tests and tests for the presence of sugar (to be compared to a simultaneous test for blood sugar), Gram stain, acid-fast stain, cultures (for anaerobes, fungi, and mycobacteria), viral studies, and cytologic studies is most important for documenting a specific causative agent.

12. Pericardial biopsy to obtain material for culture and histologic studies should be considered. For immediate diagnosis, touch preparations of a pericardial biopsy for Gram and acid-fast stains are valuable; mincing the sample before the culture increases the possibility that the cultures will be positive.

It should be remembered that the specific diagnosis of the causative agent of acute pericarditis is most commonly based on the results of diagnostic procedures that do not involve the pericardium. Because of the inherent difficulties and risks in obtaining adequate pericardial tissue for study, every effort should be made to make a diagnosis using the least dangerous method.

Idiopathic Benign Pericarditis

Idiopathic benign pericarditis is a common but inexact term that suggests the lack of an absolute diagnosis. It should not be used as a synonym for the term viral pericarditis, which should be reserved for cases of proved viral etiology; rather it should be used to imply that no cause can be found after an appropriate and complete evaluation has been made. Many cases of idiopathic benign pericarditis are probably due to undetected or undiagnosed viral infections, but other causes may also produce it. Pericardial biopsy is particularly necessary before the term idiopathic is applied. Although the course is usually benign, it may be complicated by pericardial effusion, constriction, or relapse. Pericardiectomy can benefit the patient with tamponade, constriction, or prolonged smoldering of recurrent disease.

Cardiac Tamponade (See also Chapter 14)

Cardiac tamponade is a more acute emergency because of its potential effect on cardiac function. It may be the presenting feature of pericardial disease caused by infection, tumor, trauma, or connective tissue disease. The diagnostic features of acute cardiac tamponade are listed in Table 13–5, and outlined in the following paragraphs.

Signs and Symptoms. 1. A history of acute pericardial disease or chest or heart trauma or surgery suggests the presence of cardiac tamponade.

2. Dyspnea, orthopnea, and tachypnea are the result of left-sided heart failure due to abnormal ventricular filling.

Table 13–5.   *Diagnostic Features of Acute Cardiac Tamponade*

Signs and symptoms
    History of acute pericardial disease or chest or heart trauma or surgery
    Dyspnea
    Orthopnea
    Tachypnea
    Normal, distant, or absent heart sounds and precordial movements
    Expanding precordial flatness or dullness
    Ewart's sign
    Decreased systolic pressure with narrow pulse pressure
    Pulsus paradoxus
    Elevated venous pressure and hepatic engorgement
    Exaggerated venous pulsation
    Pericardial rub (may or may not be present)
Roentgenographic and other diagnostic procedures
    Rapid enlargement of cardiopericardial silhouette (especially if lung fields are clear)
    Cardiac pulsations normal or diminished by fluoroscopy
    Positive angiocardiogram (gas or opaque)
    Positive radioisotope scan
    Positive echocardiogram
    ECG: low voltage (especially if decrease is recent), electrical alternans, S-T segment
        elevation or nonspecific T-wave changes; preceding ECG evolutionary change typical
        of pericarditis is helpful

---

3. Heart sounds may be normal, distant, or absent.

4. The usual precordial movements related to heart motion are usually absent.

5. There is expanding precordial flatness or dullness due to expanding pericardial fluid.

6. Ewart's sign is diagnostic of an acute expanding pericardial effusion.

7. Decreased systolic pressure with a narrow pulse pressure, pulsus paradoxus, elevated venous pressure, hepatic engorgement, and exaggerated venous pulsations are due to a defect in ventricular filling as a result of the external pressure on the myocardium.

8. A pericardial friction rub may or may not be present; it is not uncommon for it to disappear as the amount of fluid in the pericardial space increases.

Roentgenographic and Other Diagnostic Procedures. 1. Rapid enlargement of the cardiopericardial silhouette (especially if the lung fields are clear) is highly suggestive of a rapidly enlarging pericardial effusion; if the signs and symptoms aforementioned are present, cardiac tamponade must be seriously considered.

2. Cardiac pulsations may seem normal on fluoroscopy, but they are frequently diminished.

3. The echocardiogram is valuable in demonstrating an enlarging pericardial effusion.

4. A positive angiocardiogram result with gas or dye may demonstrate a significant pericardial effusion.

5. A positive radioisotope scan result demonstrates an enlarged pericardial effusion.

6. The ECG manifests low voltage (if the decrease is recent, an enlarging pericardial effusion should be considered), electrical alternans, S–T segment elevation, and nonspecific T-wave changes; ECG evolutionary changes typical of pericarditis are helpful.

Diagnosis. The diagnostic and therapeutic approach is similar to that for pericarditis in general, but if cardiac function is impaired, a drainage procedure should be carried out during which pericardial fluid and tissue for biopsy are obtained.

Constrictive Pericarditis

Constrictive pericarditis, usually a chronic disease, warrants discussion because of its effect on cardiac function. Although often no obvious cause is found, it may be the result of a previous bacterial infection, tuberculosis, fungous disease (especially histoplasmosis), or viral infection, as well as connective tissue disease, neoplasm, trauma, or x-irradiation. The signs and symptoms are insidious in onset, and they are usually those related to congestive heart failure. Dyspnea on exertion is common; orthopnea and paroxysmal nocturnal dyspnea less common, but abdominal and peripheral swelling are usually prominent. Physical examination may reveal an elevated venous pressure, hepatomegaly, ascites, peripheral edema, pulsus paradoxus, narrow pulse pressure, and pericardial knock. The ECG is usually characterized by low voltage, with flat or inverted T waves; there is a high incidence of atrial fibrillation. On chest roentgenogram, the lungs are usually clear and the heart normal to slightly enlarged, but pericardial calcification may be seen in over 50% of the patients. Cardiac catheterization may show no specific abnormalities, but diminished stroke volume, elevated right atrial pressure, and ventricular tracings with an early diastolic dip and an elevated diastolic plateau are common.

Treatment. Every attempt should be made to find a definitive cause before instituting therapy. The treatment of the most common infectious causes of pericarditis is outlined in Table 13–6. A variety of therapeutic regimens may be acceptable, but the choice of antimicrobial drug(s) should be based on the physician's knowledge of and experience with the individual drugs. Acute suppurative pericarditis caused by *Staphylococcus aureus, Streptococcus pneumoniae, Streptococcus pyogenes, Neisseria meningitidis, Neisseria gonorrhoeae, Salmonella* species, rickettsiae, and *Mycobacterium tuberculosis* should be treated with a

Table 13–6.   *Suggested Specific Antimicrobial Therapy for Acute Pericarditis*[a]

Bacterial
  Staphylococcus aureus (penicillin-sensitive)
    Aqueous penicillin G: 2 × 10⁶ U IV q̄ 4 hr × 14–28 days[b]
    In the penicillin-allergic patient: Clindamycin 900 mg IV q̄ 8 hr × 14–28 days
  Staphylococcus aureus (penicillin-resistant[c])
    Semi-synthetic penicillin (penicillinase-resistant), e.g., methicillin 2 g IV q̄ 4 hr × 14–28 days
    Cephalothin 2 g IV q̄ 4 hr × 14–28 days
    Clindamycin 900 mg IV q̄ 8 hr × 14–28 days
  Streptococcus pneumoniae and *Streptococcus pyogenes*
    Aqueous penicillin G: 2 × 10⁶ U IV q̄ 4 hr × 14–28 days
    In the penicillin-allergic patient: Clindamycin 900 mg IV q̄ 8 hr × 14–28 days
  Neisseria meningitidis, Neisseria gonorrhoeae
    Aqueous penicillin G: 2 × 10⁶ U IV q̄ 4 hr × 14–28 days
    In the penicillin-allergic patient: Chloramphenicol 1 g IV q̄ 6 hr × 14–28 days
  Salmonella: Chloramphenicol 1 g IV q̄ 6 hr × 14–28 days
  Mycobacterium tuberculosis: Isoniazid, ethambutol, and rifampin
Viral: None
Fungal: Amphotericin B
Rickettsial
    Chloramphenicol 1 g IV q̄ 6 hr × 10–14 days or
    Tetracycline 500 mg q̄ 6 hr × 10–14 days
Other types of infectious pericarditis should be treated with antimicrobial drugs known to be effective by sensitivity testing

---

[a] There are a variety of therapeutic regimens that are acceptable; those noted are my preferences
[b] The duration of therapy is dictated by clinical response; I feel that a minimum of two weeks' therapy is necessary
[c] Until sensitivities are available, all staphylococci should be considered to be penicillin resistant

minimum of delay in order to halt the progression of the disease, alleviate symptoms, and prevent complications.

BACTERIAL ENDOCARDITIS

Endocarditis, an infection of the endocardial surface of a valve, the ventricular wall, or septum is an infrequent but important disease entity whose recognition is of major importance because proper diagnosis and treatment have greatly reduced the morbidity and mortality characteristic of the preantibiotic era. In addition, if endocarditis is allowed to progress unabated, it may result in permanent cardiac damage or death, or it may necessitate cardiac surgery.

Although acute bacterial endocarditis and subacute bacterial endocarditis overlap considerably, the acute form is a potential cardiac emergency that necessitates rapid diagnosis and treatment to preserve cardiac integrity and to halt the unremitting infection, which may be fatal.

Acute Bacterial Endocarditis. Acute bacterial endocarditis results from bacteremia with organisms that can induce an acute, necrotizing, ulcerating lesion on the endocardial surface and, therefore, may rapidly destroy the infected structure. Infections caused by such invasive species as *S. aureus, Str. pneumoniae, Hemophilus influenzae, Str. pyogenes, N. meningitidis,* or *N. gonorrhoeae* can result in the invasion of both normal and damaged endocardium. Acute bacterial endocarditis, therefore, occurs often in persons whose hearts had been normal. Because the bacteria involved are usually highly invasive, even small numbers can invade the endocardium and establish infection.

Signs and Symptoms. The prototype and the most virulent form of acute endocarditis is that caused by *S. aureus.* The underlying event is staphylococcal bacteremia, most commonly originating from a skin infection, although any site of staphylococcal infection may be the primary source.

Fever is the most common sign, and it is usually accompanied by myalgia, arthralgia, leukocytosis, and signs of metastatic infection.

The changing cardiac murmur is typical of acute endocarditis, but a small number of patients may have no detectable murmur at the onset, the murmur first appearing during the course of the disease or even during or after therapy.

Signs of metastatic infection usually, but not always, appear. They consist of abnormalities in whatever organ system is involved by the bacteremia. The following sites of metastatic infection are common, and their involvement is helpful in making the diagnosis:

1. The meninges (staphylococcal meningitis)
2. The lungs (staphylococcal pneumonia)
3. The joints (acute staphylococcal arthritis)
4. The skin (petechiae, septic infarcts, subungual hemorrhages, and microabscesses)
5. The eyes (subconjunctival and retinal hemorrhages)
6. The kidney, liver, and brain, where multiple microabscesses may coalesce to form a large nephric or perinephric, hepatic, or brain abscess, respectively
7. The bones (staphylococcal osteomyelitis)

The most vital area involved is the heart. The endocardium, myocardium and/or pericardium may be involved, resulting in acute staphylococcal pericarditis, acute myocarditis, discrete myocardial abscesses, or acute endocarditis. The endocarditis is usually characterized by a rapidly changing murmur, which may progress to the signs and symptoms of intractable congestive heart failure secondary to valve rupture or fenestration.

Diagnosis. The diagnosis may be difficult to make on clinical grounds alone. The patient usually appears acutely ill, and he may or may not present with the signs and symptoms of the metastatic infections just listed. Any temperature elevation is usually spiking, but fever may be minimal or absent, especially in the newborn, the elderly, or the patient with altered host defense mechanisms.

Blood cultures are the most important laboratory aid; identification of the causative agent is critical not only in defining the disease but also in instituting therapy. Meticulous care must be exercised in obtaining blood cultures because contamination of the sample may result in considerable confusion and possibly inappropriate therapy, especially in staphylococcal endocarditis since *S. aureus* is a normal inhabitant of many parts of the body. At least three, and preferably six, blood cultures should be made to avoid the misinterpretation that can occur when only a single culture is made and the result is positive. At least two (and preferably three) positive culture results are needed to confirm the presence of bacteremia. In the acutely ill patient, blood for culturing should be obtained from *separate* sites as rapidly as possible so that therapy can be instituted without delay. If the patient had previously been treated with antimicrobial drugs, the pertinent information about the drug treatment should be transmitted to the laboratory. And if the patient had been treated with penicillin G, penicillinase should be added to the blood culture bottle although several commercially available types of media contain penicillinase. Occasionally the blood culture results may be negative; among the factors that may be responsible for that are (1) the previous use of antimicrobial drugs to treat febrile illnesses of undefined origin, (2) inappropriate culture techniques, (3) the presence in the blood of factors that inhibit microbial growth, and (4) right-sided endocarditis.

Other samples, including those that can be obtained from sites of obvious metastatic infection, such as sputum, spinal fluid, joint fluid, material obtained by the aspiration of skin lesions, and urine, should be similarly cultured. Recovery of the same organism from several sites is extremely helpful in documenting the diagnosis.

In the absence of material that allows a specific etiologic diagnosis to be made, bone marrow, tissue obtained by biopsy, or, rarely, samples obtained directly from the heart valve surface by catheterization may be used.

Therapy. The patient with acute endocarditis is severely ill. Left untreated, the infection may permanently damage the endocardium in a very short time; therefore therapy should be instituted when the clinical diagnosis has been made. The diagnosis can be substantiated with culture data when they become available. Thus the physician chooses the antibiotic therapy on the basis of:

1. Immediately available information, such as that obtained from the history and physical examination, and a clinical picture suggestive of acute endocarditis

2. Bacteriologic statistics that suggest the association of certain microorganisms with certain disease states

3. Examination of body fluids with Gram or other appropriate stains that frequently provide sufficient information to make a presumptive diagnosis

4. Examination of spinal fluid, joint fluid, urine, and aspirates from skin lesions.

The choice of antibiotic in the management of endocarditis is often based on the physician's personal experience. Whatever drug is used, the only requirement is that the organism be highly sensitive to it. In general, bactericidal drugs appear to be more effective than bacteriostatic ones. There is not sufficient data at present to indicate the optimal doses, duration of therapy, or route of administration of any of the antibiotics used for treating endocarditis, but it is thought that all patients should be treated for a minimum of four weeks with parenteral drugs. The regimens listed on Table 13–7 have been found to be successful.

Subacute Bacterial Endocarditis. Subacute bacterial endocarditis is usually not a cardiac emergency because it is a slowly progressive disease, with the interval from the onset of symptoms until diagnosis frequently ranging from 30 to 90 days. Nevertheless, a discussion of subacute bacterial endocarditis is appropriate here to contrast it to the acute form (Table 13–8). Untreated subacute bacterial endocarditis may result in permanent cardiac damage that will require urgent intervention. It is important to remember that the classic picture of subacute bacterial endocarditis is no longer commonly seen; rather, the disease presents insidiously and has a number of symptom complexes that may suggest illnesses other than subacute bacterial endocarditis. Diagnosis is difficult to make on clinical grounds alone because (1) the physician may not consider the possibility of subacute bacterial endocarditis, (2) the presenting manifestations are those of many other syndromes rather than the symptoms thought of as "typical" for endocarditis; and (3) the presence of the infection may be indicated by none of the special features but rather by certain combinations of often minor ones.

Etiology. The signs and symptoms related to valvular involvement are a consequence of bacteremia, and many of the subsequent signs and symptoms are a combination of those arising from a systemic infection and those related to the damage produced in the afflicted valve. Subacute bacterial endocarditis is due to infection with less invasive bacteria, such as those occurring in the oral cavity, especially in gingival crevices or apical abscesses. Those bacteria are mainly streptococci, including many

Table 13–7. Regimens for the Treatment of Bacterial Endocarditis

Organism	Sensitivity	Antibiotic	Dose per Day	Duration (wk)
Streptococcus viridans	Penicillin G sensitive (<0.2 μ/ml)	Penicillin G IM; IV	6–12 million units	4
	Penicillin G insensitive (>0.2 μ/ml)		12–20 million units	
Group A β-hemolytic streptococci Pneumococci Gonococci Meningococci		Penicillin G IM; IV	12–20 million units	4
Staphylococcus aureus *Staphylococcus epidermidis*	Penicillin G sensitive Penicillin G resistant	Penicillin G IM; IV Oxacillin IV Cephalothin IV Clindamycin IV	12–24 million units 2 g q̄ 4 hr 2 g q̄ 4 hr 900 mg q̄ 8 hr	4–6
Streptococcus faecalis		Penicillin G or ampicillin IV *and* aminoglycoside (gentamicin or tobramycin) Vancomycin	20–40 million units 12 g 5 mg/kg 3 g	4–6
*Hemophilus influenzae**		Ampicillin IV Chloramphenicol	8–12 g 6 g	4–6

*Because of the increasing incidence of ampicillin-resistant strains of *H. influenzae*, therapy should be instituted with chloramphenicol until the results of cultures and sensitivities are available.

Table 13–8. *A Comparison of the Major Features of Acute (ABE) and Subacute (SBE) Bacterial Endocarditis*

Feature	ABE	SBE
Causative agents	*Staphylococcus aureus* *Streptococcus pyogenes* *Streptococcus pneumoniae* *Hemophilus influenzae* *Neisseria meningitidis* *Neisseria gonorrhoeae*	*Streptococcus viridans* Enterococci Anerobic streptococci *Staphylococcus epidermidis* Gram-negative bacilli
Valve most commonly involved	Aortic	Mitral
Previously damaged endocardium	Unnecessary	Necessary
Valve pathology	Ulcerative; necrotizing	Indolent
Constitutional reaction	Mild to severe	Mild
WBC	N or ↑	N or ↑
Change in murmur	Rapid	Not rapid
Valve rupture	Not uncommon	Uncommon
Duration of symptoms before diagnosis	1–2 weeks	≤3 months
Primary focus	None found; wounds; skin infection	None found; teeth; genitourinary tract

nontypable strains, *Streptococcus viridans*, and microaerophilic and anaerobic streptococci; but other species, such as *Staphylococcus epidermidis* and diphtheroids, may be implicated. Subacute bacterial endocarditis may follow cardiac surgery, upper respiratory tract infection, and dental manipulation; abdominal sepsis and genitourinary infection can lead to heart valve infection with such organisms as *Escherichia coli*, *Proteus* species, *Klebsiella*, and *Pseudomonas*. Surgical procedures, urinary tract instrumentation, parturition, abortion, and trauma may also be associated with its inception. The disease produced usually evolves slowly and it has many different manifestations because it is a combination of both slowly progressive destruction and early healing in the same lesion, with the destruction exceeding the healing.

Pathogenesis. Factors involved in the development of subacute bacterial endocarditis include a combination of:

1. A previously damaged valve (not always manifested by a detectable murmur)

2. Hemodynamics that favor the deposition of a fibrin platelet clot: a high velocity flow through a small conduit (as in the regurgitant flow through a mitral valve of a ventricular septal defect) into a low pressure sink (as into the left atrium or right ventricle).

3. The development of a sterile platelet-fibrin thrombus

4. The presence of an antibody that serves to agglutinate bacteria within fibrin clots without killing them. The fact that the organisms involved are usually indigenous and that bacteremia precedes endocardial localization assures antibody development.

5. Bacteremia that establishes infection of the endocardial surface (usually asymptomatic). Whether it follows a tooth extraction, for example, is deduced by the history of such manipulation; but it is important to remember that there may have been many episodes of bacteremia rather than a single one.

6. Although rheumatic heart disease and congenital heart disease are still the most common underlying disorders on which subacute infective endocarditis is superimposed, their frequency has decreased; and arteriosclerotic heart disease has become a significant predisposing lesion. The introduction of various types of surgery of the heart has added a group of iatrogenic lesions that may serve as foci for the development of both acute and subacute valvular lesions. There has also been an increase of endocarditis in patients with acute myocardial infarction. The infection may be subacute or acute, depending on the nature of the organism involved, and it may involve either the right or the left side of the heart.

Clinical Features. 1. Fever is by far the most common sign. Under certain circumstances, the febrile response may be minimal or absent for variable periods, especially in patients with severe heart failure or uremia or in those who are receiving or have received immunosuppressive or antimicrobial therapy. The incidence of endocarditis in older persons may account for the greater frequency with which fever is absent. Repeated short courses of antibiotic therapy in patients with undiagnosed endocarditis produce a characteristic clinical pattern of repetitive episodes of remission and relapse of fever; even small quantities of antibiotic may mask the fever as well as other manifestations.

2. A cardiac murmur was once a sine qua non for the diagnosis, and the change in its quality and intensity was common in the acute but not the subacute infection. However, it is now accepted that as many as 15% of patients may have no detectable murmur when they present with endocarditis. Murmurs may first appear during therapy or some time after therapy has been completed—or they may never develop.

3. Petechiae are the most common cutaneous manifestation. They are seen in 20 to 40% of patients; in the preantibiotic era, they were seen in 85% of patients.

4. Subungual hemorrhages are also not as common as they were in the preantibiotic era.

5. Osler's nodes are seen in only 10% of cases.

6. The incidence of splenomegaly has decreased, and it is now seen in 20 to 55% of patients.

7. Roth spots, located in the retina and having the appearance of cotton wool exudates or oval- or boat-shaped hemorrhages with a central white area, are uncommon.

8. Neuropsychiatric complications are common; and if they are sought, they may be found in up to 50% of patients. Any acute unexplained neurologic syndrome or psychiatric illness arising in a patient with fever and a cardiac murmur should suggest subacute bacterial endocarditis.

9. Renal disease developing as a complication of endocarditis is not uncommon. The picture of acute glomerulonephritis is likely the result of immune complex deposition, and it is partially reversible with effective antimicrobial therapy. Renal insufficiency is seen in about 10% of patients. Hematuria occurs in 25 to 90% of patients. Uremia may develop, and it is generally accompanied by the absence of hypertension, little or no fever, and a high incidence of sterile blood cultures. Careful and frequent urinalyses early in the disease may show red blood cells, red blood cell casts, white blood cells, and albuminuria. Focal embolic glomerulonephritis and renal infarcts may also be seen as a result of subacute infective endocarditis.

10. Elevation of the sedimentation rate is the most common abnormal laboratory finding in patients with bacterial endocarditis.

11. Although the leukocyte count may be elevated and there may be a shift to the left, those findings are frequently absent.

12. An abnormality of serum proteins, namely, hyperglobulinemia with inversion of the albumin to globulin ratio, is also common, and it is accompanied by an increase in the numbers of plasma cells in the bone marrow.

13. Anemia is common, occurring in 10 to 80% of patients. The degree of anemia is generally related to the duration of infection although in more acute cases it may develop rapidly. It is usually normocytic and normochromic. The serum iron level and the total iron-binding capacity may be reduced.

14. Rheumatoid factor is present in the serum of 50% of patients; it decreases or disappears entirely after successful treatment.

15. Many patients develop higher titers of agglutinating, complement-fixing, and opsonizing antibodies specific for the invading organisms.

Diagnosis. The classic signs and symptoms—fever, murmur, anemia, and petechiae with an illness of 6 weeks' to 3 months' duration—are easily recognized and strongly suggest the diagnosis.

Clubbing, hematuria, and a history of dental disease and/or manipulation are also helpful.

The nonspecific presenting features (Table 13–9) are:

1. Prolonged, unexplained fever, especially if accompanied by a high sedimentation rate, anemia, and hyperglobulinemia. The response of

Table 13–9. *Nonspecific Presenting Clinical Features in Endocarditis*

Unexplained fever
Arrhythmias and congestive heart failure
Pulmonary infarction
Mental confusion
Sterile meningitis
Subarachnoid hemorrhage
Hemiplegia
Unexplained uremia

"fever" to short-course antibiotic trials when treatment is chosen empirically is diagnostically helpful.

2. Arrhythmias and congestive heart failure. Atrial fibrillation or cardiac failure or both, which previously rarely occurred in the early stage of subacute endocarditis, are now relatively common and are probably related to the empiric administration of short courses of antimicrobial therapy for an undiagnosed illness. Such ineffective treatment may go on for weeks or months and lead to progressive cardiac damage with the establishment of congestive heart failure and/or arrhythmias.

3. Pulmonary infarction as a direct result of bacterial endocarditis is limited almost entirely to cases involving the right side of the heart. In fact, the lung is the most common site for deposition of emboli in subacute bacterial endocarditis.

4. Mental confusion. Psychiatric changes range from minor aberrations in personality and behavior to major psychiatric breakdowns that necessitate the patient's admission to a psychiatric ward. Psychiatric complications are more common in older patients; those presenting with mental aberrations have a poorer prognosis. In some cases, abnormalities in the cerebrospinal fluid may suggest an underlying cause, but many patients who present with psychiatric features have no localizing cerebral signs and no significant cerebrospinal fluid changes. The presence of fever and a cardiac murmur should be given careful attention in such instances.

5. Sterile meningitis. Sterile meningitis is a not uncommon initial manifestation of subacute bacterial endocarditis. Because viral infections or partially treated infections of the meninges are more common causes of "sterile" meningitis, the association with endocarditis is often not considered. In fact, any unexplained neurologic syndrome, especially subarachnoid hemorrhage, in a patient with fever and a murmur should make the physician suspect subacute bacterial endocarditis.

6. Unexplained uremia. Renal failure may be a major factor in the failure to establish a diagnosis of endocarditis because the blood cultures

are often sterile and the physician may be so concerned with the kidney dysfunction that he overlooks the cardiac disease.

Blood cultures are the most important laboratory aid in establishing the etiologic diagnosis of endocarditis. The best time to draw blood for culture is as the temperature begins to rise, but that cannot always be done. Checking the temperature at 30- to 45-minute intervals, beginning at the time an increase is expected, may be helpful. Frequently, the rise in temperature can be predicted on the basis of the temperature during the previous 24 hours. Blood is cultured as soon as it is evident that fever is developing. Six separate cultures are made, with the blood being drawn at 10-to-30-minute intervals. A single positive culture, however, must be interpreted with great caution because of the possibility of contamination. This is true even when the organisms are those usually not considered contaminants. Two, and preferably three, positive blood cultures are needed to confirm the presence of significant bacteremia. One would not want to commit a patient to four to six weeks of hospitalization on the basis of one positive blood culture. All blood cultures should be incubated at 37°C; room temperature may be required for some yeasts and fungi. The cultures should be incubated for at least two to three weeks and as long as four weeks if *Brucella* is suspected. Recent studies have shown that the blood culture results are falsely negative in about 20% of patients with subacute infective endocarditis. Among the factors that may be responsible for the negative blood culture results are the use of antibiotics in etiologically undefined febrile illnesses, inappropriate culture techniques, the presence in the blood of factors that inhibit microbial growth, right-sided endocarditis, the presence of renal disease, and the prolonged duration of subacute bacterial endocarditis ("bacteria-free state").

Therapy. An acceptable outline for the treatment of subacute endocarditis is shown in Table 13–7, but the choice of antibiotic(s) for such unusual species as *Acinetobacter, Escherichia, Enterobacter, Klebsiella, Alcaligenes, Pseudomonas, Hafnia*, anaerobic diphtheroids or when resistance is known to be a problem (as with *Staphylococcus epidermidis*) is based on the in vitro sensitivity of the organism recovered from the blood. The drug chosen preferably should be bactericidal, and it should be given in maximal tolerated doses.

Amphotericin is presently the most effective drug for the management of endocarditis caused by fungi and yeast. Several dosages have been used:

1. 1.5 mg/kg every other day for the entire course of treatment
2. 0.25 mg/kg for the first day, 0.5 mg/kg for the second day, 0.75 mg/kg for the third day, and 1 mg/kg for the fourth day and for subsequent days until therapy is completed.

3. The administration of quantities of the drug necessary to produce and maintain blood levels two to four times greater than the in vitro inhibitory concentration.

In general, a total of 2 g (preferably, 3 g of amphotericin B) is desirable although larger doses may be needed.

Indications for Surgery in Endocarditis (See also Chapter 18). Surgery may be lifesaving in cases in which chemotherapy fails to produce a total cure or when potentially lethal complications develop. The indications for surgery in endocarditis are as follows:

1. Infections that fail to respond after treatment with appropriate doses of the proper antimicrobial drug(s)

2. The recurrence of infection following two or more courses of therapy with an effective antibiotic

3. A single recurrence of fungal endocarditis

4. The development of aneurysms of the sinus of Valsalva or the AV junctional tissue

5. Intractable or rapidly progressive heart failure despite specific medical therapy

6. The presence of an infected prosthetic valve or patch (if the initial treatment is followed by cure, removal of the prosthesis may not be necessary; if, however, relapse occurs after completion of one course of therapy, replacement of the intracardiac foreign body is usually indicated).

7. Recurrent systemic or pulmonary emboli (Chapter 2).

8. When surgery is otherwise indicated, the presence of active infection is not a contraindication. It is probably a mistake to wait until the infectious process seems to be under control because during the delay, tissue destruction may proceed so far that surgery becomes technically difficult or impossible. Antimicrobial therapy must be maintained before and after surgery.

Infection following Cardiac Surgery. The advent of cardiac surgery or surgery on the great vessels has introduced a new class of acute life-threatening infections involving the heart. This is particularly true in cases involving a prosthesis. Infection of an artificial valve, for example, may be a catastrophic event not only because of the infectious process per se, but because it is extremely difficult to treat the infection successfully without removing the infected foreign body. It is of paramount importance, therefore, that infection arising after cardiac surgery be diagnosed immediately and that appropriate treatment be instituted without delay to prevent infection on the prosthesis and also to insure that infection arising elsewhere is not misinterpreted as cardiac infection, giving rise to unnecessary further surgical procedures.

Infection occurring during cardiac surgery is more probably related to high-grade rather than low-grade contamination. Sources of contamination include blood transfusion, the pump-oxygenator (uncommon with the newer sterilizing techniques), devices used for pressure recordings, septic thrombophlebitis resulting from indwelling catheters, and minor or major breaks in aseptic surgical techniques. Staphylococci are the organisms most commonly involved; they may enter the operative field from the environment or from infected personnel or carriers, but usually the *patient* is the source. The prostheses may be contaminated, as may the suture materials, but newer equipment has reduced the risk. Systemic factors in the host, such as altered defense mechanisms, shock, and corticosteroid therapy may also predispose the patient to infection.

Post-cardiac–surgery infection generally occurs early (immediately or one to four weeks after surgery) or late (several months postoperatively; some of those later infections may be coincidental and unrelated to the surgical procedure).

The symptoms may be obvious or occult, with high fever and positive blood cultures being the most prominent features. The diagnosis may be difficult to make, however, when fever is low grade, especially since the characteristic features of endocarditis may be lacking.

The microbiology of post-cardiac–surgery endocarditis is varied. The most common organisms involved are *Staphylococcus aureus* (coagulase-positive) and *Staphylococcus epidermidis* (coagulase-negative); and infections caused by *S. epidermidis* are particularly difficult to treat. Though they are rare in other types of endocarditis, Gram-negative organisms, such as *Escherichia coli, Proteus* species, *Klebsiella, Enterobacter,* and *Pseudomonas aeruginosa,* are not uncommonly seen in post-cardiac–surgery endocarditis. Other uncommon bacteria that are seen occasionally and should therefore not be automatically dismissed as contaminants include species of diphtheroids, chromobacteria, flavobacteria, and even the tubercle bacillus.

Fungal endocarditis is a particularly difficult post-cardiac–surgery problem in which species of *Candida* and *Aspergillus* are most commonly involved. Although the sources of contamination are similar to those in bacterial endocarditis, antibiotic and steroid therapy and debilitation appear to be particularly important predisposing factors. Because fungal endocarditis is usually characterized by vegetations larger than those due to bacteria, embolism to large arteries is seen with impressive frequency and is, in fact, a common presenting symptom. Thus endocarditis should be suspected in any post-cardiac–surgery patient who has an embolus to a major vessel; and it is imperative that at the time of embolectomy, Gram stains and cultures be obtained to identify the offending organism. It is also of interest that fungal endocarditis generally occurs later after surgery than does bacterial endocarditis.

Because of the life-threatening nature of post-cardiac–surgery endocarditis, any patient who after surgery has unexplained fever and any of the peripheral manifestations of endocarditis just described should be rapidly and thoroughly evaluated. The appropriate blood cultures should be made, and therapy should be instituted as soon as possible. For the common organisms, therapy should be dictated by the results of the appropriate sensitivity tests. Amphotericin B therapy is the treatment of choice for fungal endocarditis, but it should be emphasized that successful therapy is the exception rather than the rule. The eradication of infection on a prosthetic valve is particularly difficult. Replacement of the prosthesis is usually necessary and it must be seriously considered unless the patient shows an immediate and obvious response to antimicrobial therapy. It is imperative that blood cultures be obtained during and after therapy to ascertain that the treatment has been effective; persistent bacteremia or fungemia during or after appropriate therapy generally indicates that infection is persisting in or on the prosthesis and that surgical replacement of the prosthesis is needed.

Table 13–10. *Etiology of Myocarditis*

Infectious
  Bacterial
    Diphtheria, *Staphylococcus aureus, Streptococcus pyogenes, Hemophilus influenzae, Salmonella, Neisseria meningitidis, Neisseria gonorrhoeae, Brucella,* tuberculosis
  Rickettsial
    Epidemic typhus, Rocky Mountain spotted fever, scrub typhus
  Viral
    ECHO, influenza, Coxsackie, rubeola, hepatitis, infectious mononucleosis, mumps, varicella, dengue, yellow fever
  Fungal
    Blastomyces, Coccidioides, Histoplasma, Torula
  Protozoan
    Chagas' disease, malaria, Toxoplasmosis
  Metazoan
    Trichinosis, schistosomiasis, echinococcosis
Non-infectious
  Myocardial disease of obscure origin
  Idiopathic cardiomyopathies
  Hemochromatosis
  Sarcoidosis
  Systemic lupus erythematosus
  Scleroderma
  Amyloidosis
  Fiedler's myocarditis
  Storage diseases
  Drug-induced myocarditis
  Hypersensitivity reactions
  Endocardial fibroelastosis
  Toxic myocarditis

MYOCARDITIS

Inflammatory lesions in the myocardium have been associated with almost every type of infectious agent, including bacteria, spirochetes, rickettsiae, viruses (especially the Coxsackie group), fungi, and parasites (Table 13–10). Although those lesions are seen frequently at careful postmortem examination, clinical myocarditis is uncommon. The frequency with which myocarditis is diagnosed depends on the degree of suspicion of its presence and on the care given to the interpretation of the serial ECGs. Myocarditis usually is first manifested as cardiac arrhythmias but it may be manifested as cardiac arrest or sudden death. Congestive heart failure in uncommon. Myocarditis may be associated with pericarditis or endocarditis.

Myocardial abscesses generally are the result of bacteremia, but they may also develop by extension from valvular lesions of bacterial endocarditis. Rarely, an abscess occurs at the site of myocardial infarction. The majority of myocardial abscesses are small and of relatively little clinical significance. Their clinical manifestations usually are overshadowed by the associated infectious process, but occasionally an abscess may cause or contribute to death.

The treatment of myocarditis depends on the causative organism; the general principles of management are those of pericarditis.

THE HEART IN SEPTIC SHOCK (See also Chapter 3)

Although septic shock per se may involve the heart directly (as outlined in Table 13–11), any pathophysiologic form of shock may directly or

Table 13–11. *Cardiac Involvement in Septic Shock*

Mechanism	Cause
Impaired cardiac function	Myocarditis
	Cardiac tamponade
	Endocarditis, e.g., ruptured valve
	Myocardial infarction
	Mechanical outflow obstruction, e.g., *Echinococcus* cyst
Impaired venous return	
Reduced blood volume	Severe diarrhea
(loss of water and electrolytes)	Adrenal insufficiency, e.g., tuberculosis
	Salt-losing pyelonephritis
	Peritonitis
	Hemorrhage
Normal blood volume	Endotoxin shock
Disturbances of arteriolar tone	Destruction of vasomotor center, e.g., bulbar polio

indirectly affect cardiac function by impairing the delivery of oxygenated blood to the myocardium. Therefore it is appropriate that any type of septic shock be considered a cardiac emergency if adequate and effective cardiac function is to be maintained. The discussion that follows, therefore, applies to septic shock as a whole, but its implications for the heart are obvious.

Septic shock is a dynamic syndrome induced by infections of various types in which inadequate perfusion of tissues with blood develops. Although the microcirculation of the capillary loop is the final determinant of the events that occur in septic shock, multiple factors are involved in the genesis and persistence of the progressive decompensation of the capillary circulation and the cells that it supports. Effective therapy of septic shock requires knowledge of its pathogenesis, anticipation and recognition of the clinical picture, the use of available bedside and laboratory techniques for assessing the nature and degree of the derangements, and rapid initiation of corrective measures.

Bacteremia is not a prerequisite for the development of septic shock; septic shock may also be due to endotoxins, exotoxins, direct bacterial invasion of a vital organ, or obstruction of blood flow to a vital organ. Although the presence of Gram-negative bacteria in the blood, with the release of endotoxin, is the most common cause of septic shock in hospitalized patients (septic shock is second only to myocardial infarction as a cause of death on many large medical services), about one-third of the cases of septic shock follow invasion by staphylococci, streptococci, and clostridia; some cases may be associated with viral or rickettsial infections.

Factors Predisposing to Endotoxic Shock

1. Endotoxic shock is most common in men over 40 years of age but is still seen in women who have had septic abortions and among neonates
2. Urinary, intestinal, biliary tract, or gynecologic manipulation or surgery
3. Transfusion of contaminated blood or intravenous fluids
4. Hepatic cirrhosis
5. Diabetes mellitus
6. Burns
7. Cancer (especially of the hematopoietic system)
8. Radiotherapy
9. The use of antimetabolites, corticosteroids, and antimicrobial drugs.

Organisms Most Commonly Associated with Endotoxic Shock

1. *E. coli*
2. *Proteus* species

3. *Pseudomonas aeruginosa*
4. *Klebsiella*
5. *Enterobacter*
6. *Bacteroides*

The Clinical Picture of Endotoxic Shock

The presence of any of the predisposing factors just listed should alert the physician to the possibility of endotoxic shock. The following signs and symptoms occurring in such a patient are highly suggestive of endotoxic shock:

1. Hypotension is present in about 80% of patients who have bacteremia with Gram-negative organisms. However, the complete syndrome of shock develops in only about 20%; the mortality in that group may range from 40 to 80%.

2. The symptom complex of shaking chills, elevated temperature, and hypotension, especially if accompanied early by hyperventilation and respiratory alkalosis, is highly suggestive of impending endotoxic shock in a susceptible host. If a high-grade fever appears in an elderly person (it does so uncommonly), a presumptive diagnosis of septic shock should be made.

3. The early phase of the syndrome when it is produced by endotoxin is often marked by "warm shock," in which the skin is warm and dry, the pulse full, and the output of urine adequate despite the hypotension. If not treated, the condition progresses to "cold shock," which is characterized by pallor, cold, clammy skin, cyanosis of the nail beds, rapid, thready pulse, collapse of veins, altered cerebral function, and reduction or total loss of urine flow.

4. In general, in the susceptible host, any alteration of the patient's clinical course (e.g., a change in mental status, appetite, or sleeping habits, vomiting or diarrhea, or unexplained urinary or gastric retention or ileus) may be the first sign of impending endotoxic shock.

Hemodynamic Abnormalities in Septic Shock

The development of any type of shock in the course of infection should precipitate an immediate assessment of the patient's condition to determine the type of hemodynamic abnormality (Table 13–11), any or all of which may be present at one time or another.

1. Cardiac failure may occur as a result of myocarditis complicating diphtheria, influenza, Coxsackie virus (type B in very young children) and other virus infections, and rickettsial disease or as a result of tamponade supervening during tuberculous, viral, and suppurative pericarditis.

2. Volume deficit may be the primary problem in severe infectious

diarrhea, salt-losing pyelonephritis, adrenal insufficiency due to tuberculosis, and infections associated with adrenal hemorrhage.

3. Peripheral vascular failure may occur when autonomic ganglia or medullary centers are injured or destroyed, as in some cases of bulbar poliomyelitis and encephalitis.

The type of shock present can be measured in a variety of ways that have been well described in the medical literature, but the ultimate goal should be the definition of the state of cardiac function and of the adequacy of total and effective circulating blood volume. Once shock has been identified and the pathophysiologic basis defined, immediate therapy is indicated.

Management of Septic Shock

At present, the management of septic shock is based on several principles:

1. Prevention and treatment of the situations known to be associated with its development. Avoiding instrumentation and manipulation, such as the use of unnecessary urinary bladder catheterization, and the early recognition and appropriate therapy for infectious or non-infectious diseases known to result in the development of septic shock are paramount.

2. Anticipation of its occurrence when predisposing factors are present.

3. Therapy of hemodynamic abnormalities and the infections with which shock is associated.

4. The most successful approach to the prophylaxis of septic shock is the rapid, intensive treatment of the infection before the shock state occurs. Early and effective chemotherapy eliminates the risk of shock in most cases.

Once septic shock is fully developed, the morbidity and mortality are significant. Prevention, therefore, is the best approach. Avoidance, if possible, of procedures that predispose to infection (such as the use of indwelling urinary bladder catheters, antimicrobial drugs, and venous catheters) is of obvious value. However, if those procedures are necessary, patients subjected to them must be studied continually for clinical and microbiologic evidence of infection, which must be treated as soon as it is detected.

Paramount to the successful management of septic shock is rapid control of the responsible infectious process, but significant airway obstruction or blood loss must be ruled out as soon as the evidence of shock becomes apparent. In many cases, a causative organism is not recovered, and the choice of treatment must be based on clinical grounds alone until the results of culture studies of blood, urine, sputum, exudates, or other body fluids, are available. Since the recognition and identification of the shock state require the institution of antimicrobial therapy before culture results are available, it is helpful to know that certain Gram-negative microorganisms are statistically associated with diseases of particular anatomic areas (Table 13–12). The choice of antimicrobial drug(s) varies from physician to physician and clinic to clinic, but it is usually possible to make a rational choice based on the available clinical data, the Gram stains of body fluids or exudates, and a knowledge of the statistical likelihood that certain organisms are present. In many cases, a combination of two drugs is desirable until cultures are available. Those combinations include an anti-staphylococcal drug and an aminoglycoside, the anti-staphylococcal drug because staphylococcal bacteremia is still a significant cause of septic shock, and the aminoglycoside because endotoxic shock is prominent as a cause of morbidity and mortality. The following combinations are commonly used:

1. Cephalothin, 2 g intravenously every 4 hours, plus gentamicin 5 mg/kg/day in three divided doses intravenously. Tobramycin (5 mg/kg/day in three divided doses intravenously) is a reasonable alternative to gentamicin. Amikacin (15 mg/kg/day in three divided doses intravenously), a newer aminoglycoside, has the distinct advantage of being useful against many organisms that may be resistant to tobramycin and/or gentamicin; in most situations, any hospital that has had a problem with gentamicin-tobramycin resistance should use Amikacin as the primary aminoglycoside until the results of cultures and sensitivities are available.

2. Clindamycin, 900 mg intravenously every 8 hours, plus gentamicin

3. Oxacillin, 2 g intravenously every 4 hours, plus gentamicin

If the organism is known, obviously the single most effective antimicrobial drug in the appropriate dose is indicated. In shock, it is always wise to use the intravenous route since the absorption of intramuscularly administered drugs may be erratic. All antimicrobial drugs excreted

Table 13–12. *Gram-Negative Sepsis: Causative Agent Suspected, by Anatomic Area*

Site of Infection	Suspected Agent
Genitourinary tract	*Escherichia coli, Klebsiella pneumoniae, Proteus* species, *Pseudomonas aeruginosa*
Gastrointestinal tract	*E. coli, Bacteroides,* other coliforms
Lower respiratory tract	*K. pneumoniae, Hemophilus influenzae*
Ear-Mastoid	*H. influenzae, P. aeruginosa*
Skin	*P. aeruginosa; Providentia* and *Proteus* species (especially in burn patients)

primarily by the kidneys must be given with extreme caution when shock is present because decreased renal function results in an accumulation of those drugs in excessive and dangerous concentrations in the blood and in the tissue fluids. It should be emphasized, however, that the *first* dose given to a patient with suspected septic shock should be a *full or normal* dose, despite the presence of renal dysfunction; after that, the interval between doses or the dose itself should be altered according to creatinine clearance.

Abscesses or other localized infections may not respond to chemotherapy alone and may require drainage. In fact, the presence of persistent bacteremia during antimicrobial therapy is most commonly a result of an undetected abscess.

Careful control of the acid-base balance is mandatory in patients with septic shock. Measurement of venous or arterial pH and serum lactate levels may prove of value; the concentration of lactic acid in the blood is an important index of severe circulatory failure.

Vasopressor drugs may be necessary in septic shock, but they are *usually not indicated.* Tissue perfusion must never be sacrificed for the sake of a rise in peripheral arterial pressure. The decision to use vasopressor drugs is based upon an overall evaluation of the patient's status.

Because urine volume is somewhat proportional to renal blood flow, it is a good index of tissue perfusion. For that reason, an adequate output (at least 30 ml per hour) usually indicates—much better than does the peripheral arterial pressure—that the blood supply to vital organs is effective and that the shock state has been reversed. Catheterization of the bladder should not be carried out, however, unless an inability to void leads to significant distention of this organ.

The use of oxygen, although safe, if of questionable value since the anoxia in septic shock is of the static type. Hypothermia and antihistamines, aldosterone, heparin, and a number of other drugs have been used in the management of experimental shock; their value in man remains to be proved. The use of suprapharmacologic doses of corticosteroids may be of value if they are given immediately and for a short period of time. The use of mannitol or other potent diuretics in the hope of maintaining urine output may be helpful but it is not mandatory. Whatever the cause of shock, the basis of treatment is prevention, if possible, and the immediate recognition, evaluation, and treatment of infection.

SUMMARY

1. Disease caused by virtually any of the known infectious agents may directly or indirectly involve the heart muscle or the membranes that line it.

2. The diagnosis and treatment of infectious heart disease demand the same great care that is needed in any other infectious or cardiac disease.

3. Because cardiac involvement by infection can be life threatening and can damage the heart permanently, the diagnosis should be made and therapy should be started with a maximum of vigor and a minimum of delay.

4. But the urgency of the situation should never be allowed to cause panic in the physician, resulting in a decision to treat without being certain that a treatable disease is present or before having obtained sufficient information to allow a rational choice of effective therapy.

SELECTED READING

Pericarditis

1. Benzing, G., III, and Kaplan, S.: Purulent pericarditis. Am. J. Dis. Child. 106:289, 1963.
2. Boyle, J. D., Pearce, M. L., and Guze, L. B.: Purulent pericarditis: Review of literature and resport of 11 cases. Medicine 41:119, 1961.
3. Clark, E.: Pericarditis. Bull. N.Y. Acad. Med. 40:511, 1964.
4. Herrman, G. R., Marchand, E. J., Grur, G. H., et al.: Pericarditis: Clinical and laboratory data of 130 cases. Am. Heart J. 43:641, 1952.
5. Rooney, J. J., Crocco, J. A., and Lyons, H. A.: Tuberculous pericarditis. Ann. Intern. Med. 72:73, 1970.
6. Wolff, L., and Wolff, R.: Diseases of the pericardium. Ann. Rev. Med. 16:21, 1965.
7. Woodward, T. E., McCrumb, F. R., Carey, T. N., et al.: Viral and rickettsial causes of cardiac disease, including the Coxsackie virus etiology of pericarditis and myocarditis. Ann. Intern. Med. 53:1130, 1960.

Endocarditis

1. Amoury, R. A., Bowman, F. O., and Malm, J. F.: Endocarditis associated with intracardiac prostheses. J. Thorac. Cardiovasc. Surg. 51:36, 1966.
2. Andriole, V. T., Kravetz, H. M., Roberts, W. C., et al.: Candida endocarditis: Clinical and pathologic studies. Am. J. Med. 32:251, 1962.
3. Belli, J., and Waisbren, B. A.: Number of blood cultures necessary to diagnose most cases of bacterial endocarditis. Am. J. Med. Sci. 232:284, 1956.
4. Bennett, I. L., and Beeson, P. B.: Bacteremia: A consideration of some experimental and clinical aspects. Yale J. Biol. Med. 26:241, 1954.
5. Block, P. C., De Sanctis, R. W., Weinberg, A. N., et al.: Prosthetic valve endocarditis. J. Thorac. Cardiovasc. Surg. 60:54, 1970.
6. Blount, J. G.: Bacterial endocarditis. Am. J. Med. 38:909, 1965.
7. Braniff, B. A., Shumway, N. E., and Harrison, D. C.: Valve replacement in active bacterial endocarditis. N. Engl. J. Med. 276:1464, 1967.
8. Conway, N., Kothari, M. L., Lockey, E., et al.: *Candida* endocarditis after heart surgery. Thorax 23:353, 1968.
9. Davis, A., Binder, M. J., and Finegold, S. M.: Late infection in patients with Starr-Edwards prosthetic valves. Antimicrob. Agents Chemother. 5:97, 1965.
10. Denton, C., Pappas, E. G., Uricchio, J. F., et al.: Bacterial endocarditis following cardiac surgery. Circulation 15:525, 1957.
11. Derby, B. M., Coolidge, K., and Rogers, D. E.: *Histoplasma capsulatum* endocarditis with major arterial embolism. Arch. Intern. Med. 110:63, 1962.
12. Felner, J. M., and Dowell, V. R., Jr.: Anaerobic bacterial endocarditis. N. Engl. J. Med. 283:1188, 1970.

13. Goodman, J. S., Schaffner, W., Collins, H. A., et al.: Infection after cardiovascular surgery: Clinical study including examination of antimicrobial prophylaxis. N. Engl. J. Med. 278:117, 1968.
14. Hall, B., and Dowling, H. F.: Negative blood cultures in bacterial endocarditis: A decade's experience. Med. Clin. North Am. 50:159, 1966.
15. Hancock, E. W., Shumway, N. E., and Remington, J. S.: Valve replacement in active bacterial endocarditis. (Editorial.) J. Infect. Dis. 123:106, 1971.
16. Hurley, E. J., Eldridge, F. C., and Hultgren, H. N.: Emergency replacement of valves in endocarditis. Am. Heart J. 73:798, 1967.
17. Kaplan, K., and Weinstein, L.: Diphtheroid infections of man. Ann. Intern. Med. 70:919, 1969.
18. Kaye, J. H., Bernstein, S., Frinstein, D., et al.: Surgical cure of *Candida albicans* endocarditis with open heart surgery. N. Engl. J. Med. 264:907, 1961.
19. Kaye, D., McCormack, R. C., and Hook, E. W.: Bacterial endocarditis: Changing pattern since introduction of penicillin therapy. Antimicrob. Agents Chemother. 37:46, 1961.
20. Kaye, J. H., Bernstein, S., Tsuji, H. K., et al: Surgical treatment of Candida endocarditis. J.A.M.A. 203:621, 1968.
21. Kerr, A., Jr.: Clinical picture: Fever, murmur, evidence of bacteremia. *In* Subacute Bacterial Endocarditis. Edited by A. Kerr, Jr. Springfield, Ill., Charles C Thomas, 1955. p. 65.
22. Lawrence, T., Shockman, A. T., and MacVaugh, H., III: *Aspergillus* infection of prosthetic aortic valves. Chest 60:406, 1971.
23. Lerner, P. I., and Weinstein, L.: Infective endocarditis in the antibiotic era. N. Engl. J. Med. 274:199, 259, 323, 388, 1966.
24. Mandell, G. L., Kaye, D., Levison, M. E., et al.: Enterococcal endocarditis. Arch. Intern. Med. 125:258, 1970.
25. Sande, M. A., Johnson, W. D., Jr., Hook, E. W., et al.: Sustained bacteremia in patients with prosthetic cardiac valves. N. Engl. J. Med. 286:1067, 1972.
26. Segal, C., Wheeler, C. G., and Tompsett, R.: Histoplasma endocarditis cured with amphotericin. N. Engl. J. Med. 280:206, 1969.
27. Shafer, R. B., and Hall, W. H.: Bacterial endocarditis following open heart surgery. Am. J. Cardiol. 25:602, 1970.
28. Walker, S. R., Shumway, N. W., and Merigan, T. C.: Management of infected cardiac valve prostheses. J.A.M.A. 208:531, 1969.
29. Weinstein, L.: Infected prosthetic valves: A diagnostic and therapeutic dilemma. (Editorial.) N. Engl. J. Med. 286:1108, 1972.
30. Weinstein, L., and Rubin, R. H.: Infective endocarditis—1973. Prog. Cardiovasc. Dis. 16:239, 1973.
31. Yeh, T. J., Anabtawi, I. N., Cornett, V. E., et al.: Bacterial endocarditis following open heart surgery. Ann. Thorac. Surg. 3:29, 1967.

Myocarditis

1. Abelmann, W. H.: Myocarditis. N. Engl. J. Med. 275:832, 1966.
2. Ryon, D. S., Pastor, B. H., and Myerson, R. M.: Abscess of the myocardium. Am. J. Med. Sci. 251:698, 1966.

Shock

1. Lillehei, R. C., Longerbeam, J. K., and Bloch, J. H.: Physiology and therapy of bacteremic shock: Experimental and clinical observations. Am. J. Cardiol. 13:599, 1963.
2. Lillehei, R. C., Longerbeam, J. K., Bloch, J. H., and Manax, W. G.: Modern treatment of shock based on physiologic principles. Clin. Pharmacol. Ther. 5:63, 1964.
3. MacLean, L. D., Duff, J. H., Scott, H. M., and Peretz, D. I.: Treatment of shock in man based on hemodynamic diagnosis. Surg. Gynecol. Obstet. 120:1, 1965.

4. McCabe, W. R., and Jackson, G. G.: Gram-negative bacteremia. I. Etiology and ecology. Arch. Intern. Med. 110:847, 1962.

5. McHenry, M. C., Martin, W. J., and Wellman, W. E.: Bacteremia due to gram-negative bacilli: Review of 113 cases encountered in five-year period 1955 through 1959. Ann. Intern. Med. 56:207, 1962.

6. Spink, W. W.: Endotoxin shock. Ann. Intern. Med. 57:538, 1962.

7. Udhoji, V. N., Weil, M. H., Sambhi, M. P., and Rosoff, L.: Hemodynamic studies on clinical shock associated with infection. Am. J. Med. 34:461, 1963.

8. Udhoji, V. N., and Weil, M. H.: Hemodynamic and metabolic studies on shock associated with bacteremia: Observations on 16 patients. Ann. Intern. Med. 62:966, 1965.

9. Weil, M. H., and Spink, W. W.: Comparison of shock due to endotoxin with anaphylactic shock. J. Lab. Clin. Med. 50:501, 1957.

10. Weil, M. H., Shubin, H., and Biddle, M.: Shock caused by gram-negative microorganisms: Analysis of 169 cases. Ann. Intern. Med. 60:384, 1964.

11. Weinstein, L., and Klainer, A. S.: Management of emergencies. IV. Septic shock—pathogenesis and treatment. N. Engl. J. Med. 274:950, 1966.

Chapter 14

ACUTE CARDIAC TAMPONADE

DAVID H. SPODICK

Cardiac tamponade is defined as the decompensated phase of cardiac compression due to an unchecked increase in intrapericardial pressure.[1] Rising pericardial pressure results from the relentless accumulation in the pericardial sac of one or more fluids—inflammatory exudate, blood, pus, chyle, or gas—that first fill and then stretch the parietal pericardium. When the elastic limit of that membrane is exceeded, the intrapericardial pressure rises and the heart is compressed, causing progressive restriction of ventricular filling. Depending on the tempo of the inciting process, sooner or later cardiac compensation fails, producing signs of severe circulatory failure. A low-grade inflammation, for example, may slowly fill the sac with from several hundred ml to one or two liters of fluid before that point is reached, because the pericardial fibrosa can stretch considerably if it is distended slowly. By contrast, brisk intrapericardial hemorrhage from a heart wound or aortic dissection can cause lethal cardiac compression by as little as 150 ml of blood in seconds to minutes.

The course of events leading to cardiac tamponade is diagrammed in Figure 14–1. The normal potential pericardial space is filled by the first 80 to 120 ml,[1] after which its elastic tissue permits the parietal pericardium to "give" as fluid accumulates (Fig. 14–1A).

COMPENSATED PHASE OF TAMPONADE

During the compensated phase, arterial and ventricular systolic pressures are fairly well maintained in the face of rising ventricular diastolic,

295

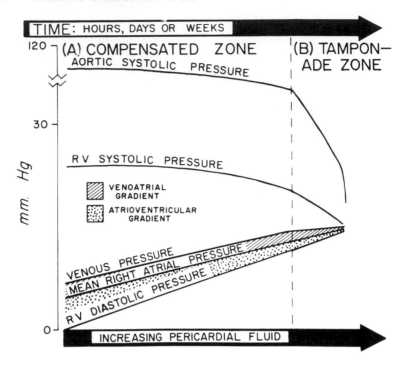

Figure 14–1. Schema of circulatory events during acute cardiac compression. A. Period of effective compensation: Increasing pericardial fluid may cause increasing intrapericardial pressure, but it does not accumulate rapidly enough to overcome adjustments of the circulation; transvalvular gradients are maintained at some level. B. Pericardial tamponade: Either intrapericardial pressure rises too rapidly to permit compensation or compensatory mechanisms have been exhausted; pressure gradients—transvalvular and venoatrial—are rapidly liquidated. (Reprinted with permission from Spodick.[1])

atrial, and venous pressures. That is possible because of the compensatory mechanisms that support atrial filling and ventricular minute output, principally (1) tachycardia, (2) arterial vasoconstriction, and (3) expansion of venous blood volume, with (4) venous hypertension.

DECOMPENSATED PHASE OF TAMPONADE

The vertical broken line in Figure 14–1 indicates the point at which compensatory mechanisms become inadequate and there is tamponade of the heart (Fig. 14–1B): rapid circulatory collapse marked by great atrial and venous hypertension, with plunging arterial and ventricular systolic pressures.

TEMPORAL ASPECTS OF TAMPONADE

Development of full-blown tamponade may take hours, days, or weeks in most forms of pericarditis or pericardial neoplasia. An important exception is rapidly developing hemopericardium, particularly in cardiac wounds, aortic dissection, and ruptured myocardial infarction or aneurysm. There, because of massive hemorrhage, the compensatory mechanisms rarely have a chance to operate. There is no time for intravenous blood volume expansion, and the heart is irretrievably compressed in seconds to minutes, with shock and no detectable venous hypertension.

CRITICAL PHASE OF TAMPONADE

In all the circumstances just mentioned, at some critical point (broken line, Fig. 14–1) during slow or rapid tamponade, quite small increments of intrapericardial contents cause disproportionate rises of pressure in the tight, low-compliance sac. The corollary to that phenomenon, with crucial therapeutic implications, is that quite small decrements in intrapericardial contents can result in marked relief of cardiac compression. Thus it is vital to recognize cardiac tamponade or impending tamponade in order to prevent or treat excessive cardiac compression with the expectation that appropriate treatment will usually give dramatic results. That is, in fact, usually the case, and the relief of cardiac tamponade is often a dramatic and rewarding experience.[1]

RECOGNITION OF CARDIAC TAMPONADE: A DIAGNOSTIC OUTLINE

The accurate diagnosis of cardiac tamponade and its differentiation from other causes of circulatory embarrassment depend on:

1. An awareness of the appropriate clinical settings: the systemic and local disorders associated with or capable of causing tamponade. Those disorders are listed in Table 14–1.

2. The recognition of any inflammatory or neoplastic pericardial disease as a potential source of tamponade[1,3]

3. The anticipation of swift tamponade during diseases that, by penetrating the heart or aortic wall, may cause rapid exsanguination into the pericardial sac—notably, dissecting aortic hematoma, acute myocardial infarction, and wounds of the chest or upper abdomen.

4. The detection of any pericardial effusion and its positive differentiation from cardiomegaly by echocardiography, cardioangiography, pneumoatriography, or radioisotope scanning.[2]

Table 14–1.   *Causative Factors in Pericardial Tamponade*

Idiopathic pericarditis (syndrome)	Diseases of contiguous or nearby structures (cont'd)
Pericarditis due to living agents	Hemopericardium of uncertain origin
Viral	Postmyocardial-infarction syndromes
Suppurative	Dissecting hematoma (aneurysm) of the aorta
Tuberculous	
Other (e.g., parasites)	Pleural and pulmonary diseases
Trauma	Pneumonia
Direct	Pleuritis
Penetrating chest or abdominal injury	Neoplasia
Surgical	Diseases of mediastinal structures
Cardiac catheterization	Inflammations and infections
Esophageal perforation	Neoplasia
Indirect	
Nonpenetrating (blunt) chest injury	Disorders of metabolism
Therapeutic irradiation of mediastinum or juxtacardiac structures	Uremic pericarditis
	Hemorrhagic states
Postmyocardial/pericardial injury syndromes	Cholesterol pericarditis
	Others
Neoplasia	Pericarditis with effusion in vasculitis-connective tissue disease group
Secondary	
Pulmonary	Lupus erythematosus
Breast	Acute rheumatic fever
Lymphoma	Rheumatoid arthritis
Other	Others
Primary (mesothelioma)	Pericarditis in hypersensitivity states
Diseases of contiguous or nearby structures	Serum sickness syndrome
Myocardial infarction	Others
Pericardial effusion from "epistenocardiac" pericarditis	Pericarditis of uncertain origin
	Certain syndromes: Reiter's, Behcet's, Löffler's
Myocardial rupture	
Hemopericardium associated (apparently) with anticoagulant administration	Pericardial effusion associated with pancreatitis
	Others

5. The detection of evidence that is more or less specific for cardiac tamponade if it occurs in appropriate clinical settings:

    a. The picture of "shock" with venous distention

    b. Central venous pressure above 180 mm H_2O, with absent y-descent in the venous and atrial pulses (except in patients with wounds of the heart or aorta who cannot have elevated venous pressure although they may have venous pulsations)

    c. Marked pulsus paradoxus: (1) an inspiratory decline or absence of the pulse or (2) an inspiratory drop in systolic blood pressure exceeding 15 mm Hg or, if the pulse pressure is less than that, equal to most or all of the pulse pressure[2,4]

    d. Inspiratory expansion of the right ventricle and compression of the left ventricle by echocardiogram

   e. Absence of a third heart sound

   f. Marked anatomic alternation of the heart by echocardiogram ("swinging" heart)

   g. Marked electric alternation of the heart, particularly if it involves the P waves as well as the QRS[4]

DEFINITIVE MANAGEMENT OF ACUTE TAMPONADE

The swift relief of acute or impending cardiac tamponade is mandatory. The pericardial contents must be evacuated as soon as possible. A few patients have overcome small-to-moderate degrees of cardiac compression, but the outlook is unpredictable, and always hanging over the patient is the threat of a sudden increment in pericardial effusion or hemorrhage, which even if small would be catastrophic in an already tight system. The specific treatment of acute cardiac tamponade is the *removal of pericardial fluid*—by needle paracentesis if possible or by surgical drainage if necessary. In the absence of significant complicating disorders (severe heart disease, true shock from exsanguination, overwhelming sepsis, underlying constrictive epicarditis[5,6]), successful pericardial drainage produces truly dramatic subjective and objective changes in the patient: (1) a rise in arterial systolic and pulse pressure, (2) a decrease in heart rate, (3) the diminution or disappearance of pulsus paradoxus, electric alternation, and venous distention, (4) the disappearance of abnormal breathing patterns, (5) the clearing of any mental confusion, and (6) a general feeling of relief. Frequently, many of those changes occur on removal of the first 50 to 150 ml of fluid[4]—the exact reverse of the "last straw" phenomenon), in which it is the last small increment of pericardial fluid that finally decompensates the cardiac response to even massive effusions. In other words, the patient's hemodynamics slide back along the pressure curves as shown in Figure 14–1 from zone B to zone A.

Indications for Pericardial Drainage

Absolute Indications. The pericardium must be drained if there is frankly critical tamponade or when signs of early cardiac compression appear to be advancing. In particular, in the presence of adequate clinical or graphic evidence of pericardial effusion and acute cardiac compression,[2] pericardial drainage is often required if any of the following occur:

   1. Cyanosis, tachypnea, a clear-cut shocklike syndrome, impaired consciousness, or (rarely) convulsions

   2. Rising peripheral venous pressure above 130 mm H_2O

   3. Pulsus paradoxus, measured by brachial sphygmomanometry to exceed 50% of the pulse pressure

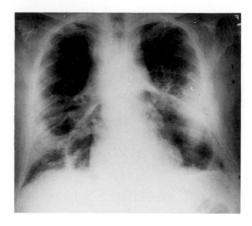

Figure 14–2.   Induced pneumohydropericardium. Patient who had cardiac tamponade due to metastases from bronchogenic carcinoma (bilateral lung lesions evident). After relief of cardiac compression by pericardiocentesis of tamponading effusion fluid, air has been insufflated into the pericardial sac through the needle used for the "tap." The heart is of normal size; the parietal pericardium is thin; there is residual fluid at the bottom of the sac.

Relative Indications. In the absence of florid tamponade, it may be desirable to drain large or increasing pericardial effusions to:
1. Forestall tamponade
2. Confirm the presence of effusion
3. Obtain fluid for etiologic diagnosis
4. Relieve intolerable chest discomfort
5. Instill certain therapeutic drugs[1]
6. Insufflate air (induced pneumohydropericardium) to demonstrate the state of the heart and pericardium[1,4,5] (Fig. 14–2).

Pericardial Paracentesis

Percutaneous needle aspiration of pericardial contents (pericardicentesis, pericardial tap) is the preferred method of drainage. In general, the distended pericardial sac can be tapped from any reasonably close location on the chest. In practice, certain "standard" points have been used (Fig. 14–3). The subxiphoid-subcostal approach (point 1, 2, or 3, Fig. 14–3) seems to be the safest one; in my experience, it has nearly always been successful. The technique for that approach, which appears to minimize the risk of cardiac injury, is as follows:
Subxiphoid-Subcostal Pericardicentesis and Catheterization. Under strict aseptic technique, the needle is inserted in the left or right xiphocostal angle or beneath the xiphoid tip perpendicular to the skin and 3 to 4 mm

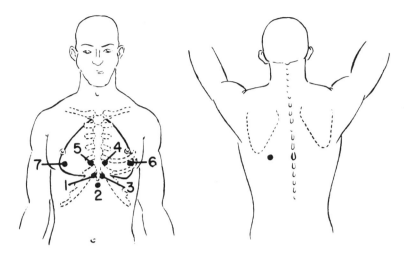

Figure 14–3.   "Standard" locations for pericardiocentesis approach. Anterior view: 1,2, and 3: Subxiphoid–subcostal approach points; 4 and 5: Fifth left and right intercostal spaces, respectively, 1 cm from sternal edge. 6: Apical. 7: Approach for major fluid accumulation on right side. Posterior view: Posterior approach. Details of subxiphoid–subcostal route are given in text. For details of other routes, see Spodick.[1] (Reprinted with permission from Spodick.[1])

below the costal margin. When the point of the needle penetrates to the level of the inner aspect of the rib cage, the hub of the needle is gently depressed so that the needle points toward the left shoulder (northeast by north). The needle is then cautiously advanced about 5 to 10 mm and its hub further depressed so that the point is only a few mm from the inner aspect of the rib cage (the hub at that point may have to be pressed into the abdominal wall if the patient has a protuberant abdomen). The needle is now cautiously advanced again by a worm gear–type turning action of the fingers until fluid is reached. (But when the parietal pericardium is punctured, there is often but not always a distinct "give.") If the epicardial surface of the heart is contacted, a definite "ticking" sensation is usually communicated to the fingers (and may even be felt on a syringe attached to the needle hub); if that occurs, the needle is immediately withdrawn a few mm, the hub is further depressed, and a new advance is attempted in a parallel axis. If fluid is not encountered and the heart not contacted, the needle should likewise be withdrawn slightly and the hub elevated for another advance in another "northeast" axis. Once in place, the needle should be replaced by a plastic catheter although quick removal of some fluid usually is desirable.

Equipment for Pericardiocentesis and Pericardial Catheterization. Except in an immediate life-or-death crisis, a 20- or 21-gauge needle should first be used to anesthetize the skin and subcutaneous tissue with procaine or an equivalent anesthetic drug.

Paracentesis is best performed with fairly large-bore needles and catheters, because proteinaceous inflammatory exudates, even those free of blood or pus, tend to congeal and because much more rapid evacuation is possible through wider lumens. A #16 Jelco- or Rochester-type needle can give good results and can be withdrawn, leaving its catheter inside the pericardial sac. For bloody or viscous fluids, a #14 thin-wall needle with obturator can be used (with extreme care). Through it, a PE-190 plastic catheter can be passed and its external end attached to a syringe or suction apparatus via a Touhey-type adapter.

When needles without attached catheters are used, soft-tip Amplatz-type "piano" wires can be passed through the needle, the needle withdrawn, and an appropriate catheter threaded over the emplaced wire.

It is desirable to use catheters that contain a radiopaque filament that permits their location to be checked by fluoroscopy or radiography.

Safeguards. Since in pericardicentesis a sharp weapon is aimed at the heart, certain protective measures are desirable:

1. The usual crashcart items should be available, including (a) pressor drugs, (b) intravenous fluids, (c) oxygen, (d) tracheal tubes, (e) a defibrillator-pacemaker, and (f) an ECG monitor.

2. A slow intravenous drip of saline or glucose in water should be started to preserve a route for intravenous therapy.

3. The shank of the paracentesis needle may be attached to the chest lead of an ECG or oscilloscope monitor by means of an insulated wire with an alligator clamp at each end. If the point of the needle contacts the ventricle, the S–T segment rises and there may be ventricular ectopic beats; when it touches the atrium, the P–R segment is elevated and atrial ectopic beats can be provoked. But even with that safeguard, the needle should be advanced slowly since there may be a delay in registering any change. Sometimes this system fails to record changes.

4. A preliminary attempt with a 20-gauge needle (it can be the needle used to deposit local anesthetic along the paracentesis route) will sometimes establish the adequacy of the route selected and the required depth of penetration. Occasionally it suffices for the removal of fluid.

5. If bloody fluid is withdrawn, it is important to know quickly whether the needle has penetrated the heart. (In tamponade, the removal of circulating blood from the heart or any vessel could be disastrous.) A microhematocrit apparatus should be available to compare the hematocrit of the first aliquot of fluid with that of the peripheral blood. If oxygen saturation is tested, intrapericardial blood may show a level below 35%. This is unlikely with intracardiac blood, even with cardiogenic shock.

Meanwhile, a drug used to estimate the circulation time may be injected. If the patient tastes the sodium dehydrocholate, saccharin, or magnesium sulfate, the needle is surely in the heart or a blood vessel. For patients unable to respond, the fluorescein-ultraviolet light technique or a radio-isotope may be used.

6. Failure of paracentesis to deliver fluid does not rule out pericardial effusion or hemorrhage; if the diagnostic criteria are strong, surgical intervention is mandatory.

Surgical Drainage of the Pericardium

When the diagnosis of pericardial effusion with tamponade is reasonably certain, failure to aspirate fluid or to successfully relieve tamponade by aspiration indicates the need for surgical drainage (pericardiotomy). A small subcostal or intercostal incision may be adequate although resection of a costal cartilage, or even thoracotomy, may be needed, especially in the case of loculated effusion. The individual situation dictates the initial surgical approach and the subsequent plan.

In tamponade due to penetrating wounds of the heart and great vessels, there is evidence favoring either:

1. Routine surgical intervention, either following an initial tap or without delay

2. Surgery only if the patient becomes worse despite a successful pericardiocentesis

The current trend in managing heart wounds is toward the more radical approach because paracentesis may not remove clots and because of late deaths and complications owing to repeated cardiac bleeding or progressive pericardial disease. Clotting is a serious problem in traumatic hemopericardium. Indeed, intrapericardial clotting can produce a false-negative echocardiogram.[7] In inflammatory and neoplastic effusions, intrapericardial blood obtained during pericardiocentesis rarely tends to clot, owing to dilution and the defibrinating effect of being constantly agitated by cardiac motion. During pure pericardial bleeding, there is no dilution, and tissue thromboplastic factors released by wounds will promote intrapericardial clotting, which tends to defeat pericardiocentesis while permitting cardiac compression to proceed.

SUPPORTIVE MANAGEMENT

If there is difficulty in draining the pericardium or if there is delay in obtaining equipment, the heart and circulation can be maintained until either successful pericardiocentesis or pericardiotomy is performed.

Supportive measures usually are unavoidable when tamponade is associated with significant blood loss. They include, particularly, the use of:

1. Intravenous fluids

2. Adrenergic stimulants, which bolster physiologic compensatory mechanisms

3. Oxygen, which may be helpful, particularly in patients with marked dyspnea, cyanosis, or psychic disturbances. But it should not be delivered by positive-pressure breathing (which raises both the intrapleural and intrapericardial pressures, thus reducing the venous return to the heart).

4. Digitalis. The place of digitalis and related substances is not clear; they may be of particular use in patients who also have heart disease.

5. Intravenously administered fluids which maintain cardiac filling by expanding the venous blood volume and maintaining the small venoatrial gradient. Glucose or saline solutions may be used, but for traumatic bleeding and in patients with severe anemias, blood is preferable.

6. Pressor drugs, particularly those with beta-adrenergic effects, produce increased myocardial stroke work per unit of effective filling pressure. They can thus support stroke volume despite cardiac tamponade. Dopamine may be the drug of choice owing to better peripheral distribution of the increased cardiac output.[8] Cardiac tamponade is one of the few disorders in which the "ideal" beta-adrenergic stimulant, isoproterenol, can be truly effective. Norepinephrine, which has both alpha- and beta-adrenergic stimulating effects, is also helpful.

SUMMARY

1. Cardiac tamponade, the decompensated phase of cardiac compression, occurs when relatively small increments in intrapericardial contents begin to cause disproportionate rises in intrapericardial pressure.

2. The accurate diagnosis of tamponade depends on (a) the awareness of the appropriate clinical settings, along with recognition of any inflammatory or neoplastic pericardial disease, (b) the detection of any pericardial effusion and its differentiation from cardiomegaly and congestive heart failure, and (c) the anticipation of swift cardiac compression associated with diseases and wounds capable of producing intrapericardial hemorrhage.

3. More or less specific indications for tamponade include (a) "shock" with venous distention (in the absence of acute hemorrhage), (b) increased venous pressure with absent y-descent in venous pulses, (c) marked pulsus paradoxus with inspiratory expansion of the right ventricle and compression of the left ventricle on the echocardiogram, (d) absence of a third heart sound, (e) marked electric alternation on the ECG, and (f) mechanical alternation ("swinging") on the echocardiogram.

4. The specific management of tamponade is evacuation of pericardial contents by needle paracentesis if possible or by surgical drainage if necessary.

5. One of those measures is absolutely indicated if the signs of cardiocirculatory embarrassment are either already marked or are moderate but detectably progressing.

6. Relative indications for one of those measures include the etiologic diagnosis of pericardial lesions, relief of symptoms (large effusions), intrapericardial administration of therapeutic drugs, and production of an induced pneumohydropericardium.

7. With the use of appropriate safeguards, pericardial paracentesis can be performed using numerous approaches, but the subxiphoid-subcostal route is preferred.

8. Insertion of an intrapericardial catheter should be routine to minimize trauma, permit continuous drainage, and obviate repeated needle punctures. The inability to remove fluid in that way mandates surgical drainage (which may be the definitive method for penetrating wounds of the heart and great vessels).

9. While paracentesis or surgical equipment is awaited, temporary relief of tamponade can be obtained by the intravenous administration of fluids and inotropic drugs, particularly dopamine.

Infectious heart disease is discussed in detail in Chapter 13, and the surgical approach to cardiac emergencies is discussed in Chapter 18.

REFERENCES

1. Spodick, D.H.: Acute Pericarditis. New York, Grune & Stratton, 1959.
2. Spodick, D.H.: Acute cardiac tamponade: Pathophysiology, diagnosis and management. Prog. Cardiovasc. Dis. 10:64, 1967.
3. Spodick, D.H.: Differential diagnosis of acute pericarditis. Prog. Cardiovasc. Dis. 14:192, 1971.
4. Spodick, D.H.: Electric alternation of the heart: Its relation to the kinetics and physiology of the heart during cardiac tamponade. Am. J. Cardiol. 10:155, 1962.
5. Spodick, D.H.: Chronic and Constrictive Pericarditis. New York, Grune & Stratton, 1964.
6. Spodick, D.H., and Kumar, S.: Subacute constrictive pericarditis and cardiac tamponade. Dis. Chest 54:62, 1968.
7. Kerber, R., and Payvandi, M.V.: Echocardiography in acute hemopericardium. (Abstr.) Circulation 56(Suppl. III):24, 1977.
8. Martins, J., Kerber, R., and Mateus, M.: Comparative effects of inotropic agents on organ perfusion in acute tamponade. (Abstr.) Circulation 56(Suppl. III):39, 1977.

Chapter 15

HYPERTENSIVE CRISIS

ALBERT N. BREST

GENERAL CONSIDERATIONS

Severe arterial blood pressure elevation may lead to a variety of clinical emergencies, including hypertensive encephalopathy, acute left ventricular failure, intracranial hemorrhage, acute coronary insufficiency, acute dissecting aneurysm of the aorta, and malignant hypertension. Such emergencies may occur during the course of either primary or secondary hypertension.

All of the various hypertensive crises demand rapid blood pressure reduction although not necessarily to normotensive levels and not necessarily with the same urgency. Thus hypertension associated with acute encephalopathy or aortic dissection requires immediate blood pressure reduction (i.e., within minutes or hours), whereas malignant or accelerated hypertension usually can be treated effectively by reduction of the arterial pressure within days. Hypertensive crises associated with impaired renal or cerebral function should be treated initially by moderate blood pressure reduction, with careful observation of the patient's subsequent clinical status to determine whether further blood pressure reduction is feasible.

There is no single level of blood pressure elevation that augurs the development of a hypertensive emergency. Instead, a moderate arterial blood pressure elevation may in certain circumstances induce hyperten-

307

sive crisis (e.g., in patients whose hypertension develops rather suddenly—children and adolescents with acute renal disease or women with the toxemia of pregnancy), whereas severe blood pressure elevation may at times occur without acute complications (e.g., in patients with longstanding hypertension).

CLINICAL ASPECTS

Acute Hypertensive Encephalopathy

Acute hypertensive encephalopathy is a dramatic clinical syndrome characterized by (1) sudden escalation of the blood pressure (i.e., an acute onset of hypertension or an acute exacerbation of previously existing hypertension), which is followed rapidly by (2) severe headache and altered consciousness. The disorder can end in death within a few days if it is not promptly recognized and rapidly reversed.

The term hypertensive encephalopathy is sometimes used loosely to designate severe blood pressure elevation by itself, without accompanying encephalopathy. However, the loose terminology is to be deplored, especially since the prognostic implications and therapeutic considerations for hypertensive encephalopathy are materially different from those for severe hypertension by itself.

Typically, diastolic blood pressure levels of 150 mm Hg or higher are encountered in acute hypertensive encephalopathy. However, lesser levels may also be associated with hypertensive encephalopathy, especially in patients with initial rather than longstanding hypertension. Accordingly, hypertensive encephalopathy may be encountered at times in patients whose diastolic blood pressure levels are no greater than 110 mm Hg (e.g., in children with acute glomerulonephritis or in pregnant women with toxemia). In addition to the hypertension, the other typical physical abnormality in hypertensive encephalopathy is found in the optic fundus, namely, extreme retinal arterial narrowing. The severe arterial spasm is often but not always accompanied by papilledema. Less commonly, retinal hemorrhage and exudates are seen.

Clinical Manifestations. Acute hypertensive encephalopathy is manifested predominantly by severe headache and altered consciousness, that is, drowsiness, stupor, disorientation, and even coma. Those manifestations may be accompanied by nausea, vomiting, visual blurring or blindness, and focal or generalized seizures. The clinical syndrome may be full blown within a few hours, or it may take a day or two to develop.

Pathology. Pathologically, cerebral edema is the most commonly encountered abnormality. At times, the cerebral pathology includes petechial hemorrhages, tiny infarcts, and arteriolar necrosis; in some cases, herniation of the medulla into the foramen magnum may account for death.

Pathophysiology. The pathophysiologic sequence of hypertensive encephalopathy appears to result from intense arterial spasm. The attendant cerebral ischemia is accompanied by increased capillary permeability, capillary wall ruptures, petechial hemorrhages, microinfarcts, and cerebral edema.

Diagnosis. The clinical diagnosis can be recognized by the abrupt onset, the usually severe blood pressure elevation, and the typical funduscopic abnormalities, in combination with the rapidly progressive encephalopathy. The ECG generally reveals focal or generalized dysrhythmias, while the cerebrospinal fluid pressure and protein content may be increased or normal. Skull X-rays, brain scan, and echoencephalogram are unremarkable in acute hypertensive encephalopathy. Prompt clinical improvement (sometimes within an hour or two) following blood pressure reduction serves to confirm the clinical impression. Obviously, the more prolonged the condition and the more severe the manifestations, the more prolonged and less complete the recovery.

Differential Diagnosis. The differential diagnosis of acute hypertensive encephalopathy includes various disorders in which blood pressure elevation and neurologic dysfunction coexist. Accordingly, the syndrome must be differentiated from certain cases of cerebral infarction and cerebral vascular insufficiency, intracerebral or subarachnoid hemorrhage, brain tumor, cerebral embolism, head injury, acute encephalitis, cerebral vasculitis, and epilepsy. The differentiation is aided if it can be shown that the blood pressure elevation had first occurred after the onset of cerebral symptoms or, in the case of preexisting chronic hypertension, if it can be shown that the exacerbation of hypertension followed the onset of clinical symptoms. Unfortunately, such information may not be available. If it is not, the overall clinical picture and (sometimes even more important) the favorable response or lack of response to emergency antihypertensive therapy may serve to confirm or disprove the clinical impression of hypertensive encephalopathy. If there is reasonable doubt about the diagnosis, prompt reduction of blood pressure should be undertaken.

In addition to the differential diagnostic considerations mentioned, clinical confusion about the diagnosis sometimes arises in conditions such as acute pulmonary edema, acute coronary insufficiency, or acute anxiety, in which dramatic (although often transient) increases in blood pressure may be encountered. However, in such instances, close examination of the total clinical picture generally serves to dispel the confusion.

General Therapeutic Approach. As indicated, hypertensive encephalopathy calls for prompt recognition and immediate reduction of blood pressure to normal or near normal levels. It is preferable to treat the patients in an intensive care unit, where changes in blood pressure, state of consciousness, convulsive activity, and airway obstruction can be monitored closely and treated promptly. Antihypertensive drugs should be administered parenterally in order to achieve the reduction of blood pressure without undue delay.

Drug Therapy. The drugs of choice in most instances are diazoxide or sodium nitroprusside. However, hydralazine may be particularly effective in controlling hypertensive encephalopathy associated with acute glomerulonephritis or toxemia of pregnancy. Reserpine and methyldopa should be used cautiously, especially since their sedative effects may lead to confusion in evaluating the patient's sensorium. Furthermore, the delayed antihypertensive response to both reserpine and methyldopa is an additional disadvantage in this emergency situation.

Acute Left Ventricular Failure

Blood pressure elevation increases the cardiac afterload, which may, in turn, result in sudden cardiac decompensation. Acute pulmonary edema is the usual clinical expression of acute left ventricular failure.

General Therapeutic Approach. It is imperative to promptly reduce the workload of the incompetent left ventricle. Accordingly, prompt reduction of blood pressure is generally more important therapeutically than the administration of digitalis, although digitalis may be useful if the patient is not already taking the drug.

Reduction of blood pressure to normal levels is indicated in the management of acute heart failure associated with uncomplicated hypertensive heart disease. However, if the patient has accompanying symptomatic coronary disease, with or without acute myocardial infarction, a less profound reduction of blood pressure is indicated; otherwise, coronary insufficiency may be invoked.

Drug Therapy. Sodium nitroprusside or ganglioplegic drugs (such as trimethaphan or pentolinium) are particularly useful in the management of acute left ventricular failure because they reduce both the cardiac afterload and the preload, thereby decreasing systemic blood pressure and right ventricular pressure simultaneously. However, diazoxide also exerts favorable antihypertensive effects in this situation. Potent diuretics (e.g., furosemide) should also be employed because they tend to enhance the blood pressure reduction and to exert favorable anticongestive effects as well.

Ancillary therapeutic measures include bed rest, oxygen administration, morphine, and dietary salt restriction.

Congestive heart failure and digitalization are discussed in detail in Chapters 1 and 7, respectively.

Intracranial Hemorrhage

Severe hypertension may be complicated by subarachnoid or intracerebral hemorrhage.

General Therapeutic Approach. Blood pressure reduction is generally indicated in intracranial hemorrhage. However, arterial spasm has been demonstrated angiographically in the area surrounding the bleeding site, and relief of the angiospasm by antihypertensive therapy may exacerbate the disorder. Accordingly, the blood pressure should be lowered cautiously, and the patient's neurologic status must be monitored carefully during the attempted blood pressure reduction. If neurologic deterioration ensues, less aggressive blood pressure lowering is indicated. Conversely, if the blood pressure reduction is well tolerated, it may be desirable to reduce the pressure to normotensive or even hypotensive levels.

Drug Therapy. The antihypertensive drugs of choice are sodium nitroprusside or the ganglioplegic drugs (such as trimethaphan or pentolinium). Each has a rapid onset and short duration of action that makes dosage titration easier by intravenous infusion than when intramuscular or bolus intravenous injections are given; furthermore, none of those drugs produces somnolence that would interfere with neurologic evaluation. Neurologic consultation should also be obtained, especially in the case of subarachnoid hemorrhage, for which surgical treatment may be more important than antihypertensive therapy.

The neurologic deficit associated with atherothrombotic stroke (cerebral infarct) is often aggravated by a drastic reduction in the blood pressure. That complication results from a decreased cerebral blood flow. Therefore if aggravation of cerebral ischemia is to be avoided, the blood pressure must be lowered cautiously. Again, the drugs of choice are sodium nitroprusside or ganglioplegic drugs.

Acute Coronary Insufficiency

Blood pressure elevation usually increases myocardial oxygen requirement, and a sharp rise in blood pressure may induce acute coronary insufficiency.

Although acute hypertension may induce coronary insufficiency, it may also happen that coronary insufficiency initiates blood pressure elevation, so that hypertension actually follows rather than precedes the coronary attack. The blood pressure rise in that circumstance may be the result of extreme anxiety with a reflexly induced blood pressure elevation; appropriate sedation will generally control the blood pressure rise.

General Therapeutic Approach. Acute coronary insufficiency that results in hypertension requires a cautious reduction in blood pressure. A drastic reduction must be avoided to prevent an undue reduction in coronary blood flow and ensuing acute myocardial infarction.

Drug Therapy. Sodium nitroprusside is valuable. However, reserpine is also useful because of its gradual antihypertensive effect, as well as its sedative action.

Acute Dissecting Aortic Aneurysm

Hypertension is the most common precursor of acute aortic dissection. Although the aorta in such a case often shows evidence of cystic medial necrosis, the degree of necrosis frequently is comparatively minor. Therefore the blood pressure elevation may be the more important factor in the pathogenesis of the disorder.

General Therapeutic Approach. Until recent years, the general impression was that acute aortic dissection had a rapid devolutionary clinical course that invariably ended in death within a few hours, days, or weeks at the most unless the lesion could be treated surgically. It is now evident, however, that acute aortic dissection can often be stabilized by hypotensive drug therapy. Thus rapid reduction of elevated arterial pressure is indicated for most patients who reach a hospital, either to prevent further dissection until surgery can be done or as the definitive, permanent measure to prevent extension of the dissection.

Drug Therapy. Medical management consists essentially of intensive monitoring and the use of drugs that decrease cardiac impulse and lower the systolic blood pressure. A suitable response can generally be achieved promptly with trimethaphan given intravenously. Unless surgery is imminent, it is advisable also to immediately begin the administration of drugs that can be maintained permanently, including a diuretic and antihypertensive drugs that decrease myocardial contractility (e.g., propranolol and guanethidine). The systolic blood pressure elevation should be maintained between 100 and 120 mm Hg. Hydralazine and diazoxide should be avoided because they tend to greatly increase the cardiac output and the stroke volume, and such effects could aggravate the aortic dissection.

Malignant and Accelerated Hypertension

Malignant hypertension and accelerated hypertension are associated with markedly elevated blood pressure and exudative retinopathy. In accelerated hypertension, the blood pressure elevation is accompanied by retinal hemorrhages and exudates, whereas in malignant hypertension, papilledema is also present.

The disorders tend to be associated with rapid systemic deterioration. Typically, the pathologic changes consist of diffuse necrotizing arteritis, which accounts for the attendant renal, cardiac, and cerebral dysfunction. In addition, acute renal ischemia usually induces the marked production of renin and secondary aldosteronism.

General Therapeutic Approach. Malignant hypertension and accelerated hypertension are semi-emergencies in that blood pressure reduction is required within days rather than within minutes or hours. Nonetheless, the rapid devolutionary course must not be underestimated.

Drug Therapy. Prompt blood pressure reduction may at times be achieved with oral antihypertensive therapy. However, to gain rapid control of hypertension, especially if oral medication is poorly tolerated because of nausea and vomiting, the use of parenterally administered antihypertensive drugs for several days may be valuable. Diazoxide, sodium nitroprusside, reserpine, trimethaphan, or pentolinium may be useful.

Hypertensive Crises Associated with Excess Circulating Catecholamines

Excess circulating catecholamines should be suspected in patients with severe blood pressure elevation associated with headache, palpitation, excessive sweating, tachycardia, facial pallor, and tremor of the hands. The syndrome may be caused by pheochromocytoma, the abrupt withdrawal of clonidine, or the ingestion of monoamine oxidase inhibitors plus tyramine-containing foods.

Drug Therapy. Phentolamine and sodium nitroprusside are the drugs of choice to control the hypertension. Also, propranolol administered intravenously may be added as needed to control any accompanying tachyarrhythmias.

ANTIHYPERTENSIVE DRUG THERAPY

Diazoxide

Diazoxide is a nondiuretic thiazide that exerts potent antihypertensive effects when administered intravenously. In contrast with the oral benzothiadiazine diuretics, the drug promotes sodium retention. Nonetheless, diazoxide is a potent and rapidly acting antihypertensive drug. It acts directly on the arterioles, with a resultant decrease in peripheral vascular resistance. Its antihypertensive effect is accompanied by an increase in heart rate and cardiac output, but the fall in blood pressure is not ordinarily accompanied by significant reduction in the renal blood flow or the glomerular filtration rate.

Administration. To be effective, diazoxide must be given rapidly (in 10 to 15 seconds) by intravenous push from a syringe without diluting the commercial preparation. The usual effective dosage is 300 mg. Blood pressure falls steeply, with a maximal effect achieved in 3 to 4 minutes. The effect may persist for 12 hours or longer.

Side Effects. Diazoxide causes sodium and fluid retention, and therefore if the drug must be used for more than two or three days, oral or parenterally administered diuretics should also be used. Because diazoxide induces hyperglycemia, the drug should be used with appropriate caution in diabetic patients. In addition, because diazoxide may cause abrupt cessation of labor, its use is limited in the toxemia of pregnancy. Diazoxide should be avoided in the medical treatment of acute dissection of the aorta because its enhancement of cardiac output may provide additional stress at the site of intimal tear.

When used in the standard manner of administration (a 300 mg intravenous bolus), diazoxide may be associated with cardiovascular complications, such as angina pectoris, myocardial infarction, and stroke. Hence, in patients with symptomatic coronary or cerebral vascular insufficiency or renal failure, mini-bolus (a 50 to 100 mg intravenous bolus) injections of the drug may be a useful alternative to provide gradual reduction of blood pressure. The mini-bolus injections may be repeated at 15-minute intervals until the diastolic blood pressure falls below 100 mm Hg.

Sodium Nitroprusside

Sodium nitroprusside, like diazoxide and hydralazine, is a direct vasodilator. However, in contrast to the other two vasodilators, sodium nitroprusside also relaxes venous smooth muscle, and the consequent venodilation results in decreased venous return and diminished cardiac output. The renal blood flow and the glomerular filtration rate usually remain constant because the renal vascular resistance falls about as much as the arterial pressure does. The drug is instantly and consistently effective.

Administration. The fall in arterial pressure during the intravenous administration of sodium nitroprusside depends on the rate of infusion. Blood pressure lowering occurs within seconds, and the hypotensive effect dissipates within a few minutes after the infusion is stopped. Therefore, the drug is best administered with an infusion pump; careful monitoring of the patient is also essential to prevent undesirable fluctuations in arterial pressure. Individual sensitivity varies, and infusion rates from 0.3 to 6 μg/kg/min may be required for adequate blood pressure control. Tolerance to the hypotensive action of sodium nitroprusside occurs very rarely if fluid retention is prevented with a diuretic. Because of the precipitous fall in blood pressure it can cause, the infusion should be titrated with particular care in patients with coronary or cerebrovascular insufficiency.

Side Effects. Since the nitroprusside ion is converted to thiocyanate, the serum levels of thiocyanate should be determined every other day if the infusion must be continued for longer than 72 hours. To avoid an acute toxic reaction, the infusion should be discontinued if the serum concentration of thiocyanate exceeds 12 mg/100 ml. The many manifestations of thiocyanate intoxication range from weakness, nausea, and tinnitus to hypothyroidism and psychosis.

Ganglioplegic Drugs

The ganglioplegic drugs are potent antihypertensive drugs, but their usefulness in the treatment of hypertensive emergencies is necessarily limited by the fact that their greatest effect is exerted when the patient is in the upright position. The ganglioplegic drugs are particularly indicated in instances of severe congestive heart failure in which blood pressure elevation is sudden, in acute dissecting aortic aneurysm, and in cases of severe hypertension complicated by intracranial hemorrhage. As therapeutic blockade is established, venous tone is reduced, with a resultant decrease in venous pressure, a decrease in right atrial pressure, and an increase in cardiac output. To obtain maximum benefit from ganglioplegic drugs, the patient should be in a semi-recumbent position, and the head of his bed should be elevated 10 to 12 inches on blocks.

Administration. Like sodium nitroprusside, trimethaphan must be administered by intravenous infusion under constant supervision. Usually, 1000 mg of trimethaphan is added to 1000 cc of a 5% solution of glucose in water. The adult dosage requirement ranges from 1 to 15 mg/min. When pentolinium is given by continuous intravenous infusion for hypertensive emergencies, 50 to 200 mg is placed in 1000 cc of a 5% solution of glucose in water. The drug is infused at a moderate rate until the blood pressure begins to fall, and then the rate of infusion is adjusted so as to maintain an adequate blood pressure reduction. For intramuscular injection, an initial dose of 5 mg is used and subsequent doses can be progressively increased (at 1 to 2 hour intervals) until the reduction is adequate or a maximum dose of 50 mg of pentolinium is being given. Response is rarely greater with larger doses. Because of the ensuing salt and water retention, diuretics should be added to the regimen whenever ganglioplegic drugs are administered for more than 24 hours.

Side Effects. Continuous parenteral use of the ganglioplegic drugs often leads to the development of ileus and urinary retention. Foley catheters are nearly always required for elderly men who receive ganglioplegic drugs for any significant period. Cathartics should be used freely for the relief of constipation, and cholinergic drugs are sometimes even more effective.

Reserpine

Parenteral reserpine is a potent antihypertensive drug that is effective in most hypertensive emergencies. Equally important is the fact that its antihypertensive effect is manifested when the patient is in the recumbent as well as the upright position, an attribute of particular importance when the patient is acutely ill and bedfast. However, following either the intravenous or intramuscular administration of the drug, there is a latent period of one to two hours before the blood pressure decreases. If immediate reduction of blood pressure is desirable, a more rapidly acting drug must be administered.

Administration. The initial recommended dose of parenteral reserpine is 1 to 2.5 mg. Thereafter, the dose may be increased by 2.5 mg increments until an adequate blood pressure reduction is achieved; however, at least two hours must be allowed between doses in order to observe the maximum response to any one dose. If necessary, subsequent doses of 5 or even 10 mg may be given, but individual doses should rarely exceed 10 mg and the total dose should not exceed 20 mg per day.

After the proper dose has been established, the patient can be placed on a schedule, usually 2.5 to 5 mg of reserpine every 6 to 12 hours. The dosage and the interval between doses depend on the blood pressure response and are adjusted so as to maintain the desired blood pressure level.

Side Effects. The side effects of reserpine tend to become more prominent as the dose or the frequency of administration is increased. Prolonged daily administration of more than 10 mg depresses cerebration and may cause a Parkinson's-like syndrome. The latter manifestations are temporary, however, and they tend to disappear several days after discontinuation of the drug. Reserpine may also activate peptic ulcers, leading to acute gastrointestinal bleeding. However, the major disadvantage of the drug is its tendency to cause profound somnolence. The soporific effect is particularly troublesome in cerebral hemorrhage or hypertensive encephalopathy, because it interferes with the clinical evaluation of the sensorium, which is so important in assessing the progress of the patients.

Hydralazine

Hydralazine, like diazoxide, reduces blood pressure by direct arteriolar dilator effects. Its use is commonly accompanied by reflex-mediated increases in the cardiac output and the heart rate. When administered alone, the drug occasionally aggravates or precipitates coronary insufficiency and congestive heart failure. In short-term use, hydralazine increases the renal blood flow. For that reason, the drug is especially effective in the management of hypertensive encephalopathy complicating acute or chronic glomerulonephritis or eclampsia. The onset of blood pressure reduction (15 to 20 minutes) is more rapid after the administration of hydralazine than after the administration of reserpine. However, the best results are often obtained when the two drugs are used in combination, hydralazine producing the more rapid action and reserpine allowing a more sustained effect. If hydralazine is administered over several days, tolerance to its hypotensive effect may necessitate a rapid increase in dosage or the addition of a diuretic.

Administration. An initial dose of 10 to 20 mg can be given intravenously as a single injection over a five-minute period, or a dose of 10 to 50 mg may be given intramuscularly. Then 100 mg may be placed in 1000 cc of a 10% solution of glucose in water and administered by continuous intravenous injection. The rate of infusion should be adjusted according to the blood pressure response. In other instances, blood pressure reduction may be maintained by giving hydralazine intramuscularly in doses ranging from 10 to 50 mg as often as every four hours.

Phentolamine

Phentolamine is an alpha-adrenergic blocking drug. Its use in hypertensive crises is recommended only for patients with excess levels of circulating catecholamines. The drug is ineffective in managing hypertensive crises arising from other causes. The effect of phentolamine is short lived, usually lasting less than 15 minutes. It may be desirable to administer phentolamine by constant intravenous infusion after the blood pressure has been controlled initially by rapid intravenous injection of 5 to 15 mg from a syringe.

The beta-adrenergic mediated effects of catecholamines are not blocked by phentolamine. Hence, accompanying tachyarrhythmias must be treated separately by intravenously administered propranolol. However, patients with excess circulating catecholamines should not be treated with a beta-adrenergic drug unless an alpha-adrenergic drug has already been used; otherwise, the hypertension may be exacerbated. Blocking only the vasodilator (beta-receptor) action of catecholamines leaves the vasoconstrictor (alpha-receptor) action unopposed, and a severe rise in blood pressure may ensue.

Methyldopa

Methyldopa reduces peripheral vascular resistance with only a modest fall in cardiac output (or none at all) and no reduction in renal blood flow. Intravenously administered methyldopa has a delayed onset of action (4 to 6 hours), which limits its effectiveness in hypertensive emergencies. The drug is less consistently effective than is reserpine. Furthermore, like reserpine, methyldopa may also cause sedation, thereby interfering with evaluation of the patient's sensorium. Thus the drug is usually avoided in patients with hypertensive encephalopathy or stroke. Methyldopa should be administered intravenously by intermittent infusion over a 30 to 60-minute interval; the usual dose is 250 to 1000 mg.

Diuretics

The antihypertensive action of all the antihypertensive drugs discussed is enhanced by the concomitant administration of a diuretic. The diuretic drugs of choice are furosemide or ethacrynic acid because (1) they can be given intravenously, (2) they are rapidly effective, and (3) they do not cause an acute decline in the glomerular filtration rate (unlike the thiazide diuretics).

The usual dose of furosemide is 40 to 80 mg, whereas ethacrynic acid is given in a dose of 50 to 100 mg. Larger doses may be required in patients with impairment of renal function. Both furosemide and ethacrynic acid may cause nerve deafness when rapidly infused intravenously in large doses in azotemic patients.

OVERALL THERAPEUTIC APPROACH

An outline for the drug treatment of hypertensive emergencies is given in Table 15–1. The useful attributes of individual drugs are listed in Table 15–2. Quick appraisal of the state of renal compensation is extremely important, as is evaluation of the patient's cardiac and cerebral status. Evaluation of renal function can best be done by measurement of the serum creatinine level. When the creatinine level is elevated, serial values should be measured every two or three days while the blood pressure is being regulated. When evidence of a rising creatinine level is observed, the blood pressure should be allowed to increase slowly by reducing the

Table 15–1. *Outline for Parenteral Drug Treatment of Hypertensive Emergencies*

Emergency	Preferred Drug(s)	Drug(s) to Avoid or to Use with Caution
Acute hypertensive enceph- alopathy	Diazoxide Sodium nitroprusside	Reserpine Methyldopa
Acute ventricular failure	Sodium nitroprusside Trimethaphan Pentolinium	Hydralazine
Intracranial hemorrhage	Sodium nitroprusside Trimethaphan Pentolinium	Reserpine Methyldopa
Acute coronary insuffi- ciency	Sodium nitroprusside Reserpine	Hydralazine
Acute dissecting aortic aneurysm	Trimethaphan	Hydralazine Diazoxide
Malignant and accelerated hypertension	Diazoxide Sodium nitroprusside Reserpine Trimethaphan Pentolinium	
Excess circulating catecholamines	Phentolamine Sodium nitroprusside	All others

dose of antihypertensive agent until the creatinine again decreases to pretreatment levels.

Should undue reduction of blood pressure occur during treatment, a direct pressor drug, such as levarterenol bitartrate (4 mg/L), may be used to treat the drug-induced hypotension. However, discontinuation of the infusion usually suffices when short-acting depressor drugs, such as sodium nitroprusside or trimethaphan, are used. Replenishment of plasma volume by infusions of saline solution, whole blood, or low-molecular-weight dextran is important when diuretic drug therapy has induced oligemia.

After the hypertensive emergency is controlled and the blood pressure and general status of the patient have been stabilized for three to seven days, oral antihypertensive drugs should be substituted for the parenteral drugs.

SUMMARY

1. A variety of hypertensive crises may be encountered during the course of primary or secondary hypertension. Those emergencies include

Table 15–2. Drugs Commonly Used in Hypertensive Emergencies

Drug	Route	Usual Dosage	Onset of Action	Major Side Effects
Vasodilators				
Diazoxide (Hyperstat)	IV rapidly	300 mg	3–5 min	Hyperglycemia, flushing, nausea, vomiting
Sodium nitroprusside (Nipride)	IV drip	50–150 mg/liter	Immediate	Nausea, vomiting, muscle twitching, possible thiocyanate toxicity
Hydralazine (Apresoline)	IM or IV	10–50 mg	IV:10 min IM:30 min	Palpitation, tachycardia, flushing, headache, angina
Sympathetic inhibitors				
Trimethaphan (Arfonad)	IV drip	1000 mg/liter	Immediate	Urinary retention, ileus, dry mouth, loss of accommodation
Phentolamine (Regitine)	IM or IV	5–15 mg	Immediate	Flushing, tachycardia
Reserpine (Serpasil)	IM or IV	1–5 mg	1–3 hr	Drowsiness, stupor
Methyldopa (Aldomet)	IV	250–1000 mg	2–6 hr	Drowsiness, liver abnormalities
Diuretics				
Furosemide (Lasix)	IM or IV	40–80 mg	1–5 min	Cramps, hypokalemia
Ethacrynic acid (Edecrin)	IV	50–100 mg	1–5 min	Cramps, hypokalemia

acute hypertensive encephalopathy, acute left ventricular failure, intra-cranial hemorrhage, acute coronary insufficiency, acute dissecting aortic aneurysm, malignant hypertension, and excess circulating catechol-amines.

2. Each of those emergencies requires prompt recognition and rapid reduction of blood pressure although not necessarily to normotensive levels and not necessarily with the same urgency.

3. Preferably, such patients are treated initially in an intensive care unit, where changes in blood pressure, state of consciousness, convulsive activity, and airway obstruction can be monitored closely and treated promptly.

4. Antihypertensive drugs are administered parenterally, and the selection of a particular drug is determined by the specific emergency and by the patient's overall clinical condition (especially his cardiac, renal, and cerebral status).

5. After the hypertensive emergency is controlled and the patient's blood pressure and general status have been stabilized for three to seven days, oral antihypertensive drugs should be substituted for the parenteral drugs.

SUGGESTED READINGS

1. AMA Committee on Hypertension: The treatment of malignant hypertension and hypertensive emergencies. J.A.M.A. 228:1673, 1974.
2. Bhatia, S.K., and Frohlich, E.D.: Hemodynamic comparison of agents useful in hypertensive emergencies. Am. Heart J. 85:367, 1973.
3. Finnerty, F.A., Jr.: Hypertensive encephalopathy. Am. J. Med. 52:672, 1972.
4. Freis, E.D.: Hypertensive crisis. J.A.M.A. 208:338, 1969.
5. Gifford, R. W., Jr., and Richards, N.G.: Hypertensive encephalopathy. Stroke 5:43, 1970.
6. Hypertension Study Groups: Resources for the management of emergencies in hypertension. Circulation 43:A157, 1971.
7. Koch Weser, J.: Current concepts: Hypertensive emergencies. N. Engl. J. Med. 290:211, 1974.
8. Mroczek, W.J., Davidov, M., Gavrilovich, L., et al.: The value of aggressive therapy in the hypertensive patient with azotemia. Circulation 40:893, 1969.
9. Vaamonde, C.A., David, N.J., and Palmer, R.F.: Hypertensive emergencies. Med. Clin. North Am. 55:325, 1971.
10. Richardson, D.W., and Raper, A.J.: Management of complicated hypertension including hypertensive emergencies. Cardiovasc. Clin. 9(1):227, 1978.

Chapter 16

DIGITALIS INTOXICATION

EDWARD K. CHUNG
LISA S. CHUNG

GENERAL CONSIDERATIONS

Cardiac glycosides have probably been the most valuable drugs available for treatment of heart disease since 1785, when the British physician William Withering introduced digitalis.[1] It is well documented that cardiac glycosides are essential to the management of congestive heart failure, regardless of the underlying heart disease and of various supraventricular tachyarrhythmias, particularly atrial fibrillation with rapid ventricular response.[2]

In recent years, however, the incidence of digitalis intoxication has increased because of the frequent use of potent purified cardiac glycosides in conjunction with potent diuretics, which predisposes the patient to the development of hypokalemia. The incidence of digitalis intoxication in general hospitals has been estimated to be approximately 20%.[2] Digitalis intoxication is often unavoidable, because the margin between therapeutic and toxic doses is relatively narrow. The margin is further reduced in elderly and seriously ill patients and those with various modifying conditions, such as hypokalemia, myxedema, electrolyte imbalance, hypoxia, renal failure, and pulmonary disease. It has been shown that the therapeutic dose is approximately 60% of the toxic dose.

Although cardiac glycosides are indispensable to the treatment of heart failure and various supraventricular tachyarrhythmias, they are no longer beneficial to a patient who has developed manifestations of digitalis intoxication. Frequently, digitalis intoxication may develop in a patient after a relatively small dose that is either therapeutic or inadequate for other patients. That is especially true when there are various modifying conditions, such as those just listed. Consequently, the digitalis requirement varies from patient to patient and from time to time in the same patient. The use of the standard dosage for digitalization without adjusting to the individual response is a common cause of digitalis intoxication. It is not uncommon for digitalis to reach intoxicating levels without having the desired therapeutic effect, especially in patients with intractable congestive heart failure. In retrospect, apparently inexplicable death in patients with refractory congestive heart failure can often be attributed to digitalis intoxication.

Although digitalis is one of the oldest and most commonly used drugs, it is not possible for physicians to determine precisely the optimal therapeutic dosage. The determination of serum digoxin or digitoxin levels is widely used at many institutions to assess the therapeutic and toxic doses of digitalis.[3,4] Markedly increased serum digitalis levels usually indicate digitalis intoxication, whereas very low serum digitalis levels often indicate underdigitalization. The determination of serum digitalis levels is extremely valuable in patients suffering from intractable congestive heart failure or complex cardiac arrhythmias when little or no information regarding previous digitalization is available. (The determination of serum digitalis levels is discussed in detail on pp. 335 to 337.)

The most common manifestations of digitalis intoxication are gastrointestinal disturbances, various cardiac arrhythmias, aggravation of preexisting congestive heart failure or the development of new congestive heart failure, neurologic disturbances, and visual disturbances.[2] Common and uncommon manifestations of digitalis intoxication are listed in Table 16–1.

GASTROINTESTINAL SYMPTOMS

Anorexia is often the earliest sign of digitalis intoxication, and it is usually followed by nausea and vomiting in two or three days if digitalization is continued. The nausea and vomiting are considered to be central rather than gastric in origin.

Diarrhea is a rather uncommon manifestation of digitalis intoxication, and constipation and abdominal pain have also been reported rarely. Gastrointestinal symptoms are often not clearly evident in elderly patients, probably being masked by the severity of the congestive heart

Table 16–1. *Manifestations of Digitalis Intoxication*

Symptoms	Common	Uncommon
Gastro-intestinal	Anorexia, nausea, vomiting	Abdominal pain, constipation, diarrhea, hemorrhage
Cardiac	Worsening of congestive heart failure, ventricular premature contraction, paroxysmal atrial tachycardia with block, nonparoxysmal AV junctional tachycardia, AV block, sinus bradycardia	Atrial fibrillation, atrial flutter, ventricular tachycardia, ventricular flutter, sinus arrest, SA block, atrial premature contraction, AV junctional premature contraction
Visual	Color vision (green or yellow) with halos	Blurring or shimmering vision, scotoma, micropsia or macropsia, amblyopia
Neurologic	Fatigue, headache, insomnia, malaise, confusion, vertigo, depression	Neuralgia, convulsions, paresthesia, delirium, psychosis
Nonspecific	—	Allergic reaction, idiosyncrasy, thrombocytopenia, gynecomastia

failure and cerebral insufficiency. It is well documented that most of the purified glycosides produce nausea and vomiting much less frequently than does digitalis leaf. Thus digitalis-induced arrhythmias are frequently the earliest manifestation of digitalis intoxication with the purified glycosides. When nausea and vomiting develop, and the possibilities of overdigitalization and underdigitalization are almost equal, digitalis should be discontinued immediately and the patient should be reevaluated.

VISUAL AND NEUROLOGIC MANIFESTATIONS

Green or yellow color vision with colored halos has for many years been considered to be a pathognomonic feature of digitalis intoxication.[2] Other visual disturbances include scotoma, blurring, shimmering vision, and, less commonly, micropsia and temporary or permanent amblyopia.[2] Those visual manifestations may easily go unrecognized unless the physician asks specifically about them.

Cardiac glycosides may produce various neurologic symptoms, including headache, fatigue, lassitude, insomnia, malaise, depression, confusion, delirium, and vertigo and, less commonly, convulsions, neuralgias, especially trigeminal neuralgia and paresthesia. Visual and neurologic manifestations usually develop later than gastrointestinal symptoms or cardiac arrhythmias, and the symptoms just mentioned (except the color vision disturbances) are less specific for digitalis intoxication than are the gastrointestinal manifestations and the arrhythmias. Furthermore, neurologic symptoms are often difficult to evaluate in elderly people because those symptoms may be due to many other conditions, such as cerebrovascular accidents and chronic brain syndrome.

RARE MANIFESTATIONS

Allergic manifestations, such as urticaria and eosinophilia, and idiosyncrasy are *not* true manifestations of digitalis intoxication.[2,5] Similarly, unilateral or bilateral gynecomastia that develops during digitalis therapy does not seem to be a manifestation of digitalis intoxication although some investigators consider it to be so. Those investigators have seen several patients who have shown no other toxic manifestations after the development of gynecomastia in spite of continued digitalis therapy.[2] Therefore gynecomastia due to an estrogen-like activity of digitalis is most likely *not* a toxic manifestation.[6] Furthermore, digitalis-induced gynecomastia seems to be duration dependent rather than dosage dependent since it usually develops when patients receive cardiac glycosides for more than two years.

A rare occurrence of digitoxin-induced thrombocytopenia has been reported, and it was considered to be a specific sensitivity reaction to digitoxin bound to the gamma globulin fraction of the serum.[7]

CARDIAC MANIFESTATIONS

The two major cardiac manifestations of digitalis intoxication are alteration of contractility and digitalis-induced arrhythmias. They often occur simultaneously.[2]

Alteration of Contractility

A worsening of preexisting congestive heart failure or the development of new heart failure during digitalization is a not uncommon manifestation of digitalis intoxication.[2,5] Indeed, intractable or refractory congestive heart failure is frequently due to digitalis intoxication, a relationship that may be much more common than is recognized. Regardless of the fundamental mechanism involved, all patients with intractable congestive heart failure should be carefully reevaluated for possible digitalis intoxication.

Digitalis-Induced Cardiac Arrhythmias

Although cardiac glycosides are often essential to the treatment of most supraventricular tachyarrhythmias, they may produce almost every known type of cardiac arrhythmia by altering impulse formation or conduction or both.[2] Recognition of digitalis-induced arrhythmias is extremely important because various cardiac arrhythmias may be not only the earliest but also the only sign of digitalis intoxication. The use of purified glycosides in recent years has led to an increased incidence of cardiac arrhythmias without other symptoms of intoxication. Furthermore, hypokalemia induced by the frequent use of potent diuretics predisposes the patient to the development of digitalis-induced cardiac arrhythmias.[2]

It has been estimated that some form of cardiac arrhythmia occurs in 80 to 90% of patients with digitalis intoxication.[2,8] Various combinations of cardiac arrhythmias are commonly observed in patients with advanced digitalis intoxication; it is not uncommon for cardiac arrhythmias to change from one type to another in the same ECG tracing.[2]

It should be emphasized that the classic digitalis effect (S–T segment and T wave changes) in the ECG during digitalis therapy is completely unrelated to digitalis intoxication.[2,8] The digitalis effect in the ECG may be absent in about two-thirds of the cases of digitalis toxicity, and, by the same token, striking S–T segment and T wave changes are frequently observed in the absence of any evidence of digitalis intoxication. Other ECG findings during digitalis therapy, such as a shortening of the Q–T interval, increased amplitude of the U waves, and peaking of the terminal portion of the T waves, also are not indicative of digitalis toxicity.[2]

Ventricular bigeminy or trigeminy is probably the most common digitalis-induced cardiac arrhythmia. Almost equally common are AV junctional arrhythmias, especially in the presence of preexisting atrial fibrillation.[2]

Almost all types of cardiac arrhythmias may be induced by digitalis, but some arrhythmias do not seem to be related to cardiac glycosides. Nondigitalis-induced cardiac arrhythmias include Mobitz type II AV block, parasystole, nonparoxysmal ventricular (idioventricular) tachycardia or parasystolic ventricular tachycardia, bilateral bundle branch block of varying degree, sinus tachycardia, and paroxysmal AV junctional tachycardia.

Disturbances of Sinus Impulse Formation and Conduction. Minor toxic effects of digitalis may induce sinus bradycardia (Fig. 16–1), which may lead to more serious arrhythmias, such as sinus arrest and sinoatrial (SA) block if digitalization continues. A sudden reduction of the heart rate to below 50 beats per minute in an adult during digitalization should raise the suspicion of digitalis intoxication (Fig. 16–1). A pulse rate below 100 per minute in an infant has the same clinical significance. SA block with or without the Wenckebach phenomenon is not uncommon in digitalis intoxication, especially in children.[2] Indeed, digitalis may be the most

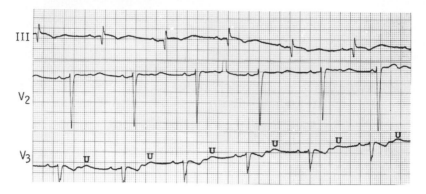

Figure 16–1.   Sinus bradycardia (49 beats per minute). Note the prominent U waves due to hypokalemia.

common cause of SA block. Sinus tachycardia does not seem to be induced by digitalis. However, it should be noted that some patients with congestive heart failure may have persisting sinus tachycardia even after full digitalization. That happens when the congestive heart failure is associated with other diseases, such as chronic pulmonary diseases, hyperthyroidism, obesity, and anemia.

Spontaneous sinus bradycardia, sinus arrest, or SA block, particularly in elderly people, is often due to the sick sinus syndrome (Chapter 9).

Atrial Arrhythmias. It is well documented that various atrial tachyarrhythmias may be produced by digitalis, even though digitalis is the drug of choice in the treatment of most atrial tachyarrhythmias.

Atrial Tachycardia. Atrial tachycardia is the most common digitalis-induced atrial arrhythmia, and it is frequently associated with varying degrees of AV block[2,9] (Fig. 16–2). The condition is called paroxysmal atrial tachycardia (PAT) with block. Although the frequent occurrence of digitalis-induced PAT with block is often emphasized, it actually accounts for only about 10% of digitalis-induced cardiac arrhythmias.[2]

It has been said that carotid sinus stimulation frequently terminates PAT with block not due to digitalis intoxication but is ineffective when digitalis is the cause.[8] However, the danger of applying carotid sinus stimulation to patients with suspected digitalis intoxication cannot be overemphasized. It has been shown that some patients have died from ventricular fibrillation during or after carotid sinus stimulation.[10,11] All of those patients had been critically ill and had received cardiac glycosides. Based on those observations, carotid sinus stimulation should be avoided if at all possible in patients who are taking even small amounts of digitalis.

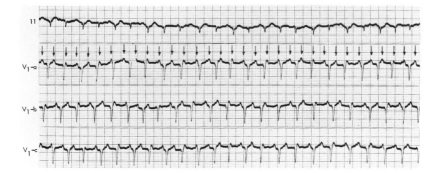

Figure 16–2.   Leads V₁-a, b, and c are continuous. The arrows indicate P waves. The rhythm is atrial tachycardia (atrial rate: 210 beats per minute) with varying degrees of Wenckebach AV block (ventricular rate: 145 to 165 beats per minute).

As for the fundamental mechanism responsible for the production of atrial tachycardia, the refractory period of the atrial musculature is markedly shortened by an indirect vagal stimulating action of digitalis. Thus increased conductivity within the atrial muscle can produce various atrial tachyarrhythmias. A combination of the depressive effect on the AV conduction and the shortening effect on the atrial refractory period results in atrial tachycardia with varying degrees of AV block.[2]

Atrial Fibrillation or Flutter. Atrial fibrillation or flutter may be produced by digitalis, but its occurrence is very rare indeed. It is not clear why digitalis-induced atrial fibrillation or flutter is so rare in comparison with atrial tachycardia.

Atrial Premature Contractions. Although atrial premature contractions are not as common as ventricular ones, when they do occur the ectopic P waves are frequently not conducted to the ventricles (nonconducted or blocked atrial premature contractions) in spite of relatively long coupling intervals. The combination of impaired AV conduction and the increased excitability in the atria results in frequent nonconducted atrial premature contractions.

AV Junctional Arrhythmias. As mentioned on page 327, the incidence of various AV junctional arrhythmias in digitalis intoxication is probably as high as the incidence of ventricular premature contractions.[2] Digitalis induces various AV junctional arrhythmias, due either to passive impulse formation resulting in AV junctional escape rhythm (Fig. 16–3) or to enhancement of AV junctional impulse formation resulting in non-paroxysmal AV junctional tachycardia (Fig. 16–4).

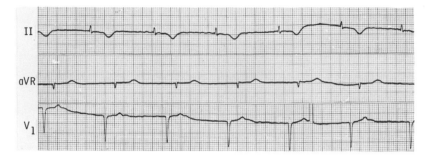

Figure 16–3.   Atrial fibrillation with AV junctional escape rhythm (46 beats per minute) due to complete AV block.

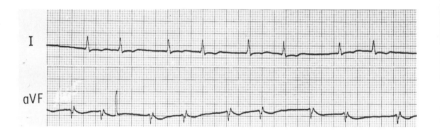

Figure 16–4.   Nonparoxysmal AV junctional tachycardia with 3 : 2 Wenckebach exit block in the presence of atrial fibrillation, producing complete AV dissociation.

Nonparoxysmal AV Junctional Tachycardia. Nonparoxysmal AV junctional tachycardia is probably the most common digitalis-induced cardiac arrhythmia, particularly in the presence of underlying atrial fibrillation (Fig. 16–4). For that reason, digitalis intoxication should be considered as the first probable cause when one is dealing with unexplainable non-paroxysmal AV junctional tachycardia. It should be emphasized that paroxysmal AV junctional tachycardia is *not* observed in patients with digitalis intoxication.

In advanced digitalis intoxication, exit block of varying degree may develop around the AV junctional pacemaker, and the ventricular cycle may become slower and/or irregular. When the exit block is Wenckebach type, the ventricular cycle may show regular irregularity (Fig. 16–5). Ventricular tachycardia may be closely simulated by AV junctional tachycardia with aberrant ventricular conduction, especially in the presence of preexisting atrial fibrillation. On rare occasions, double AV junctional rhythm or tachycardia may be produced by digitalis; the phenomenon is a rare form of AV dissociation (Fig. 16–6). It should be

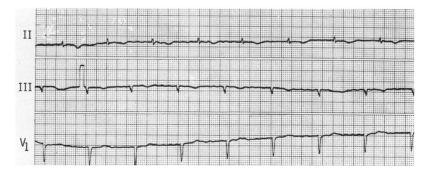

Figure 16–5. Nonparoxysmal AV junctional tachycardia (68 beats per minute) in the presence of atrial fibrillation producing complete AV dissociation.

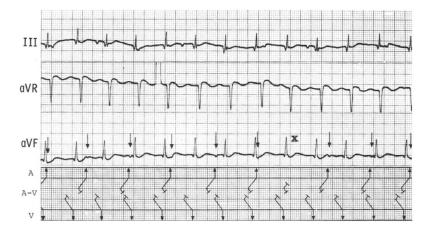

Figure 16–6. Double AV junctional tachycardia. The rate of the AV junctional tachycardia (75 beats per minute) controls the atria in a retrograde fashion (indicated by arrows), whereas another AV junctional tachycardia activating the ventricles produces a faster rate (100 beats per minute). Retrograde block is most likely responsible for the absence of a P wave in lead aVF (marked X).

emphasized that the basic rhythm is frequently atrial fibrillation when digitalis-induced AV junctional arrhythmias develop (Figs. 16–4 and 16–5). At times, the atrial mechanism may be atrial flutter or tachycardia in the presence of AV junctional tachycardia (Fig. 16–7), leading to double supraventricular tachycardia.

AV Junctional Escape Rhythm. AV junctional escape rhythm is much less common than nonparoxysmal AV junctional tachycardia in digitalis

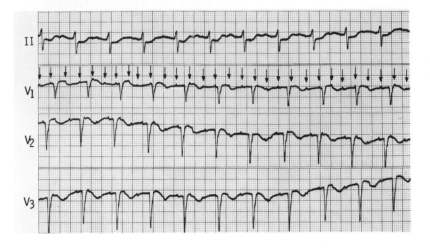

Figure 16–7.   The arrows indicate atrial activity. The rhythm is atrial tachycardia (atrial rate: 220 to 240 beats per minute) with nonparoxysmal AV junctional tachycardia (94 beats per minute), producing complete AV dissociation (double supraventricular tachycardias).

intoxication. Again, the underlying rhythm is often atrial fibrillation, and the electrophysiologic mechanism that produces AV junctional escape rhythm is usually high-degree (advanced) or complete AV block (AV nodal block, Fig. 16–3).

AV Conduction Disturbances. Digitalis may produce various degrees of AV block resulting from both the direct and indirect actions of the drug.[2] Those actions are, needless to say, essential to the management of various supraventricular tachyarrhythmias, especially atrial fibrillation. The degree of AV block in digitalis intoxication depends largely on the dosage of the drug, underlying heart disease, preexisting AV conduction disturbances, and electrolyte imbalance.

First-Degree AV Block. Although first-degree AV block is one of the earliest manifestations of digitalis intoxication, some investigators do not include it among the toxic manifestations of the drug. However, digitalis-induced second- or higher-degree AV block is often followed by first-degree AV block when digitalis is stopped. Therefore, first-degree AV block during digitalization should definitely be considered a manifestation of digitalis intoxication.

Second-Degree AV Block. The average incidence of second-degree AV block in different series is estimated to be 11%.[2,8] Among second-degree AV blocks, Wenckebach (Mobitz type I) AV block is more common than is 2:1 AV block. On the other hand, Mobitz type II AV block has not been reported as a manifestation of digitalis intoxication. It

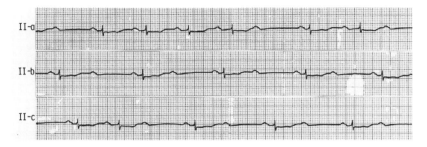

Figure 16–8.   Leads II-a, b, and c are *not* continuous. The tracing shows sinus rhythm (atrial rate: 66 beats per minute) with 2:1 AV block and varying degrees of intermittent Wenckebach AV block.

is common to observe that Wenckebach AV block and 2:1 AV block often coexist in the same ECG tracing (Fig. 16–8).

High-Degree or Complete AV Block. High-degree (advanced) or complete AV block is very common in digitalis intoxication when the underlying rhythm is atrial fibrillation (Fig. 16–3). It has been said that digitalis intoxication is the second most common cause of complete AV block.[2]

Ventricular Arrhythmias. *Ventricular Premature Contractions.* Ventricular premature contractions, particularly ones that are multifocal in origin, are the most common and often the earliest manifestation of digitalis intoxication in adults. The incidence has been reported to be approximately 50% of all digitalis-induced arrhythmias. It has been known for many years that ventricular bigeminy (Fig. 16–9) is a hallmark of digitalis-induced arrhythmia.[2,8] The diagnostic probability of digitalis intoxication is 100% when ventricular bigeminy coexists with nonparoxysmal AV junctional tachycardia or AV block, especially in the presence of atrial fibrillation (Fig. 16–9).

In children and in healthy adults, supraventricular arrhythmias and AV conduction disturbances are more common than are ventricular premature contractions.[2,8] Ventricular bigeminy or trigeminy induced by digitalis occurs frequently in the presence of a diseased myocardium, particularly in the aged. Ventricular premature contractions may originate from a single focus, or they may be multifocal. Multifocal ventricular premature contractions are more pathognomonic for digitalis intoxication than are unifocal ones.

Ventricular Tachycardia and Fibrillation. When ventricular premature contractions are frequent, particularly multifocal or bidirectional ones, ventricular tachycardia may develop, producing unidirectional or bidirectional tachycardia or even ventricular fibrillation. The average incidence of ventricular tachycardia has been estimated to be 10% of all digitalis-induced arrhythmias.[2,8] If ventricular tachycardia persists, there is always the possibility of the development of ventricular fibrillation and sudden death. The mortality of patients with digitalis-induced ventricular tachycardia is extremely high (68 to 100%).

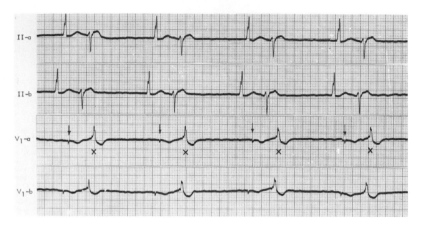

Figure 16–9.   Leads II-a and b are continuous, as are leads V_1-a and b. The rhythm is atrial fibrillation with AV junctional escape rhythm (indicated by arrows) due to complete AV block and ventricular bigeminy (marked X).

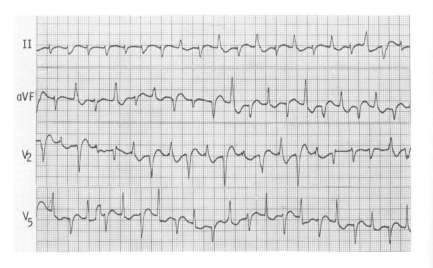

Figure 16–10.   Tracing taken from a 70-year-old man with cor pulmonale and thyrotoxicosis who died soon after this ECG was recorded. The serum digoxin level was more than 10 ng/ml. The rhythm is atrial fibrillation with bidirectional ventricular tachycardia (176 beats per minute), producing complete AV dissociation.

Bidirectional ventricular tachycardia (Fig. 16–10) is considered to be more pathognomonic for digitalis intoxication than is the unidirectional entity.[2] Bidirectional ventricular tachycardia is more common in advanced heart disease, and frequently the basic atrial mechanism is atrial fibrillation, flutter, or tachycardia (Fig. 16–10).

It should be emphasized that nonparoxysmal ventricular (idioventricular) tachycardia (accelerated ventricular rhythm) and parasystolic ventricular tachycardia are *not* due to digitalis intoxication (Chapter 7).

Except for idioventricular rhythm, the mechanism of ventricular tachycardia or fibrillation is most likely similar to that responsible for the production of ventricular premature contractions. Enhancement of automaticity is probably responsible for most digitalis-induced ventricular arrhythmias.

DETERMINATION OF SERUM DIGITALIS LEVELS BY RADIOIMMUNOASSAY

In the past 10 years, various methods of determining the levels of serum cardiac glycosides in order to assess an optimal therapeutic dosage and to diagnose digitalis intoxication with accuracy[3,4] have been proposed. The radioimmunoassay method most commonly used at present was first employed by Oliver and his co-workers[12] to determine serum digitoxin levels. Later, Smith and his co-workers[3] developed a radioimmunoassay method for measuring serum digoxin levels.

The clinical importance of serum cardiac glycoside levels rests in the reasonably close correlation between blood content and tissue content of digitalis. The blood levels reflect total body and myocardial concentrations.[4] That relationship was first noted by Doherty and his co-workers, who observed a relatively constant ratio between blood and myocardial levels of digoxin in animals as well as in man.[4]

At present, it is generally agreed that patients with unequivocal digitalis intoxication have significantly higher serum or plasma levels of digoxin or digitoxin than have non-intoxicated patients. Nevertheless, there is substantial overlap between toxic and nontoxic serum or plasma cardiac glycoside levels, particularly in patients suffering from intractable congestive heart failure or various complex arrhythmias. As has been emphasized repeatedly, the dosage of digitalis varies not only from patient to patient but also from time to time in the same patient. Similarly, toxic and nontoxic serum or plasma digitalis levels may differ from patient to patient because of various modifying factors, including electrolyte imbalance, thyroid disease, renal disease, acute or chronic lung disease, and, particularly, the nature and severity of the underlying heart disease.

In a prospective study by Beller and his co-workers of 931 consecutively studied patients with digitalis intoxication, serum concentrations of digoxin and digitoxin in intoxicated patients were 2.3 ± 1.6 ng/ml and 34 ± 18 ng/ml, respectively.[13] On the other hand, serum concentrations of digoxin and digitoxin in non-intoxicated patients were 1 ± 0.5 ng/ml and 20 ± 11 ng/ml, respectively, in the same study. Clearly, there is significant overlap of values in the two groups.

In general, serum digoxin levels of 2 ng/ml or below and serum digitoxin levels of 20 ng/ml or below are considered to be nontoxic, even though intoxicated patients may have serum levels below those values.[3,4,12,13] Very low serum cardiac glycoside concentrations (digoxin levels below 0.4 ng/ml or digitoxin levels below 10 ng/ml) usually indicate under-digitalization.[3,4,12,13] Values that low are, as a rule, not observed among intoxicated patients.

The radioimmunoassay methods are extremely valuable when the serum cardiac glycoside levels are evaluated in conjunction with the total clinical picture and ECG findings. Determination of the serum digitalis level is useful when little or no information is available about the patient's previous use of digitalis. Once the serum digitalis level in such a patient is known, the subsequent additional digitalis dosage may be determined much more accurately. Determination of serum digitalis levels is also valuable in patients in whom various modifying factors dictate the daily regulation of the digitalis dosage. Another use of the determination of serum digitalis levels is in the assessment of underdigitalization, which may be difficult or even impossible to ascertain clinically or electro-cardiographically, especially in the presence of sinus rhythm.

The most important use of the determination of serum digoxin or digitoxin levels by radioimmunoassay methods is in establishing the optimal dosage for a given patient. It is to be hoped that those methods will enable many physicians to prescribe cardiac glycosides more effectively and more appropriately so that the risk of digitalis intoxication can be minimized or even eliminated.

DETERMINATION OF SALIVA ELECTROLYTES

Recently it has been shown that the electrolyte content of the saliva is closely related to digitalis intoxication. Wotman and his co-workers[14] demonstrated that patients with digitalis intoxication have disproportionately high concentrations of potassium and calcium in their saliva. There was some overlap between intoxicated and non-intoxicated groups although mean values of saliva potassium and calcium were significantly higher in the group with digitalis intoxication. Further clinical evaluation is needed to assess the value of the saliva test.

Evaluation of the total clinical condition of each patient during digitalis therapy is essential; the results of any single laboratory test must not be used as the basis for diagnosis or treatment.

MANAGEMENT OF DIGITALIS INTOXICATION (See also Table 16–2)

Unfortunately, there is no known drug that is an antagonist to digitalis. Various drugs have been tried in the treatment of digitalis intoxication with varying success; diphenylhydantoin and potassium have proved to be the most effective in terminating various digitalis-induced tachyarrhythmias.

The most important treatment for digitalis intoxication is immediate withdrawal of the drug, not merely a reduction in dosage.[2] Most patients with mild digitalis intoxication (showing such effects as sinus bradycardia, first-degree AV block, and occasional ventricular premature contractions) can recover from digitalis intoxication if the drug is discontinued for several days. Generally, in patients with digitalis intoxication, emotional stress and physical activity should be restricted, and all other factors that may aggravate the intoxication should be eliminated. Any patient with advanced digitalis intoxication, particularly serious cardiac arrhythmias, should be treated in a cardiac care unit or a room similarly equipped. Various drugs can be given orally, intramuscularly, or intravenously, depending on the clinical situations.

Potassium

Potassium is one of the most effective drugs for abolishing various atrial and ventricular tachyarrhythmias in digitalis intoxication.[2,15]

Administration and Dosage. The amount of potassium to be administered depends on the severity of the intoxication, the degree of suspected potassium deficiency in the myocardium, and the response to potassium therapy. Potassium in the form of potassium chloride may be administered orally in doses of 20 to 80 mEq/L/day or by a slow intravenous infusion in doses of 40 or 60 mEq/L over a 2 to 3 hour period initially. Intravenous administration is preferred because the exact amount received by the patient can be controlled and the drug can be discontinued at any time.[2] Oral administration is widely used for milder cases of digitalis intoxication when hypokalemia is suspected or is known to be present. During the intravenous administration of potassium, continuous ECG monitoring is essential to prevent hyperkalemia or cardiac arrhythmia.

Table 16–2. *Treatment of Digitalis Intoxication*

Drugs and Other Methods	Mild Intoxication	Severe Intoxication	Contra-indications
	IMMEDIATE WITHDRAWAL OF DIGITALIS!		
Potassium	1–2 g KCl q̄ 4 hr	40–60 mEq/liter KCl in 500 ml 5% D/W IV injection (2–3 hr period) under ECG monitor and periodic serum K⁺ determination	Hyperkalemia, uremia, second and third degree AV block, SA block
Diphenylhydantoin (Dilantin)	100 mg tid or qid by mouth	125–250 mg IV injection (2–3-min period) under ECG monitor. Same dosage may be repeated q̄ 5–10 min.	Second- and third-degree AV block, SA block, marked sinus bradycardia
Lidocaine (Xylocaine)	—	1 mg/kg body wt. IV injection q̄ 20 min. Maximum dose: 750 mg	Similar to diphenyl-hydantoin (see above)
Propranolol (Inderal)	10–30 mg tid or qid before meals and at bedtime	1–3 mg slow IV injection (not to exceed 1 mg/min) under ECG monitor. Second dose may be repeated after 2 min. Additional medication should be withheld for at least 4 hr.	Bronchial asthma, allergic rhinitis, marked sinus bradycardia, SA block, second- and third-degree AV block, cardiogenic shock, heart failure, pulmonary hypertension
Procainamide (Pronestyl)	250–500 mg q̄ 3–4 hr by mouth	50–100 mg q̄ 2–4 min slow IV injection or 1 g in 200 ml 5% D/W IV drip (30–60-min period) under ECG monitor. Maximum dose: 2 g	Similar to diphenyl-hydantoin (see above)
Quinidine	300–400 mg qid by mouth	0.6 g in 200 ml 5% D/W IV drip (30–60 min period) under ECG monitor	Similar to diphenyl-hydantoin (see above)
Magnesium sulfate	Slow (1 cc/min) IV infusion (20 cc of 20% solution) under continuous ECG monitoring		
Sodium EDTA	Not recommended for clinical use		
Direct current counter-shock	Not recommended except as a last resort after all available measures have been exhausted		
Artificial pacemaker	Temporary demand pacemaker is indicated for third-degree AV block and occasionally for second-degree AV block or SA block		

Precautions and Contraindications. Potassium is absolutely contraindicated in the presence of renal failure and hyperkalemia. Potassium is also relatively contraindicated in the presence of second-degree or complete AV block unless the serum potassium level is very low. Frequent determination of the serum potassium level is also indicated.

Needless to say, potassium is most effective when a significant degree of hypokalemia is present (Fig. 16–1).

Diphenylhydantoin (Dilantin)

Clinical investigations have demonstrated that diphenylhydantoin is effective in treating digitalis-induced arrhythmias, including paroxysmal atrial tachycardia, AV junctional rhythm, wandering atrial pacemaker, ventricular bigeminy, multifocal ventricular premature contractions and AV junctional or ventricular tachycardia[2,15-17] (Fig. 16–11).

Administration and Dosage. Most patients respond in 3 seconds to 5 minutes to the intravenous administration of diphenylhydantoin. The duration of response varies from 5 minutes to 4 to 6 hours. The initial intravenous dose is 125 to 250 mg for 1 to 3 minutes given under ECG monitoring. The same dose may be repeated every 5 to 10 minutes until the effect is established.

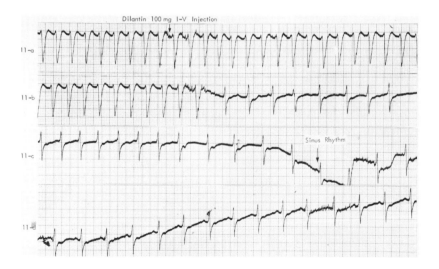

Figure 16–11.   Leads II-a, b, c, and d are continuous. Ventricular tachycardia (155 beats per minute) has been converted to sinus rhythm by the intravenous administration of 100 mg of diphenylhydantoin.

After conversion to sinus rhythm or after digitalis-induced arrhythmias have been terminated, an oral maintenance dosage (200 to 400 mg) given in divided doses is sufficient.

Side Effects and Toxicity. Toxic manifestations or side effects of diphenylhydantoin include respiratory arrest, skin reaction (urticaria, purpura), drowsiness, depression, nervousness, arthralgia, gingival hyperplasia, transient eosinophilia, and transient hypotension. Those manifestations are rare and usually not serious.

Prophylactic Value in Post-cardioversion Arrhythmias. It has recently been shown that diphenylhydantoin is of prophylactic value before direct current shock in a digitalized patient. The drug is capable of preventing arrhythmias induced by cardioversion[2] by increasing the threshold of the excitability of the heart by counteracting the electrophysiologic actions of digitalis. Diphenylhydantoin is probably the safest and most effective drug for the treatment of all types of digitalis-induced tachyarrhythmias.

Beta-Adrenergic Blocking Drugs

Propranolol is the most commonly used beta-adrenergic blocking drug.[18,19]

Administration and Dosage. The usual intravenous dose of propranolol is 1 to 3 mg given under continuous ECG monitoring. The drug should be administered slowly, at a rate not exceeding 1 mg (1 cc) per minute. Sufficient time should be allowed to enable a slow circulation to carry the drug to its site of action. A second dose, if needed, may be repeated after two minutes. Additional medication should be withheld for at least four hours. Propranolol may be given orally as soon as cardiac arrhythmias are abolished or are markedly improved.[18,19] Intravenous atropine (0.5 to 1 mg) may be needed if marked bradycardia occurs. In non-urgent situations, propranolol may be given orally in doses of 10 to 30 mg, three to four times a day, before meals and at bedtime. The same dosage is also recommended for long-term use and for prophylaxis.

Precautions and Contraindications. Propranolol is probably contraindicated for patients with bronchial asthma and allergic rhinitis (especially during the pollen season), marked sinus bradycardia, second- or third-degree AV block, SA block, sinus arrest, cardiogenic shock, and significant congestive heart failure.[18,19] The drug is also contraindicated in patients receiving anesthetics that produce myocardial depression, such as chloroform and ether. Patients receiving adrenergic-augmenting psychotropic drugs (including MAO inhibitors) also should not receive the drug. Propranolol may be given with caution after the two-week withdrawal period from such drugs. It should be emphasized that ECG monitoring is mandatory during the intravenous administration of propranolol. In our experience, propranolol has not been as effective as potassium or diphenylhydantoin for the treatment of digitalis intoxication.

Side Effects and Toxicity. The most common side effect of propranolol is slowing of the sinus rate. At times, propranolol may produce marked sinus bradycardia. Other untoward effects include production or aggravation of congestive heart failure, bronchial asthma, and hypotension. Recently, it has been emphasized that cardiopulmonary resuscitation is often difficult in patients who are receiving large amounts of propranolol, particularly during major cardiac surgery. Thus it is advised that the drug be discontinued or the dosage be significantly reduced at least a few days before surgery as the clinical circumstance permits.

Procainamide (Pronestyl) and Quinidine

Procainamide and quinidine may be effective in abolishing supraventricular and ventricular tachyarrhythmias induced by digitalis.[2] Procainamide may be used if potassium, diphenylhydantoin, and propranolol are ineffective or contraindicated. Quinidine has been less widely used because of the frequent occurrence of hypotension during parenteral administration. Its effect is unpredictable and often hazardous.

Administration and Dosage. Procainamide may be given intravenously in a slow drip not exceeding 50 to 100 mg every 2 to 4 minutes, or orally in a dose of 250 to 500 mg every 3 to 4 hours. The usual dosage of quinidine is 0.3 to 0.4 gm every 6 hours orally. Parenteral administration of quinidine is seldom used at present because it has significant side effects.

Precautions and Contraindications. During the parenteral administration of either procainamide or quinidine, ECG monitoring and frequent blood pressure determinations are indicated. A vasopressor drug should be readily available.

Side Effects and Toxicity. The therapeutic effects of quinidine and procainamide include prolongation of the Q–T interval, widening and notching of the P waves, flattening or inversion of the T waves, and depression of S–T segments. If patients exhibit toxic manifestations of those drugs, the ECG will show varying degrees of AV block, progressive intra-atrial and intraventricular block, and atrial standstill. In severe cases, ventricular fibrillation or tachycardia may develop.

The lupus erythematosus-like syndrome that is induced by procainamide is relatively common and is well known. Both procainamide and quinidine are contraindicated in the presence of AV or intraventricular block.

Lidocaine (Xylocaine)

Like procainamide, the antiarrhythmic mechanism of lidocaine is related to the drug's ability to raise the diastolic stimulation threshold of the ventricles.[20,21] Lidocaine penetrates the tissues more rapidly than does procaine or procainamide, but its action is often transient. Lidocaine may be effective for the treatment of digitalis-induced ventricular arrhythmias.[20,21]

Administration and Dosage. Lidocaine may be given in doses of 1 to 2 mg/kg intravenously for 1 to 2 minutes. The same dose may be repeated at 20-minute intervals if needed. A constant intravenous drip is often necessary following the administration of a direct intravenous bolus of lidocaine since the duration of the antiarrhythmic effect is relatively brief (10 to 20 minutes). Although most adult patients require 75 to 150 mg of the drug, as much as 750 mg of lidocaine has been safely used in anesthetized patients during the first hour of administration.

Side Effects and Toxicity. The side effects of lidocaine include hypotension, depression of the central nervous system, and convulsions.[20,21]

Precautions and Contraindications. Lidocaine is contraindicated in the presence of AV block, SA block, intraventricular block, and hypotension. The drug is, of course, contraindicated in patients who show hypersensitive or idiosyncratic reactions.

Chelating Agents

Sodium EDTA (ethylenediaminotetraacetate) is occasionally of value in the treatment of digitalis-induced ventricular arrhythmias and AV block.[22,23] The chief advantage of the drug is its rapid onset of action; its disadvantages include its transient effect and the hypotension and renal damage that occasionally follow large doses. Chelating drugs may be used when potassium and diphenylhydantoin are contraindicated or ineffective. In general, chelating drugs are not recommended for clinical use because many superior drugs are now available.

Magnesium Sulfate

Recent clinical and experimental investigations have shown that hypomagnesemia predisposes one to digitalis intoxication. Therefore, magnesium sulfate should be administered when digitalis intoxication is associated with hypomagnesemia.[24,25] The drug may be given by slow (1 cc/min) intravenous infusion (20 cc of a 20% solution) under continuous ECG monitoring.

Clinically, hypomagnesemia and hypokalemia often coexist, and hypomagnesemia is frequently encountered in patients with alcoholic cardiomyopathy.

Carotid Sinus Stimulation

Although carotid sinus stimulation has been frequently used in the differential diagnosis of various tachyarrhythmias (Chapter 7), including those that are digitalis induced, the procedure should be avoided in patients with digitalis intoxication. Carotid sinus stimulation in the presence of digitalis intoxication may induce more serious cardiac arrhythmias, particularly ventricular fibrillation, ventricular standstill, and even death.

Direct Current Shock

Cardioversion should not be attempted on patients with suspected or proved digitalis-induced arrhythmias because the procedure frequently induces more serious and irreversible arrhythmias, such as ventricular tachycardia or fibrillation[2,26] (Fig. 16–12). If cardioversion is definitely needed, the prophylactic administration of diphenylhydantoin or potassium may prevent the occurrence of serious arrhythmias. It is essential to discontinue cardiac glycosides before cardioversion. If a short-acting preparation has been given, the procedure should be postponed for at least 24 to 48 hours; if long-acting preparations have been used, the procedure should be delayed for at least three to five days.

In general, when treating the digitalis-induced tachyarrhythmias, cardioversion should be attempted only as a last resort, after all other available measures have failed.[2]

Artificial Pacemakers

The primary indication for an artificial pacemaker is the sick sinus syndrome (Chapter 9) and AV block associated with the Adams-Stokes syndrome. Although digitalis intoxication is reported to be the second most common cause of complete AV block, the Adams-Stokes syndrome as a manifestation of digitalis overdose has been found to be rare since the ventricular rate in digitalis-induced complete AV block tends to be faster than that in complete AV block due to other causes.[2] The main reason is that digitalis-induced AV block is a block in the AV node (intranodal block), so that the escape pacemaker is located in the AV junction, *not* in the infranodal areas. Digitalis-induced AV block is usually reversible.

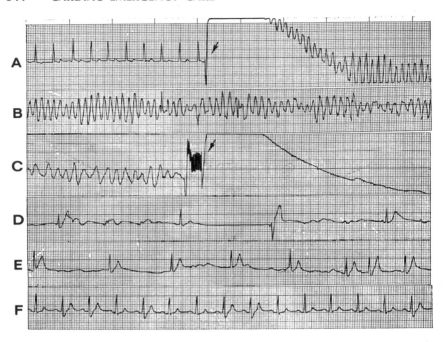

Figure 16–12.   The rhythm strips A, B, C, D, E, and F are continuous. Direct current shock is applied for atrial fibrillation, but ventricular fibrillation is provoked by the procedure (arrow in strip A). Direct current shock-induced ventricular fibrillation is successfully terminated by the second application of direct current shock (arrow in strip C). Note that a long period of slow and unstable cardiac rhythm follows the second direct current shock until a stable sinus rhythm is restored (strip F). It is obvious to recognize intermittent right bundle branch block during sinus rhythm (strip F).

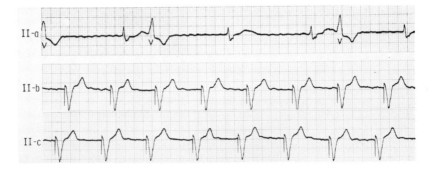

Figure 16–13.   Leads II-b and c are continuous. A temporary demand pacemaker was inserted (leads II-b and c) for the treatment of symptomatic high-degree AV block in the presence of atrial fibrillation and frequent ventricular premature contractions (marked V) shown in lead II-a.

Therefore, simple withdrawal of digitalis is often sufficient treatment. However, if the underlying rhythm is atrial fibrillation, the incidence of Adams-Stokes seizures increases. When the Adams-Stokes syndrome develops as a result of digitalis intoxication, use of a temporary demand pacemaker is quite suitable because the AV block induced by digitalis is often transient and intermittent (Fig. 16–13). The use of an artificial pacemaker with a fixed-rate is not recommended because of the danger of provoking a pacemaker-induced parasystolic rhythm that competes with the patient's own basic rhythm or ectopic rhythm, resulting in ventricular tachycardia or fibrillation. Implantation of a permanent pacemaker for the treatment of digitalis-induced AV block is rarely called for unless there are other coexisting causes of AV block.

SUMMARY

1. Once a patient develops digitalis intoxication, digitalis is no longer beneficial, even in the presence of congestive heart failure.

2. The most important therapeutic approach to digitalis intoxication is immediate withdrawal of the drug, not simply reduction of the dosage.

3. Almost every known type of cardiac arrhythmia may be induced by digitalis. The most common digitalis-induced arrhythmias are ventricular premature contractions, particularly those that are multifocal in origin, and nonparoxysmal AV junctional tachycardia, especially in the presence of atrial fibrillation.

4. Mild forms of digitalis-induced arrhythmias usually disappear after the withdrawal of digitalis. However, treatment of advanced and more serious tachyarrhythmias involve the use of drugs as well as the withdrawal of digitalis.

5. The most effective drugs are diphenylhydantoin (Dilantin) and potassium.

6. Digitalis-induced bradyarrhythmias usually improve after the withdrawal of digitalis. In rare cases of high-degree or complete AV block, especially when the underlying rhythm is atrial fibrillation, a temporary demand pacemaker may be required. A permanent pacemaker is almost never indicated.

7. It should be reemphasized that the dosage of digitalis varies not only from person to person but also from time to time in the same person, depending on various modifying factors, such as the status of underlying heart disease, the presence or absence of hypokalemia and hypoxia, and the status of renal and thyroid function.

8. Determination of the serum digitalis level is extremely useful, but that value should be interpreted carefully in conjunction with the clinical background and the ECG findings.

9. Cardiac glycosides are the most useful and essential drugs for the treatment of heart disease, but they may produce serious untoward effects and even death from digitalis intoxication.

10. The serious manifestations of digitalis intoxication can be avoided if all physicians make themselves thoroughly familiar with this most valuable drug, particularly with its toxicity.

11. Direct current shock or carotid sinus stimulation should be avoided because they may produce serious cardiac arrhythmias and even death.

REFERENCES

1. Withering, W.: An Account of the Foxglove and Some of Its Medical Uses with Practical Remarks on Dropsy and Other Diseases. London, M. Swinney, 1785 (Reproduced in Med. Classics, 2:30, 1937).
2. Chung, E.K.: Digitalis Intoxication. Baltimore, Williams & Wilkins Co., 1969.
3. Smith, T.W., and Haber, E.: Current techniques for serum or plasma digitalis assay and their potential clinical application. Am. J. Med. Sci. 259:301, 1970.
4. Doherty, J.E., Perkins, W.H., and Flanigan, W.J.: The distribution and concentration of tritiated digoxin in human tissues. Ann. Intern. Med. 66:116, 1967.
5. Somylo, A.P.: The toxicology of digitalis. Am. J. Cardiol. 5:523, 1960.
6. Navab, A., Koss, L.G., and LaDue, J.S.: Estrogen-like activity of digitalis. J.A.M.A. 194:30, 1965.
7. Young, R.C., Nachman, R.L., and Horowitz, H.I.: Thrombocytopenia due to digitoxin. Am. J. Med. 41:605, 1966.
8. Irons, G.V., Jr., and Orgain, E.S.: Digitalis-induced arrhythmias and their management. Prog. Cardiovasc. Dis. 8:539, 1966.
9. Lown, B., Wyatt, N.F., and Levine, H.D.: Paroxysmal atrial tachycardia with block. Circulation 21:129, 1960.
10. Alexander, S., and Ping, W.C.: Fatal ventricular fibrillation during carotid stimulation. Am. J. Cardiol. 18:289, 1966.
11. Hilal, H., and Massumi, R.: Fatal ventricular fibrillation after carotid-sinus stimulation. N. Engl. J. Med. 275:157, 1966.
12. Oliver, G.C., Jr., Parker, B.M., Brasfield, D.L., et al.: The measure of digitoxin in human serum by radioimmunoassay. J. Clin. Invest. 47:1035, 1968.
13. Beller, G.A., Smith, T.W., Abelmann, W.H., et al.: Digitalis intoxication. A prospective clinical study with serum level correlations. N. Engl. J. Med. 284:989, 1971.
14. Wotman, S., Bigger, J.T., Mandel, I.D., and Bartelstone, H.J.: Cardiologists hear about rapid saliva test for digitalis toxicity. J.A.M.A. 215:1068, 1971.
15. Lyon, A.F., and DeGraff, A.C.: Reappraisal of digitalis. X. Treatment of digitalis toxicity. Am. Heart J. 73:835, 1968.
16. Ruthen, G.C.: Antiarrhythmic drugs. IV. Diphenylhydantoin in cardiac arrhythmias. Am. Heart J. 70:275, 1965.
17. Conn, R.D.: Diphenylhydantoin sodium in cardiac arrhythmias. N. Engl. J. Med. 272:277, 1965.
18. Irons, G.V., Jr., Ginn, W.N., and Orgain, E.S.: Use of a beta adrenergic receptor blocking agent (propranolol) in the treatment of cardiac arrhythmias. Am. J. Med. 43:161, 1967.
19. Stock, J.P.P.: Beta adrenergic blocking drugs in the clinical management of cardiac arrhythmias. Am. J. Cardiol. 18:444, 1966.
20. Jewitt, D.E., Kishon, Y., and Thomas, M.: Lignocaine in the management of arrhythmias after acute myocardial infarction. Lancet 1:266, 1968.
21. Harrison, D.C., Sprouse, J.H., and Morrow, A.G.: Antiarrhythmic properties of lidocaine and procaine amide: Clinical and physiologic studies of their cardiovascular effects in man. Circulation 28:486, 1963.

22. Rosenbaum, J.L., Mason, D., and Sever, M.J.: The effect of disodium EDTA on digitalis intoxication. Am. J. Med. Sci. 240:111, 1960.
23. Cohen, B.D., Spritz, N., Lubash, G.D., and Rubin, A.L.: Use of a calcium chelating agent (Na EDTA) in cardiac arrhythmias. Circulation 19:918, 1959.
24. Seller, R.H., and Moyer, J.H.: Magnesium and digitalis toxicity. Heart Bull. 18:32, 1969.
25. Kim, Y.W., Andrews, C.E., and Ruth, W.E.: Serum magnesium and cardiac arrhythmias with special reference to digitalis intoxication. Am. J. Med. Sci. 242:87, 1961.
26. Kleiger, R., and Lown, B.: Cardioversion and digitalis. II. Clinical studies. Circulation 33:878, 1966.

Chapter 17

CARDIOPULMONARY EMERGENCY CARE IN INFANCY AND CHILDHOOD

GEORGE H. KHOURY

GENERAL CONSIDERATIONS

The basic pathophysiology of cardiopulmonary emergencies is similar in the adult and child. However, in children the incidence, causes, clinical manifestations, and management differ according to the various age groups. The immediate recognition and treatment of various emergencies in children, particularly in young infants, are essential to improving the morbidity. In this chapter, congestive heart failure, cyanotic spells, cardiac arrhythmias, respiratory failure, and cardiac arrest are discussed in detail.

CONGESTIVE HEART FAILURE

The incidence of congestive heart failure due to congenital heart disease is high during the first six months of life and is usually associated with a high morbidity.[1-8] The causes of heart failure can be classified into three main categories: (1) pressure-overloading lesions, such as obstruction of either the aortic or pulmonary valve, coarctation of the aorta and complete transposition of the great vessels, (2) volume-overloading lesions, such as large ventricular septal defect, patent ductus arteriosus, valvular insufficiency, and severe anemia, (3) diffuse myocardial disease, such as endocardial fibroelastosis and myocarditis, and anomalous origin of the left coronary artery from the main pulmonary artery.

Clinical Manifestations and Diagnosis

Infancy. In the newborn period, the diagnosis of congestive heart failure is often subtle. Several studies have demonstrated that there is a correlation between the type of cardiac defect and the age of the child at onset of heart failure (Fig. 17–1). The correlation is helpful to clinicians in making an exact diagnosis of the underlying cardiac lesion. During the first week of life, the most common cause of heart failure is hypoplastic left-sided heart syndrome, for which the outlook is bleak. In children eight days old to one month of age, coarctation of the aorta and complete transposition of the great vessels are the leading causes of heart failure. The prognosis for that lesion is improving with continuing advances in surgical treatment. In infants older than one month of age, a frequent cause of heart failure is large ventricular septal defect. In each age group, there is a group of miscellaneous causes, including AV canal defect, pulmonary atresia, cerebral arteriovenous fistula, and paroxysmal atrial tachycardia.

The clinical presentation of heart failure in infants is more subtle than in older children. In infants, its presence should be suspected when a sudden change in feeding habits or color occurs.

The cardinal indicators of heart failure are:
1. Dyspnea and tachypnea
2. Tachycardia

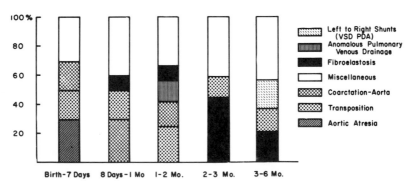

Figure 17–1.   Causes of heart failure from birth to 6 months as found in a study of 161 infants. (VSD = ventricular septal defect; PDA = patent ductus arteriosus.)

3. Hepatomegaly

4. Venous congestion, as indicated by congested neck veins or swollen veins on the dorsum of the hand or in the scalp

Those signs and symptoms occur in various degrees, depending on the severity of the lesion. In the newborn, one has to rely more on the presence of dyspnea and hepatomegaly than on the degree of tachycardia because the heart rate in the healthy newborn infant is rapid, with a wide range of normal variation. Other common symptoms of heart failure in young infants are poor feeding, vomiting, cough, irritability, and excessive perspiration on the forehead.

The diagnosis of heart failure is usually not difficult to make when a typical clinical picture is present. However, the condition has frequently been either overlooked or overdiagnosed.

When the only manifestation is increased respiratory activity (i.e., tachypnea) the differential diagnosis should include primary pulmonary disorders, such as respiratory distress syndrome, pneumonia, and bronchiolitis. A chest roentgenogram is very helpful in differentiating those conditions from congenital heart disease (Figs. 17–2 and 17–3). On the other hand, overdiagnosis of heart failure is often made in patients with cyanotic congenital heart disease in which the patient is subject to anoxic, blue, or paroxysmal dyspneic spells.

Older Children. In older children, the most common cause of heart failure is myocarditis of either viral or rheumatic origin, but there may be other causes, such as acute glomerulonephritis, chronic lung disease, and

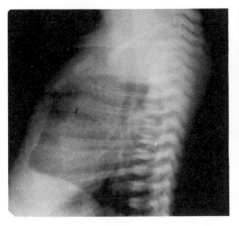 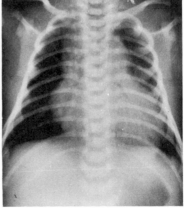

Figure 17–2.   Chest roentgenogram of a 3-day-old baby who, at autopsy, was found to have "hypoplastic left-heart complex." Notice the gross cardiomegaly with bilateral venous congestion. In the lateral view, the posterior cardiac border is straight.

anemia. The onset is usually sudden, and the manifestation is usually that of pulmonary edema. The diagnosis is made on the basis of sudden dyspnea and tachypnea with air hunger. The chest roentgenogram is usually classic (Fig. 17–4). It shows bilateral venous congestion that is

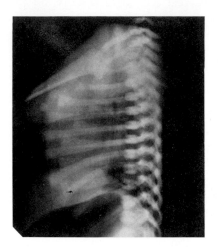 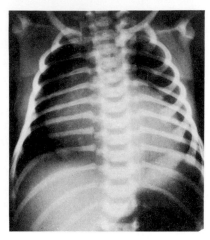

Figure 17–3.   Chest roentgenogram of a 2-day-old baby with "hypoplastic right-heart complex," which consists of pulmonary atresia, tricuspid stenosis, and right ventricular hypoplasia. Notice the large right atrial shadow. The pulmonary vascular markings are decreased. In the lateral view, the lower retrosternal space is clear.

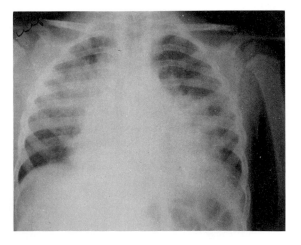

Figure 17–4.   Chest roentgenogram of a 2-year-old boy who was admitted to the hospital with severe pulmonary edema. The heart is enlarged. Note the bilateral hilar pulmonary infiltrate with venous congestion.

denser in the hilar area. Immediate recognition of the problem is mandatory if the child is to be saved.

Medical Treatment

Therapy for heart failure has four main components: (1) digitalis, (2) diuretics, (3) oxygen, and (4) low salt diet.

Digitalis. The guidelines for digitalis therapy must be followed (see Chapter 7). It is improper to digitalize acutely ill patients without careful clinical and ECG monitoring. There are many preparations of digitalis available, but the physician should become accustomed to one type; for children, digoxin (Lanoxin) is considered the safest preparation. Digoxin may be administered either orally or parenterally (see Chapter 7). The parenteral route is usually preferred if the infant or child has severe congestive heart failure or if there is a history of vomiting. Dosage may be prescribed in different ways, as shown in Table 17–1. The order must be written clearly and precisely. Every physician should be familiar with the usual digitalizing methods (see Chapter 7). Therapy can be monitored by obtaining a determination of the blood digitalis level. Digitalis intoxication is manifested by vomiting and diarrhea followed by various cardiac arrhythmias, mainly ventricular ectopic beats, supraventricular tachycardia, and varying degrees of AV block (Chapter 16). The earliest sign of digitalis intoxication in infants is usually vomiting.

Diuretics. The diuretics most commonly used in acute congestive heart failure are furosemide (Lasix) and ethacrynic acid (Edecrin). Ethacrynic acid should only be given intravenously. Furosemide could be given orally, intramuscularly, or intravenously. The dose is 1 to 2 mg/kg.[10] When using diuretics, one should be alert to the possibility of hypochloremia, hyponatremia, and hypokalemia, which make the patient

Table 17–1. *Digoxin Dosages*

Digitalizing Dose	Age of Child (yr)	
	<2	>2
Oral	0.07 mg/kg	0.04 mg/kg
IM or IV	0.05 mg/kg	0.03 mg/kg
Oral	0.03 mg/lb	0.02 mg/lb
IM or IV	0.02 mg/lb	0.015 mg/lb
Oral	1.6 mg/m²	1.0 mg/m²
IV	0.9 mg/m²	—

Maintenance dose: ⅓ to ⅕ of the digitalizing dose.

less responsive to digitalis and predisposes him to digitalis intoxication (Chapter 16). Thiazide diuretics are usually used once the acute episode is over.

Surgical Treatment

Surgical treatment is sometimes indicated when there is no response to the medical decongestive measures. A notable example is in coarctation of the aorta or transposition of the great vessels. One can only stress that severe congestive heart failure in infants should be considered an emergency, because a delay in either medical or surgical treatment may result in death.

CYANOTIC SPELLS

Etiology, Clinical Manifestations, and Diagnosis

Cyanosis is an alarming symptom, particularly when it is associated with respiratory distress and when it manifests itself in the first few days of life. First, it must be determined whether the cause of cyanosis is cardiac or noncardiac. That determination is made with the aid of a carefully taken history and physical examination, in conjunction with a chest roentgenogram, an ECG, a blood gases analysis, and an echocardiogram. When a cyanotic congenital heart disease is suspected, an aggressive approach should be adopted, since a delay in diagnosis and treatment may be disastrous.

People with cyanotic heart disease and decreased pulmonary blood flow, such as tetralogy of Fallot, are susceptible to cyanotic spells. (Those spells are also known as paroxysmal dyspneic spells, blue spells, and anoxic spells.) The cyanotic spells are characterized by a sudden hyperpnea, marked cyanosis, generalized limpness, and fainting. Occasionally, the patient may develop severe convulsion resulting in death.

The incidence of those spells in people suffering from cyanotic heart disease is from 20 to 40%.[11-12] The spells are usually triggered by crying or tachycardia, which results in an increase in right to left shunt, producing a sudden alteration in arterial oxygen and carbon dioxide tension and hydrogen ion concentration. Those manifestations in turn stimulate the respiratory center and cause the hyperpnea, which perpetuates the cycle.

Treatment

The treatment consists of:
1. The immediate administration of oxygen

2. Sedation, in the form of morphine, 0.1 mg/pound
3. Propranolol, which has been used at a dosage of 1 to 2 mg/kg orally in cases of tetralogy of Fallot with infundicular stenosis

Frequent spells dictate early surgical correction of the lesion.

In addition to cyanotic spells, one must be aware of other complications in cyanotic heart disease, such as acidosis, hypocalcemia, and hypoglycemia.

To improve the salvage rate of patients with cyanotic heart disease, one should refer them to a fully equipped medical center where an accurate diagnosis can be established and proper management can be instituted before complications develop.

CARDIAC ARRHYTHMIAS

Cardiac arrhythmias are encountered less frequently in children than in adults. The causes of the cardiac arrhythmias seen in children are as follows:
1. Idiopathic causes
2. Congenital heart disease
3. Familial causes
4. Autonomic immaturity
5. Hypoxia
6. Infections (e.g., myocarditis)
7. Cardiac tumors
8. Iatrogenic causes (cardiac surgery, cardiac catheterization, drugs, anesthesia)

Serious arrhythmias commonly seen in children are those that produce clinical symptoms, including supraventricular tachycardia, atrial flutter, congenital AV block, and postsurgical arrhythmias.

Supraventricular Tachycardia

Clinical Manifestations and Diagnosis. Supraventricular tachycardia is the most common serious arrhythmia occurring in children two weeks to six months of age. The true incidence is unknown, but an estimate of 1:25,000 was given by Keith, Rowe, and Vlad.[13] The onset of the arrhythmia is usually sudden, and it is precipitated by infection, commonly pneumonia. The infant may be asymptomatic in the early stages, in which case the only abnormal finding is the tachycardia itself. However, if the tachycardia persists, the infant usually develops congestive heart failure and presents with peripheral vascular collapse. The infant is usually ashen gray or cyanotic, clammy, and cold. Respiration is rapid and labored. The heart rate may vary from 180 to 300 beats per minute

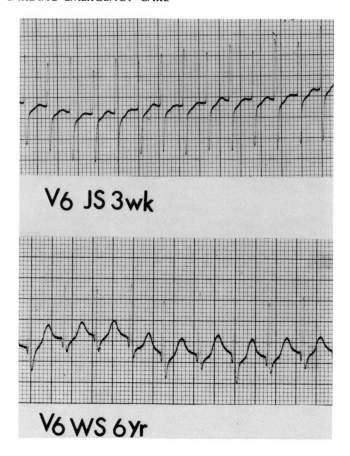

Figure 17–5.   The top tracing shows supraventricular tachycardia with a ventricular rate of 280 beats per minute in a 3-week-old baby. The bottom tracing shows paroxysmal supraventricular tachycardia with a ventricular rate of 180 beats per minute in a 6-year-old boy.

(Fig. 17–5). Peripheral pulses are usually weak and thready. In 15 to 20% of patients, the ECG during sinus rhythm exhibits the Wolff-Parkinson-White syndrome. The paroxysms that occur before six months of age are more common in boys than in girls, and the recurrence rate is very low. In older children, supraventricular tachycardia usually has less effect on cardiovascular hemodynamics, and the main symptom is usually palpitation.

Treatment. The treatment usually consists of rapid intravenous or intramuscular digitalization (Chapter 7). However, in severe heart failure, immediate termination of the tachycardia is desirable, and direct current cardioversion is the treatment of choice (Chapter 10). The longer the duration of tachycardia, the higher the incidence of heart failure. Propranolol, in combination with digoxin, provides effective prophylaxis for recurrent supraventricular tachycardia (Chapter 7). Various antiarrhythmic drugs (Chapter 7) have been used in adults, but they are of little value in children.

Congenital Atrioventricular Block

Clinical Manifestations and Diagnosis. The clinical picture in congenital AV block differs from that of AV block in adults[14] (Chapter 8). The cardiac output is usually normal because of increased stroke volume. The majority of patients are asymptomatic except for easy fatigability and subnormal exercise tolerance. When symptoms do occur, the prognosis is usually less favorable. The two most common symptoms of congenital AV block are congestive heart failure and Adams-Stokes attacks in the form of fainting spells or convulsions or both. Those symptoms are likely to occur in patients with a slow ventricular rate, usually below 30 to 40 beats per minute, and a wide QRS complex, which indicates that the block is in the lower part of the His bundle. When the ventricular rate is faster than 60 beats per minute, the diagnosis may be missed, especially when an ECG is not taken (Fig. 17–6). On auscultation, a systolic ejection murmur

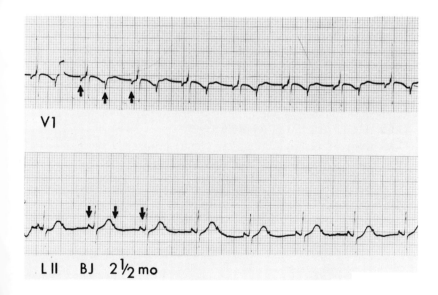

V1

L II   BJ   2½ mo

Figure 17–6. The electrocardiogram shows 2:1 AV block with atrial rate of 160 beats per minute and ventricular rate of 80 beats per minute.

in an infant with a heart rate of 60 beats or less per minute is a clinical sign that strongly suggests complete AV block.

Treatment. The indications for cardiac pacing in congenital AV block are:
1. Persistent heart failure in spite of therapy with digitalis and diuretics
2. The occurrence of the Adams-Stokes syndrome
3. A ventricular rate below 40 beats per minute with symptoms on exercise (Chapter 11). A His bundle recording is of value in delineating the level of the block and in clarifying the prognosis in individual cases. The use of artificial pacemakers is discussed in detail in Chapter 11.

Atrial Flutter

Atrial flutter in infancy is very rare. It may occur in a congenital form, which can usually be predicted before the child is born.[15] The presenting symptoms of atrial flutter with 1:1 AV response are heart failure or repeated bouts of vomiting or both (Fig. 17–7). Therapy consists of cardioversion (Chapter 10) or the use of antiarrhythmic drugs, particularly diphenylhydantoin (Dilantin) and quinidine (Chapter 7).

Postsurgical Arrhythmias

Postsurgical arrhythmias in children commonly occur following open-heart surgery, but they can occur during anesthesia. The common arrhythmias include AV junctional tachycardia, atrial flutter, complete AV block, premature ectopic beats, and ventricular tachycardia.

In dealing with postsurgical arrhythmias, one must answer the following questions:
1. Is the patient symptomatic or asymptomatic?
2. What is the status of the patient's cardiovascular hemodynamics?
3. Does the patient have hypotension?
4. Does the patient have congestive heart failure?

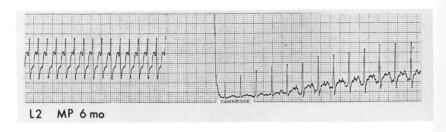

L2   MP 6 mo

Figure 17–7.   Atrial flutter with 1:1 AV response (ventricular rate: 360 beats per minute). Sinus rhythm with a rate of 150 beats per minute was restored by direct current cardioversion.

In other words, one must determine the urgency of termination of the arrhythmia. Antiarrhythmic drugs (Table 17–2) should be used judiciously, with continuous ECG monitoring. A detailed description of antiarrhythmic therapy is found in Chapter 7.

Table 17–2. *Dosages of Antiarrhythmic Drugs*

Quinidine gluconate
    IM: 2 mg/kg as initial test dose; then 5–10 mg/kg every 6 hours as needed
    IV: 0.5 mg/kg given slowly over 10–15 minutes with ECG monitoring; stop if bradycardia
       develops
    PO: 10–30 mg/kg/day
Propranolol (Inderal)
    PO: 1–2 mg/kg
Diphenylhydantoin (Dilantin)
    PO: 2–5 mg/kg/day in two or three doses
    IV: 3–5 mg/kg injected slowly over 5 to 10 minutes
Lidocaine (Xylocaine)
    IV: 0.15–1 mg/kg every 20 to 60 minutes as needed

RESPIRATORY FAILURE

Acute respiratory distress is an emergency that requires immediate recognition and prompt, multidisciplinary management. Respiratory failure may occur in any patient who has a severe pulmonary, cardiac, or central nervous system disorder.[16] In children, the causes, clinical presentation, and management of respiratory failure vary with the child's age (Table 17–3).

Table 17–3. *Common Causes of Acute Respiratory Failure*

Age	Cause
Newborn	Respiratory distress syndrome due to:
	Hyaline membrane disease
	Pneumonia
	Atelectasis
	Pleural effusion, bilateral
	Diaphragmatic hernia
	Congestive heart failure, severe
	Central nervous system disorders
Infancy and childhood	Acute bronchiolitis
	Epiglottitis
	Status asthmaticus
	Bronchopneumonia with tenacious secretions
	Cardiac surgery
	Infectious polyneuritis
	Drowning
	Septic shock

Hyaline Membrane Disease

In the newborn, hyaline membrane disease (HMD) is the leading cause of respiratory failure, and hence it merits discussion. HMD is primarily a disease of premature infants, but it can occur in full-term infants born by cesarean section or to diabetic mothers. The principal cause of HMD is a deficiency of pulmonary surfactant, a lipoprotein complex consisting of two molecules, lecithin and sphingomyelin. The lack of pulmonary surfactant leads to collapse of the alveolar sacs and ducts, with deposition of an eosinophilic membrane along the inner lining of the terminal bronchioles and alveolar sacs and ducts.

Suspected HMD can be confirmed before the child's birth by examining the amniotic fluid for the lecithin-sphingomyelin (L-S) ratio.[17] The clinical diagnosis of HMD depends on the presence of characteristic findings, which consist of tachypnea, expiratory grunting, subcostal and intercostal retractions, nasal flaring, cyanosis, and poor muscle tone. However, those signs could be indicative of other causes of respiratory distress, including pneumonia, pneumothorax, pleural effusion, pulmonary hemorrhage, atelectasis, diaphragmatic hernia, and ascites. The diagnosis of HMD is usually confirmed by radiographic demonstration of a reticulogranular pattern usually described as a ground-glass appearance of both lungs and an air bronchogram extending beyond the cardiac shadow.

Clinical Manifestations and Diagnosis

The signs and symptoms that should alert the physician to the possibility of impending respiratory failure are tachypnea, dyspnea, erratic breathing, chest wall retraction, cyanosis, generalized hypotonia with depressed reflexes and systemic hypotension or hypertension. Those findings should be corroborated by the analysis of arterial blood gases at room air and after breathing 100% oxygen for 10 to 15 minutes. Biochemically, the patient with respiratory failure has combined metabolic and respiratory acidosis.

Laboratory Findings

The blood gas indices of respiratory failure and of the need for assisted ventilation also vary according to the cause of the failure. However, in general, hypoxemia (PO_2 50 mm Hg or less for newborns after breathing 100% oxygen and less than 100 mm Hg in older children) and hypercarbia (PCO_2 75 mm Hg or over) should alert the physician to the need for assisted ventilation.

Management

In the management of respiratory failure in infants, adequate caloric intake should be maintained. Body temperature should be regulated to prevent hypothermia. Complications, such as sepsis, bleeding, vascular problems due to vessel catheterization, and oxygen intoxication, should be prevented.

CARDIAC ARREST

Etiology and Clinical Manifestations

Cardiac arrest means an abrupt cessation of the circulation of the blood due to either ventricular fibrillation or ventricular standstill. In association with cardiac arrest, the respiratory efforts are ineffective and hence pulmonary ventilation is poor. Cardiac arrest may occur at any age, and it is often unexpected. Its cause is any condition leading to hypoxia, myocardial depression, or arrhythmia, drug poisoning, anesthesia, electrolyte imbalance, and any condition leading to shock.

Cardiopulmonary Resuscitation (See also Chapter 12)

The success of cardiopulmonary resuscitation depends on many factors, including primary causative disease, adequacy and timing of emergency treatment, and adequacy of drug therapy in conjunction with the use of defibrillator as needed.

In cardiopulmonary resuscitation, the following principles must be kept in mind:

1. The cardiac output must be maintained by closed cardiac massage.

2. The most efficient type of artificial ventilation is expired ventilation using the mouth-to-mouth method or a mask and bag tightly applied to the mouth.

3. Acidosis often develops rapidly after cardiac arrest, and it must be treated promptly.

Phase 1. 1. The exact time of the arrest should be recorded if it is known.

2. A sharp blow should be delivered to the precordium, and help should be summoned.

3. For mouth-to-mouth breathing to be effective, the airway should be opened by tilting the person's head backward, and a tight seal should be applied over his nose and mouth. (Tracheal intubation should be performed only by skilled personnel.)

Table 17–4.   *Drugs Used for Cardiopulmonary Resuscitation*

Drug	Dosage
Sodium bicarbonate	2 mEq/kg every 10 minutes (monitor pH)
Epinephrine	0.1–0.5 mg IC or IV
Calcium gluconate (10%)	3–5 cc IV
Isoproterenol (Isuprel)	Initial dose 0.5 mg diluted in 10 ml 5% D/W IV or IC. Then slow IV drip 1 mg in 250 ml 5% D/W (discontinue if tachycardia or arrhythmias occur)
Metaraminol bitartrate (Aramine)	IV drip 0.3 mg/kg in 250 ml 5% D/W

4. Closed cardiac massage should follow ventilation; the pressure point in infants and young children is on the lower half of the breast plate, just above its soft lower end. In infants, the chest should be held with both hands and the thumbs held exactly over the breast plate. In older children, the heel of one hand should be placed over the lower sternum. Compression should be in the form of rhythmic pressure of 1 to 1.5 inches at a rate of 100 to 120 per minute. The effectiveness of the cardiac massage should be evaluated by noting the patient's color, size of pupils, pulse, and cardiac action.

Phase 2. Phase 2 is the period during which

1. An ECG should be recorded to determine the type of electrical activity; it may be asystole (i.e., total absence of electrical activity) or ventricular fibrillation.

2. An intravenous infusion should be started immediately; information about the drugs and dosages frequently used in cardiopulmonary resuscitation is summarized in Table 17–4.

Phase 3. Phase 3 refers to the care of the patient after (1) cardiac action has been restored and (2) an adequate cardiac output has been established with or without adrenergic drugs. The patient is then moved to the intensive care unit, where he is carefully monitored, since cardiac arrest may recur. Every effort should be made to eliminate the possible causes of arrest.

The success of cardiopulmonary resuscitation depends on a disciplined and organized team effort. Cardiopulmonary resuscitation is described in detail in Chapter 12.

SUMMARY

1. The incidence, causes, clinical manifestations, and management of cardiopulmonary emergencies in children are different from those in adults.

2. The immediate recognition and treatment of various emergencies,

particularly in young infants, are essential to a successful outcome and an improved salvage rate.

3. The incidence of heart failure due to congenital heart disease is high during the first six months of life, and it is usually associated with a high morbidity.

4. The cardinal clinical features indicating the presence of heart failures are dyspnea, tachycardia, hepatomegaly, and venous congestion. Other common symptoms include poor feeding, vomiting, cough, irritability, and excessive perspiration on the forehead.

5. The initial therapy for heart failure is medical, but surgical therapy is indicated in such conditions as coarctation of the aorta and transposition of the great vessels when there is no response to decongestive measures.

6. Cyanotic spells, known also as paroxysmal dyspneic spells, are characterized by a sudden hyperpnea, marked cyanosis, generalized limpness, and fainting. The incidence of those spells ranges from 20 to 40% in patients with cyanotic heart diseases associated with decreased pulmonary blood flow. The treatment consists of immediate administration of oxygen and sedation with morphine or phenobarbital. Frequent spells dictate early surgical correction of the cardiac lesion.

7. Cardiac arrhythmias are encountered less frequently in children than in adults. The most common arrhythmias are supraventricular tachycardia and post-surgery arrhythmias. The use of antiarrhythmic drugs varies according to the specific type of rhythm disturbance. They should be used judiciously and with constant ECG monitoring.

8. Acute respiratory distress is an emergency that requires immediate recognition and prompt, multidisciplinary management. The causes, clinical presentation, and management of respiratory failure vary with the person's age and with the cause.

9. Hyaline membrane disease is the leading cause of respiratory failure in the newborn, and its diagnosis is usually confirmed by the radiographic demonstration of a reticulogranular pattern described as a ground-glass appearance of both lungs and an air bronchogram that extends beyond the cardiac shadow.

10. Cardiac arrest, from whatever cause, requires prompt cardiopulmonary resuscitation. The principles of cardiopulmonary resuscitation for children are the same as those for adults (Chapter 12), but the technique differs somewhat. The success of cardiopulmonary resuscitation depends on a disciplined, organized team approach.

REFERENCES

1. Keith, J.D.: Congestive heart failure. Pediatrics 18:491, 1956.
2. Nadas, A.S., and Hauck, A.J.: Pediatric aspects of congestive heart failure. Circulation 21:424, 1960.

3. Neill, C.A.: Recognition and treatment of congestive heart failure in infancy: I. Diagnosis. Mod. Concepts Cardiovasc. Dis. 28:499, 1959.
4. Neill, C.A.: Recognition and treatment of congestive heart failure in infancy: II. Treatment. Mod. Concepts Cardiovasc. Dis. 28:507, 1959.
5. McCue, C.M., and Young, R.B.: Cardiac failure in infancy. J. Pediatr. 58:330, 1961.
6. Engle, M.A.: Cardiac failure in infancy: Recognition and management. Mod. Concepts Cardiovasc. Dis. 32:825, 1963.
7. Lambert, E.C., Canent, R.V., and Hohn, A.R.: Congenital cardiac anomalies in the newborn. A review of conditions causing death or severe distress in the first month of life. Pediatrics 37:343, 1966.
8. Khoury, G.H., and Hawes, C.R.: Congestive heart failure in infancy: Pitfalls in diagnosis and management. Med. Times 97:142, 1969.
9. Hauck, A.J., Ongley, P.A., and Nadas, A.S.: The use of digoxin in infants and children. Am. Heart J. 56:443, 1958.
10. Sparrow, A.W., Friedberg, D.Z., and Nadas, A.S.: The use of ethacrynic acid in infants and children with congestive heart failure. Pediatrics 42:291, 1968.
11. Morgan, B.C., Guntheroth, W.G., Bloom, R.S., and Fyler, D.C.: A clinical profile of paroxysmal hyperpnea in cyanotic congenital heart disease. Circulation 31:66, 1965.
12. Guntheroth, W.G., Morgan, B.C., and Mullins, G.: Physiologic studies of paroxysmal hyperpnea in cyanotic congenital heart disease. Circulation 31:70, 1965.
13. Keith, J.D., Rowe, R.D., and Vlad, P.: Heart Disease in Infancy and Childhood. 2nd ed. New York, The Macmillan Co., 1967.
14. Paul, M., Rudolph, A., and Nadas, A.S.: Congenital complete atrioventricular block: Problems of clinical assessment. Circulation 18:183, 1958.
15. Landtman, B., and Kassila, E.: Auricular flutter in infancy. Acta Paediatr. Scand. 44:272, 1955.
16. Downes, J.J., Fulgencio, T., and Raphaely, R.C.: Acute respiratory failure in infants and children. Pediatr. Clin. N. Am. 19:423, 1972.
17. Gluck, L., Kulvoich, M.V., Borer, R.C., et al.: Diagnosis of the respiratory distress syndrome by amniocentesis. Am. J. Obstet. Gynecol. 109:440, 1971.

Chapter 18

THE SURGICAL APPROACH TO CARDIAC EMERGENCIES

STANLEY K. BROCKMAN

There are a number of conditions for which an emergency cardiac operation is the treatment of choice. (Those conditions are enumerated in Table 18–1.) The emergency operative approach to the heart requires that the surgical team be familiar not only with standard methods but also with techniques of extracorporeal circulation and circulatory assist devices. A

Table 18–1. *Types of Conditions Requiring Emergency Cardiac Surgery*

Trauma
Penetrating
Nonpenetrating
Dissecting hematoma (aneurysm) of the aorta
Cardiac tumors
Valvular heart disease
Ischemic heart disease
Complications of myocardial infarction
Ventricular aneurysm
Ventricular septal defect
Mitral regurgitation
Cardiogenic shock
Pericarditis
Arrhythmias
Congenital heart disease

fully equipped emergency room, operating room, and postoperative care unit, all with personnel trained in the care of complicated cardiac problems, are required.

In the discussion in this chapter, emphasis has been put on the practices and techniques in use at our institution as well as elsewhere.

CARDIAC TRAUMA

Cardiac trauma continues to grow as a source of mortality and morbidity paralleling advances in our mechanized society and the increased incidence of man raising weapons against his fellows. Approximately two-thirds of people killed in automobile accidents have some cardiac trauma. Stab wounds of the heart continue to occur with regularity. In some localities, gunshot wounds of the heart continue to increase at an alarming rate. In many instances, cardiac trauma is not isolated but is associated with massive chest trauma or trauma involving multiple organ systems.

Penetrating Cardiac Trauma

Historical Aspects and Perspectives. Most penetrating wounds are caused by sharp instruments, such as knives or ice picks, or by gunshot wounds. Penetrating trauma compromises circulation and may cause death by producing cardiac tamponade, hemorrhage, or an ineffective heart beat. The first successful suture closure of an actively bleeding wound of the human heart was done by Rehn (in 1897).[1] The first successful closure of a cardiac wound in the United States was performed by Hill (in 1902).[2] In 1920, Tuffier[3] reviewed 305 cases of cardiac trauma and reported a recovery rate of approximately 50%, which confirmed the use of cardiorrhaphy as the treatment of choice for penetrating wounds of the heart. In 1943, Blalock and Ravitch[4] suggested pericardial aspiration as an alternative method of treatment of tamponade associated with penetrating wounds of the heart. Open operation was reserved for wounds that were not immediately fatal in which pericardiocentesis alone would not suffice. The conservative approach of pericardiocentesis has been used with claims of good results. However, during the last 15 years many inadequacies of pericardiocentesis have been recognized. The comparison of immediate operation with pericardiocentesis has been somewhat misleading since patients treated by pericardiocentesis are carefully selected and those with massive hemorrhage and severe wounds have been omitted from most studies. Almost all surgeons now clearly prefer early thoracotomy with pericardiotomy and cardiorrhaphy as the most effective method of treating patients with penetrating wounds of the heart.

Emergency operation to avoid recurrent tamponade, infection, pseudo-aneurysm formation, and death has again emerged as the treatment of choice for penetrating wounds of the heart.

Pathology. More than 50% of the people with penetrating cardiac wounds do not reach the hospital alive. The survival depends largely on the severity of the wound, so that patients with massive injuries, particularly gunshot wounds, are least likely to reach the hospital alive. Approximately 70% of penetrating injuries to the heart occur in the ventricle, and the right ventricle is involved more frequently than the left. Ten per cent of the wounds are in the atrium, and 20% involve the pulmonary artery, vena cava, coronary vessels, intrapericardial aorta, or the pericardium alone.[5-8] Sugg and his co-workers[8] demonstrated that wounds of the left ventricle have the highest mortality. Only 8% of patients with isolated left ventricular wounds reached the hospital alive.

Pathophysiology. The pathophysiology is essentially the production of acute hemopericardium with cardiac tamponade. Were it not for the unyielding presence of the tough, fibrous pericardium, most patients would suffer hopeless hemorrhage and immediate death. The restraining force of the pericardium, with its consequent pericardial tamponade, enables the patient to survive long enough to reach the hospital and the operating room. In surviving patients, there is a balance between the lifesaving effect of the pericardial tamponade and its lethal effects. The limitation of diastolic expansion of the ventricle caused by the pericardial tamponade decreases cardiac filling. Cardiac output and blood pressure fall, venous pressure rises, and the clinical picture of low cardiac output leading to shock evolves. Acute hemopericardium (150 to 200 ml of blood) can cause severe shock and death as a result of the tamponade. At those levels, pericardial aspiration of small amounts of blood may mean the difference between life and death.

Diagnosis and Clinical Status. Most patients are admitted to the emergency room with obvious trauma, and in most instances the nature of the weapon is known. The most important factor in the diagnosis of penetrating wounds of the heart is the physician's high index of suspicion. When the physician has a high index of suspicion, he should assume that there is a penetrating wound of the heart unless proved otherwise. The majority of patients are in shock that is out of proportion to the severity of the wound or any obvious loss of blood. Almost 50% of the patients have low or no detectable blood pressure when they are first seen in the emergency room. Approximately 23% of the patients have a systolic blood pressure of 40 mm Hg or less, and approximately 31% of the patients have a systolic blood pressure of 70 mm Hg or above.[8] Other clinical signs of shock, such as a dull sensorium, agitation, disorientation, rapid, thready pulse, and cold, clammy skin, are frequently present. The neck veins may be distended, the heart sounds muffled and difficult to hear; and a falling or absent blood pressure with a rising or elevated venous pressure confirm the diagnosis of pericardial tamponade. As soon as the diagnosis is suspected, emergency pericardiocentesis should be performed for diagnostic and therapeutic purposes. When blood is removed from the pericardium, the diagnosis is certain. Even when blood is not aspirated, at least 15% or more of the patients still have hemopericardium. In patients with massive trauma without pericardial tamponade who survive to reach the hospital, the clinical manifestations are predominantly those of shock due to massive blood loss. In addition, those patients have signs and symptoms of associated trauma, such as pneumothorax, hemothorax, or tension pneumothorax, adding to the picture of shock. Chest roentgenograms (Chapter 19) may help by showing enlargement of the cardiac shadow or associated hemothorax and pneumothorax. The roentgenogram may show the location of a bullet and aid one in plotting its course to determine what organs may have been damaged. In many patients, however, the time necessary for obtaining a chest roentgenogram might be better used in the operating room. The ECG usually shows S–T and T-wave changes,[6] but it is not of great help in diagnosing or determining the severity of a penetrating wound of the heart. If the patient's condition is stable, the ECG can be obtained, but if his condition is even slightly unstable, an operation should not be delayed. Within a few days after injury, most patients demonstrate some elevation of the S–T segments, which may be followed by inversion of the S–T segments in some of the leads. Those changes may be temporary or permanent. If they are permanent, they should not be mistaken later for ischemic heart disease.

Treatment (See also Chapter 14). Before 1965, most penetrating wounds of the heart were treated by pericardiocentesis and observation, with surgery reserved for patients for whom pericardiocentesis proved unsuccessful. Since 1965, pericardiocentesis has been used less and less and only to confirm the diagnosis or to decompress the tamponade while the patient is being prepared for operation. The results of pericardiocentesis have been enigmatic, and reports have been misleading since massive injuries with exsanguinating hemorrhage have frequently not been included. In patients with large pericardial lacerations and penetrating injuries of the heart, brisk hemorrhage occurs, requiring prompt cardiorrhaphy. Pericardiocentesis alone has the following disadvantages: (1) there may be persistent or recurrent tamponade, (2) the patient may deteriorate rapidly during an observation period, (3) thrombi may be present and cannot be removed, (4) secondary hemorrhage may occur hours or days later, (5) constrictive pericarditis may eventually result from clotted blood, (6) rarely, traumatic ventricular aneurysm may result,

(7) damage may be done to the heart by the probing needle, and (8) infection may result from trapped, clotted blood.[5-8,74] Current medical practice dictates that any patient strongly suspected of having penetrating cardiac injury with tamponade be moved to the operating room as rapidly as possible for thoracotomy or sternotomy, pericardiotomy, and direct repair of the wound. Time is spent in the emergency room and enroute to the operating room only for typing and cross-matching blood, beginning intravenous infusions, establishing an airway, inserting a Foley catheter, and performing diagnostic and therapeutic pericardiocentesis. Diagnostic studies, such as roentgenograms, measurement of venous pressure, and ECG, may be performed when the patient is stable and when it is certain that the loss of time will not jeopardize the patient's health. Patients with any degree of low cardiac output, particularly those having shock and anoxia, may be prone to cardiac arrest during induction of anesthesia; for such patients, emergency and rapid thoracotomy or sternotomy is required. Most penetrating wounds of the heart are best approached through a left anterolateral thoracotomy via the fourth or fifth intercostal space. The incision may be extended across the sternum for additional exposure of the right side of the heart. When the wound of entrance is on the right side of the heart, a right-sided thoracotomy may be done. In some instances, a median sternotomy may be the preferred incision, particularly when cardiopulmonary bypass is likely to be used. The pericardium is widely incised, blood clots are rapidly evacuated, and the point of bleeding is controlled by direct digital pressure. Release of the cardiac tamponade and control of hemorrhage are the crucial points of the operation. When digital control of bleeding under direct vision has been achieved, blood and fluid replacement is achieved to establish normal circulation before the definitive repair of the wound is made. If the heart is asystolic, it may be advantageous to close the wound rapidly prior to cardiac massage and resuscitation. Circulation must be restored as soon as possible to prevent irreversible cerebral damage. The wound is closed by suture repair beneath the occluding finger, and each suture is tied before the next suture is placed until the wound is completely closed. In some instances, small pledgets of Teflon and Dacron felt may be helpful. When the wound is adjacent to a coronary vessel, the suture may be passed beneath the coronary vessel in mattress fashion to avoid obstruction of the coronary flow. When there are extensive cardiac wounds or when there are posterior wounds that are difficult to expose, emergency cardiopulmonary bypass may be lifesaving. For some patients with massive hemorrhage, the use of an autotransfusion device may be helpful. Finally, a circulatory assist technique, such as intra-aortic balloon pumping, may help the patient through a period of depressed circulation that would otherwise be fatal. Wounds of the atrium may be best handled by

the use of noncrushing vascular clamps rather than digital pressure because of the thin and yielding nature of the atrial wall. It should be stressed that careful examination of the heart in the operating room is required and the wound of exit as well as the wound of entrance be located. Cases have been reported in which the wound of exit has been missed, with tragic results.

Complications. The complications of penetrating wounds of the heart that may require further therapy are constrictive pericarditis, the post-pericardiotomy syndrome, congestive heart failure from valvular damage, ventricular septal defect, aorto-ventricular fistula, and ventricular and coronary artery aneurysms. Early operative management of penetrating wounds of the heart should prevent the occurrence of late constrictive pericarditis by the removal of all blood and clots from the pericardium, along with the establishment of good postoperative drainage. There may be an occasional case in which continued small leaks in the immediate postoperative period could produce constrictive pericarditis. The development of a ventricular or coronary artery aneurysm should be prevented by adequate initial repair, but theoretically one could develop with a leak through the ventricular suture line or a missed coronary artery wound. The post-pericardiotomy syndrome occurs in a small percentage of patients with or without operation; if therapy is required, salicylates or steroids are used. When valvular insufficiency, ventricular septal defect, or other intracardiac defects are produced, they are rarely if ever corrected at the time of the initial operation. The corrective operation is usually performed electively weeks after the original injury and after cardiac catheterization and angiography have precisely defined the nature and severity of the defect.[17,18]

Results. In general, the results of surgery reflect the severity of the injury. Most of the deaths are of patients who enter the emergency room with irreversible shock and severe injuries. The mortality for penetrating wounds of the heart with cardiac tamponade treated by pericardial aspiration alone has ranged up to 25%.[9-15] Beall and his co-workers[9] reported a mortality of 5.5% in 78 patients treated by pericardiocentesis. In 23 patients who did not respond to pericardiocentesis, the mortality was 26.7% when thoracotomy and cardiorrhaphy were carried out almost immediately, but that figure more than doubled when significant delays were permitted. In a more recent report, the same group now advocates the aggressive operative management of penetrating chest trauma.[13] Mortality figures similar to those for pericardiocentesis have been reported for emergency thoracotomy and range up to 36%.[5-8,29-31,74] It is significant that the mortality has been reduced since 1965 by early thoracotomy, an approach that was championed by Naclerio in 1964.[6] In 1968, Sugg and his co-workers[8] reported a mortality of 36% in patients treated before 1966. Of 18 deaths, 10 were due to secondary and recurrent tamponade; the authors felt that the wounds involved could have been repaired by thoracotomy. The same group reported a mortality of only 5% after 1966, when early thoracotomy was adopted. In 1970, Borgia and his co-workers[7] reported a mortality of 16.6% in 54 patients with stab wounds of the heart that were treated by early thoracotomy from 1951 through 1968. Of the deaths in that group, two patients died from transfusion reaction after having been given unmatched blood, three patients died of cardiac arrest in the recovery room, and one patient died from a myocardial infarction following obstruction of the left anterior descending coronary artery caused by an inappropriately placed suture. One patient was clinically dead on arrival at the operating room, and one patient died from exsanguination, with irreversible brain damage. Thus the deaths could not be ascribed to the use of thoracotomy as compared with pericardiocentesis. In 1971, Hutchinson and his co-workers[19] reported on 34 patients with penetrating cardiac wounds from 1967 to 1970, of whom 31 were in severe shock at the time of admission. There were only eight deaths among these patients. Three deaths were the result of severe gunshot wounds, and seven of the eight patients who had died had no recordable blood pressure when they were admitted to the operating room. The excellent results are attributed to early thoracotomy. Balanowski and his co-workers[16] reported a mortality of 15% in 34 patients with stab wounds of the heart and a mortality of 60% in those with gunshot wounds of the heart. All those patients were treated by immediate thoracotomy. In 1972, Carrasquilla and his co-workers[21] reported on a series of patients having penetrating wounds of the heart, almost 50% (27) of which were caused by gunshot. Twenty of the 27 patients survived, and their survival is largely attributed to early thoracotomy. In that group, the protective effect of tamponade strikingly demonstrated the fact that all the deaths occurred in patients without tamponade. Until that report, survival after gunshot wounds of the heart was thought to be uncommon. One of the better survival rates (64.5%) had been reported by Ricks and his co-workers.[20] Thirteen of the patients had no recordable blood pressure on admission and five of those thirteen died. Of the 14 patients who had a systolic pressure exceeding 50 mm Hg, only two died. Of the 14 patients who had tamponade, only two died. In contrast, of the 13 patients who did not have tamponade, five died. In 1977, Szentpetery and Lower[74] reported on 30 consecutively studied patients treated by emergency thoracotomy. The patients had 12 stab wounds and 18 gunshot wounds. Four of them died, giving a mortality of 13%. Those excellent results also support the need for emergency thoracotomy.

In all those reports, postoperative morbidity was mainly that of pulmonary dysfunction, including atelectasis and pleural effusion. Occasionally there was pericarditis and the post-pericardiotomy syndrome, as well as the intracardiac defects just mentioned, which were handled later by elective cardiopulmonary bypass.

Nonpenetrating Cardiac Trauma

The types of injury that may be produced by blunt cardiac trauma are listed in Table 18–2 and discussed in the following paragraphs.

Myocardial Contusion. Nonpenetrating cardiac trauma frequently produces contusion of the heart in patients who survive. The contusion can be treated by bedrest and medications designed to relieve pain; it does not require operative management.

Myocardial Rupture. In some instances, patients with massive blunt cardiac trauma, particularly rupture of the myocardial chamber, survive long enough to allow emergency correction of the defect. In 1958, Parmley and his co-workers[22] presented a review of 546 autopsied cases of nonpenetrating traumatic injuries to the heart. Cardiac contusion and laceration were the two most common lesions of blunt trauma in the series. Ventricular rupture was common, and it was usually associated with immediate death, except for one patient who lived for four hours until massive exsanguination caused death. Thirteen patients with atrial rupture (19% of the patients with atrial ruptures) survived the initial injury and might have been saved by emergency operation. In the series of blunt cardiac injuries reported by Bright and Beck,[23] 14 of 66 patients with rupture of the atrium survived long enough to be operated on. In a review by Kohn and his co-workers[24] there were 79 patients with atrial rupture, and 19 of them survived long enough to permit operation. It is clear that approximately 20% of people with atrial ruptures secondary to blunt injury of the heart survive long enough to undergo an emergency operation. It is assumed that those who die of exsanguination have an associated large pericardial tear that produces early exsanguination and death rather than cardiac tamponade, which would allow longer survival.

Rupture of the Ventricular Septum. Rupture of the ventricular septum was found in 30 patients in Parmley's series,[22] and in five of those 30 the

Table 18–2. *Types of Cardiac Injury from Nonpenetrating Trauma*

Myocardial contusion
Myocardial rupture
Rupture of the ventricular septum
Disruption of the AV valve
Disruption of the aortic valve

septal rupture was the sole cardiac lesion. Both immediate and delayed rupture of the intraventricular septum following nonpenetrating cardiac trauma has been documented. The defect usually occurs in the muscular septum near the apex, but it may occur at any site. Delayed septal defects are most likely due to necrosis of previously contused muscle. Some of those patients may survive long enough for operative correction. Ventricular septal defects secondary to blunt trauma of the heart rarely require emergency operation if they are the only lesion. Those lesions are usually identified by cardiac catheterization and angiography, and they are operated on electively at a later date. Patch closure of the defect and the muscular septum is recommended.

Disruption of the Atrioventricular Valve. Disruption of the AV valve was the most common valvular injury in Parmley's series, but there was usually enough associated myocardial injury that the patient did not survive long enough for operative correction. There have been two successful valve replacements for traumatic insufficiency of the tricuspid valve.[30-31] I have successfully corrected one instance of traumatic disruption of the mitral valve by valve replacement in a patient two years after blunt trauma. The lesions of the tricuspid and mitral valve did not constitute an emergency and they were repaired electively under extracorporeal circulation.

Disruption of the Aortic Valve. Of greater interest to the surgeon are the four cases of aortic valvular rupture in Parmley's series since there have been a number of reports of successful operative correction of such a rupture. Traumatic disruption of the aortic valve results when nonpenetrating trauma to the chest occurs during the diastolic phase of the cardiac cycle. The left and/or noncoronary aortic leaflets are the ones most commonly perforated or detached. The diagnosis is usually suggested by the high-pitched musical aortic diastolic murmur, and it may be confirmed by aortography. The physician must be extremely sensitive to the lethal nature of the lesion and if it is suspected, an immediate operation for cardiopulmonary bypass and aortic valve replacement must be performed. The classic description of traumatic rupture of the aortic valve, including a review of 113 cases, is that of Howard (1928).[26] In 1955, Leonard and his co-workers[27] reported the first operative correction, which was achieved by inserting a Hufnagle plastic valve into the descending aorta. The first successful total correction after insertion of a ball valve was reported by Beall and Shirkey (1964).[28] A number of survivals following operative correction have been reported.[26-29]

The principles of treatment described for penetrating cardiac trauma apply to nonpenetrating cardiac trauma, particularly when there is a rupture of the atrium. At least nine successful repairs of atrial ruptures have been reported.[24,25] Most of those were repaired by direct suture without the need for extracorporeal circulation.

DISSECTING HEMATOMA (ANEURYSM) OF THE AORTA

Anatomy and Pathology

Dissecting hematoma of the descending aorta is a true cardiac emergency that will tax the judgment of the cardiac surgeon and cardiologist. Cystic medial necrosis is the most common pathologic finding of the ascending aorta. Most patients with that condition have hypertension. Approximately one-third of the patients also have Marfan's syndrome. In some instances, atherosclerosis alone may be a causative factor. A number of other conditions, including coarctation of the aorta, patent ductus arteriosus, pheochromocytoma, and Cushing's disease, may be associated with dissecting hematoma of the aorta.

There are three types of dissecting hematoma of the aorta.[32] Type I accounts for at least two-thirds of the dissecting hematomas. It begins in the ascending aorta and propagates distally for varying distances. Type II is rare; it may be found in Marfan's syndrome. It remains confined to the ascending aorta. Type III originates at or just beyond the origin of the left subclavian artery, and it progresses distally for varying lengths. Approximately one-fifth to one-third of the patients seen will have type III dissecting hematoma. It is unusal for type III to extend proximally although such an extension has been observed.

Natural History of Dissecting Hematoma

In untreated acute aortic dissecting hematoma, death occurs in approximately 20% of the patients within 24 hours, two-thirds within two weeks, and 90% within three months due to rupture of the aorta with hemorrhage and/or cardiac tamponade. Since so-called healed dissecting hematoma of the aorta has been reported as an incidental autopsy finding in later life, survival without treatment is possible.

Diagnosis

The diagnosis of dissecting hematoma of the aorta is usually made or its presence is suspected on the basis of typical symptoms of severe, tearing chest pain, which may be associated with hypertension and weak or absent pulse in one or more of the extremities. Once there is a high index of suspicion and a presumptive diagnosis has been made, it must be confirmed by thoracic and abdominal aortography within a few hours to precisely define the site of the intimal tear as well as the extent of the dissecting hematoma and the involvement of the aortic branches.

Treatment

There is still controversy about treatment, particularly about emergency operation. I agree with the concepts set down by Wheat and his co-workers,[33,34] who consider drug therapy the treatment of choice for the immediate management of patients with acute dissecting hematoma of the aorta, except in certain instances. If drug treatment is chosen, the systolic blood pressure is reduced to 100 to 120 mm Hg with carefully selected antihypertensive medication. The patient is carefully observed in the intensive care unit in regard to his urine output, pulses, ECG, blood pressure, blood urea nitrogen, and sensorium. The antihypertensive medication should not be used or its use should be abandoned when (1) pain is not alleviated, indicating progression and extension of the dissection, (2) the blood pressure cannot be brought under control although the patient's urine output, blood urea nitrogen, and sensorium remain adequate, (3) there is insufficiency of the aortic valve, (4) there is roentgenographic evidence of enlargement of the aneurysm (Chapter 19), (5) there is suspicion that the dissecting hematoma is leaking or that rupture is imminent, (6) patients who respond well to hypotensive drug therapy enter a chronic stage, developing an acute saccular aneurysm or aortic insufficiency. Approximately 20 to 30% of patients in that last group require operation. (Antihypertensive drug therapy is discussed in detail in Chapter 15.)

When there is obstruction of a major branch of the aorta, a local operative procedure, such as segmental replacement, may suffice. Thus the combination of hypotensive drug therapy with operative intervention when required best serves the overall interests of the patient with a dissecting hematoma of the aorta. In general, type I and type II dissecting hematomas of the aorta are associated with valvular insufficiency, and they are usually satisfactorily treated by emergency operative intervention.[35-37]

From a technical point of view, the operative approach has gone through a number of changes, beginning with palliative "fenestration" operation, together with segmental excision with end-to-end anastomosis. In 1961, DeBakey reported on 72 cases of dissecting aneurysm of the aorta treated operatively with good results.[38] Many of DeBakey's patients had some type of graft replacement for aneurysm and it was difficult to ascertain what procedures were done on an emergency basis and what were done at a later stage.

In type I dissecting hematoma, extracorporeal circulation is used. The ascending aorta is transected just above the aortic valve, and the proximal and distal double-barreled lumens are oversewn and reapproximated with or without a prosthetic tubular graft. The procedure resuspends the aortic valve leaflets and abolishes the insufficiency in most instances. In those cases in which the aortic leaflets are still insufficient, a prosthetic valve may be required. The operative approach for a type II aneurysm is essentially the same as that for a type I aneurysm. Most type III aneurysms are successfully treated by antihypertensive drug therapy. When antihypertensive therapy fails, operation is undertaken with partial extracorporeal circulation by femoro-femoral bypass or by left atrial-to-femoral artery bypass. The aneurysm is isolated and excised. The double-barreled lumens are oversewn proximally and distally, and the two ends are connected by a Dacron prosthesis. Recently, Ablaza and his co-workers[75] introduced a new surgical technique. The basic technique consists of inserting a woven tubular Dacron graft with grooved rings at each end into the true lumen of the dissected aorta and circumferentially ligating the aorta against the grooves in the ring at each end. The technique stabilized the aorta and corrected the aortic insufficiency in two patients. The technique, which is intriguing, requires further clinical trial.

The complications of operation are postoperative hemorrhage, congestive heart failure, arrhythmia, and myocardial infarction. In general, there has been an operative mortality of 10 to 25% with type I and type II dissecting hematomas of the aorta.[35–37] There is a late mortality of as much as 20% in patients who survive operation. Hypotensive drug therapy also has untoward effects, largely due to poor tissue perfusion. Those untoward effects also include tubular necrosis of the kidney, duodenal ulcer associated with reserpine therapy, depressed sensorium with confusion and lethargy due to partial hypotension, and occasionally drug-induced jaundice.[33,34]

CARDIAC TUMORS

Cardiac myxomas may require emergency excision because of the threat of sudden death or disabling sequelae following embolism of the tumor. Seventy-five percent of all cardiac neoplasms are benign. Myxoma accounts for approximately 50% of all cardiac neoplasms and is of prime interest to the surgeon. Myxomas arise in the left atrium in 70 to 80% of the cases, with most of the remainder arising in the right atrium. A number of myxomas have been discovered in and removed from the right and left ventricles. Myxomas vary in size and configuration, and they are usually attached by a narrow pedicle to the atrial septum in the area of the fossa ovalis. The tumor may have a ball valve effect, passing back and forth from atrium to ventricle when the pedicle is long enough to intermittently obstruct the mitral valve. In other instances, the tumor may produce no clinical symptoms, and it may be an incidental finding. The clinical symptoms of myxoma are due to embolism, obstruction of blood flow at the level of the valve, with congestive heart failure and certain constitutional effects, including arthralgia, weight loss, anemia, fever, and hyperglobulinemia. The constitutional effects are poorly understood. The diagnosis may be made by echocardiography and confirmed by catheterization and angiography.

The clinical course of myxoma may be quite uncertain with severe disabling features due to peripheral emboli, progressive deterioration of valvular function, and severe heart failure. In some instances, sudden death may occur. It may follow near total obstruction of the AV orifice. Thus a myxoma is considered an indication for emergency operation as soon as possible after the diagnosis is made. Under extracorporeal circulation, the myxoma is removed, along with a small portion of the adjacent atrial septum. Although many operations have been done without removing a portion of the atrial septum, there have been reports of recurrence.[39,40] The mortality has been low following excision of atrial myxoma. Patients who survive operation for removal of atrial myxoma are usually asymptomatic, and they can lead normal lives.

VALVULAR HEART DISEASE

Operations on the aortic valve are almost always performed on an elective basis when significant symptoms of congestive heart failure, syncope, or angina pectoris occur. There are occasions, however, in which the clinical symptoms indicate that the patient is at extreme risk for sudden death, and the operation is then performed on an urgent or emergency basis. That is particularly true when acute severe aortic valve insufficiency occurs and the hemodynamic derangement becomes so severe as to rapidly lead to heart failure and death. Such acute valve insufficiency may follow acute dissecting hematoma of the aorta, blunt trauma, or infective endocarditis.

The emergency operative approach to acute aortic insufficiency following dissecting hematoma of the aorta or blunt trauma has already been discussed. An urgent or emergency operation may be required for patients with infective endocarditis and severe aortic insufficiency. Because of the success of antibiotics, aortic valve perforation with severe cardiac failure has become the leading cause of death in patients treated for infective endocarditis. When cardiac failure is present, it may be extremely difficult to "sterilize" the patient who has bacterial endocarditis. When progressive and intractable cardiac failure occurs with aortic valve insufficiency, there is no alternative to urgent or emergency replacement of the aortic valve, even when a full course of antibiotic therapy has not been completed or even if the antibiotic therapy has just been started. There have been a number of reports of operation for bacterial endocarditis with cardiac valve involvement and cardiac failure in which aortic valve replacement has been performed with excellent results under urgent or emergency conditions without a previous course of antibiotics.

Operations on the mitral valve are almost always performed on an elective basis. One exception is for rupture of an entire papillary muscle as a complication of myocardial infarction; emergency operative correction must be rapidly undertaken since death will rapidly occur following the acute hemodynamic derangement. That problem is discussed with the complications of myocardial infarction (pp. 380, 381 and 382).

ISCHEMIC HEART DISEASE (See also Chapter 5)

Aortocoronary saphenous vein bypass has emerged as the operative procedure of choice in patients with ischemic heart disease. Chronic angina pectoris that cannot be satisfactorily treated by medical means is the main indication for aortocoronary bypass on an elective basis. Urgent or emergency operative treatment of ischemic heart disease has been advocated in (1) unstable angina pectoris, (2) selected instances of acute evolving myocardial infarction, and (3) critical obstruction of the left main coronary artery.

Unstable Angina Pectoris

The development of a clear-cut treatment program for patients with unstable angina pectoris is still impeded by lack of a precise definition of the syndrome. The different terms used to describe those patients include unstable angina pectoris, crescendo angina, acute coronary insufficiency, pre-infarction angina, impending myocardial infarction, intermediate syndrome, coronary failure, and rest angina. Some workers include in the syndrome angina of recent origin, angina occurring for the first time, increasing severity of stable angina that becomes increasingly severe, angina lasting for a long time, angina not relieved by rest or nitrates, and angina that begins again in a person who had a myocardial infarction. There are no changes in the ECG or serum enzymes that are diagnostic of myocardial infarction. Although the natural history of patients with unstable angina pectoris is still somewhat enigmatic, it has been reported that up to 40% may experience myocardial infarction within three months, with a relatively high mortality.[41-43] Operative treatment of patients with unstable angina pectoris is strongly recommended by many workers; and some workers consider the condition an acute emergency that requires immediate cardiac catheterization and surgery for optimal therapeutic result.[46,47,76,77] A review of over 2000 patients operated on for impending myocardial infarction shows an operative mortality of 3 to 8% and averaging approximately 5 to 6%.[44-47,76,77] At present, we agree with the approach advocated by Langou and his co-workers,[77] in which approximately 48 hours after the initiation of maximum medical therapy in the coronary care unit the patients are classified into two groups according to their response to medical therapy. Those that respond to medical therapy may undergo elective cardiac catheterization and surgery later, at an appropriate time. In patients whose anginal symptoms were not controlled with medical therapy, urgent or emergency cardiac catheterization followed by aortocoronary saphenous vein bypass can be carried out. Many of those patients may benefit from the use of intra-aortic balloon pumping to minimize the risk of operation and perioperative infarction. Wiener and his co-workers[49,56] have attempted to improve case selection by making a metabolic evaluation of coronary sinus efflux to determine the patient's operability. Those workers consider the patient with impending myocardial infarction a strong candidate for operation if he had an abnormality of lactate metabolism (that is, increased lactate production). Wiener and his co-workers reason that the increased lactate production is a sign of an ischemic but still viable myocardium and that the optimal time for operation is during the early creatinine phosphokinase (CPK) efflux in the coronary sinus blood before systemic CPK elevation occurs.

Acute Myocardial Infarction

The use of emergency aortocoronary bypass grafts for acute myocardial infarction is still controversial but the operation may have application in selected instances. The justification for emergency operation in those instances is based on the improvement of oxygen delivery to the area of myocardium adjacent to the area of necrotic contraction, the "twilight zone" of ischemic tissue. Salvage of the potentially reversible ischemic myocardium would reduce the size of the infarct. The overall experience of emergency operations for acute myocardial infarction remains limited and the operative mortality remains higher than that for patients with stable angina pectoris or impending myocardial infarction. Patients who suffer myocardial infarction during coronary angiography are in a separate category. An emergency operation for those patients may be justified, and the results have been gratifying.[48] Several centers have reported small numbers of emergency operations for acute myocardial infarction that have had satisfactory results,[58-62] while other groups with similar numbers of patients have reported more discouraging results.[53-55] Such contradictory results emphasize the controversy that surrounds emergency operations in acute myocardial infarction. Patients having chest pain at rest soon after myocardial infarction have a clinical syndrome of unstable angina pectoris superimposed on their acute evolving myocardial infarction. Those patients are at increased risk for extension of their myocardial infarction, and they may be considered emergency candidates for bypass surgery. Frequently, intra-aortic balloon pumping is instituted on those patients prior to cardiac catheterization. The operative risk is related largely to the underlying hemodynamic state rather than to the ischemic myocardium, and it is gratifying when significant impairment of left ventricular function has not occurred.

Stenosis of the Left Main Coronary Artery

Patients with left main coronary artery obstruction treated medically have a five-year survival rate of less than 57% and a 10-year survival rate of 25%.[57,78] The Veterans Administration perspective randomized study showed a survival rate of approximately 60% in three years for patients treated medically and a survival rate of 83% in three years for patients treated surgically.[79] The cumulative survival rate of patients with left main coronary artery stenosis at the end of three years is over 80%,[58,60,79] clearly indicating that operation is the treatment of choice. Because of the high risk for those patients despite good medical management, urgent or emergency operation seems justified.

COMPLICATIONS OF MYOCARDIAL INFARCTION
(See also Chapter 5)

Ventricular Aneurysm

Left ventricular aneurysm following myocardial infarction has been reported to occur in 5 to 35% of patients. From the surgeon's point of view, a ventricular aneurysm is a thick scar replacing a portion of the left ventricular wall. It is usually adherent to the pericardium, and it may contain thrombi on the endocardial surface. Differences in the interpretation of left ventriculograms may account for the varying reports of the incidence of the condition. Most left ventricular aneurysms are in the anterior or apical portions of the heart, and the rest are in the posterior portion. Most posterior aneurysms involve the mitral valve mechanism, causing death from severe mitral insufficiency. Among patients with myocardial infarction who also develop left ventricular aneurysms, the survival rate is approximately one-third the rate among those who do not develop an aneurysm.[61] Most of the deaths are accounted for by congestive heart failure that follows a mechanical dysfunction produced by the aneurysm.[61,62] A significant percentage of the deaths result from arrhythmias, and peripheral embolism may be troublesome in 5 to 10% of the patients. Most operations for left ventricular aneurysm are performed on an elective basis because of the presence of refractory congestive heart failure. In some instances, the presence of emboli may be the indication for operation. In a small percentage of patients, the presence of refractory ectopic tachyarrhythmias is the indication for operation, and it is in those patients that an emergency operation may be required. Cardiac arrythmias have ranged from supraventricular to ventricular tachycardias and have included conduction disturbances, such as intraventricular block (bundle branch block and bifascicular or trifascicular block) and frequent ventricular extrasystoles. In a number of instances emergency operation has been performed successfully for intractable arrhythmias, particularly ventricular tachycardia. There have also been instances of a successful emergency operation performed for severe, life-threatening congestive heart failure.[62-64] Patients who survive the operation usually have a satisfactory postoperative course, with greatly improved ventricular performance and, usually, disappearance of the arrhythmia once the mechanical deficits and ventricular irritability secondary to the aneurysm have been removed.

Post-Infarction Ventricular Septal Defect

Post-infarction ventricular septal defect is not common. One to 2% of patients dying of acute myocardial infarction have experienced ventricular septal defect. In two-thirds of those patients, the defect is in the apical portion of the septum, and in a few it is in the posterior, middle, or superior portion of the septum. Occasionally, multiple perforations may be found. Perforation of the ventricular septum usually occurs five to 15 days after the myocardial infarction and coincides with the time of maximal degeneration of the muscular tissue. Since one-third of the patients have an associated left ventricular aneurysm, that aneurysm should always be suspected in the presence of an acquired ventricular septal defect. Once a perforation of the ventricular septum occurs, 25% of the patients die within 24 hours and two-thirds of them die within two weeks. At the end of one year, less than 10% of the patients are alive. The resulting congestive heart failure is usually refractory to conservative management because of the burden of the left-to-right shunt superimposed on the already damaged myocardium. An operation is performed on the patient whose condition is deteriorating despite medical management. In many instances, the operation is an emergency, life-saving procedure. In those instances in which the diagnosis is uncertain and other conditions, such as mitral insufficiency, are suspected, the Swans-Ganz catheter may be used for confirmatory diagnosis at the bedside.[65] The results are best if the operation can be delayed for three to six weeks after the occurrence of the ventricular septal defect to allow fibrous edges to develop so that a secure repair can be performed. Nevertheless, an emergency operation may be performed if the patient's condition is rapidly degenerating. Among 26 patients who were operated on within two weeks of infarction, the operative mortality was 56%.[66] Of the patients who were operated on less than six weeks after infarction, only 9% were alive at the end of one year, whereas of the patients who were operated on six weeks or more after the occurrence of the ventricular septal defect, at least 35% were alive after one year. In a report from the Mayo Clinic,[66] there was a 54% survival rate at the end of one year or more when the operation was performed three weeks or more after the occurrence of the ventricular septal defect. When a patient has a rapid downhill course after acute myocardial infarction and acquired intraventricular septal rupture, the emergency introduction of the intra-aortic balloon pump followed by emergency cardiac catheterization and operation may be lifesaving. In such patients the operative mortality remains high despite that approach. Nevertheless, the surgical results are far more successful than the medical results in those very high risk patients.

Post-Infarction Mitral Regurgitation

Rupture of the papillary muscle is also somewhat rare, accounting for about 1% of the deaths that follow myocardial infarction. The posterior papillary muscle is usually involved, and the infarction is located in the diaphragmatic surface of the heart. Most patients have widespread diffuse coronary vessel disease. Intractable left ventricular failure follows papillary muscle rupture. Over two-thirds of the patients die within 24 hours, and almost 90% of them die within two weeks. Operative intervention for papillary muscle rupture is almost always undertaken as an emergency measure in the acute post-infarction period. There are a few reports of successful mitral valve replacement in mitral insufficiency due to post-infarction rupture of the papillary muscle. The most important prognostic criteria are the extent of the infarct and the quality of the remaining muscle. Concomitant aortocoronary saphenous vein bypass will improve results. The intra-aortic balloon pump should be used prior to cardiac catheterization and operation in an attempt to slow down the deterioration of the patient's condition, permitting successful study and operation. The first successful operative correction with valve replacement was performed in 1965.[67] When patients have enough viable myocardium to sustain life following mitral valve replacement and/or aortocoronary saphenous vein bypass, the results are satisfactory, but the mortality remains high.

Cardiogenic Shock (See also Chapter 3)

Cardiogenic shock still has a high mortality despite all methods of treatment. Diastolic augmentation with the intra-aortic balloon pumping may allow the patient to survive for hours or days, but it may not of itself alter the eventual outcome. It will permit cardiac catheterization and an emergency operation to be performed if indicated.

Emergency bypass operation in cardiogenic shock, a desperate condition, is controversial, but in selected instances when survival is theoretically possible, it may be the only alternative to certain death. In 10 reports of a total of 80 operations, there was a 39% survival following emergency operation.[68] In general, the surviving patients were those who had adequate amounts of viable myocardium. They were those who received prompt treatment and who had had cardiogenic shock for no longer than 12 hours. In one study of 42 patients who had intra-aortic balloon pumping for 36 hours to 14 days, five patients are reported to have survived on a long-term basis.[68] Emergency operation was performed on 16 of those patients. Fourteen patients had aortocoronary bypass grafts, eight had infarctectomy and bypass grafts, two had infarctectomy alone, and two had mitral valve replacements. At the end of one month to one year, seven of those patients were alive. Although the mortality is extremely high, salvage of these patients by operative intervention on an emergency basis is justified in selected cases.

PERICARDITIS (See also Chapters 13 and 14)

The operative treatment of pericarditis, including chronic pericardial effusion, acute inflammation of the pericardium, and chronic constrictive pericarditis, is usually performed on an elective basis when it becomes clear that the impairment has produced an increase in the venous volume and pressure proximal to the ventricle in both the systemic and pulmonary circulation, causing low cardiac output. There are a few instances in which emergency operation may be appropriate, particularly in purulent pericarditis and uremic pericarditis. Open drainage of the pericardium, pericardiotomy, or pericardiostomy may be required in purulent pericarditis, particularly when repeated needle aspirations are unsatisfactory. The principle of the operative procedure is based on the classic surgical principle of incision and drainage of an abscess in a closed space under pressure. The type of operative technique must be selected for each patient. Tube pericardiostomy is the treatment of choice in some cases, while the more radical procedure of open drainage of pericardiotomy can be performed when required. Emergency operation may also be required for patients with uremic pericarditis, particularly those who may later have renal transplantation. Almost 50% of the patients undergoing chronic dialysis will have pericarditis with effusion (usually bloody), with or without tamponade. That can usually be treated by pericardiocentesis or by tube pericardiostomy. If those procedures fail, urgent or emergency pericardiotomy may be required.

CARDIAC ARRHYTHMIAS (See also Chapters 7–9)

Certain arrhythmias may benefit from urgent or emergency operative treatment. The operative approach to refractory tachyarrhythmias in the Wolff-Parkinson-White (WPW) syndrome has been established.[69,70,80] The indication for operation is drug-resistant supraventricular tachyarrhythmias, particularly atrial fibrillation. Sealy and his co-workers[69,70,80] have described an excellent technique that requires electronic mapping and an incision, which is later sutured, around the mitral or tricuspid valve and carried through the anulus fibrosus. In that manner, the accessory Kent bundle may be located and divided, whether the WPW syndrome is type A or type B. Sealy and his co-workers[80] have operated on 50 patients for tachyarrhythmias associated with Kent bundles. The indications for operation were refractory or life-threatening tachyarrhythmias. The division of the Kent bundle was successful in 31 patients; two deaths occurred from cardiomyopathy. His bundle interruption was required on seven patients for control of the supraventricular tachycardia. Eight patients continued to have delta waves in the postoperative period, and drugs were required for control of the supraventricular tachycardia in those patients. There were three failures.

Ventricular tachyarrhythmias continue to be the most common cause of death in patients with coronary artery disease, and antiarrhythmic drugs may not prevent sudden death. Aortocoronary saphenous vein bypass grafting has been suggested by a number of workers as a logical treatment for ventricular tachyarrhythmias since myocardial ischemia appears to be the primary cause. At present, it appears that revascularization bypass operation alone is not effective in preventing recurrent ventricular tachyarrhythmias. Urgent or emergency operation for recurrent, potentially lethal ventricular tachyarrhythmias should be performed only when the left ventricular aneurysm, amenable to resection, can be demonstrated in preoperative studies. Ventricular aneurysmectomy may be an effective means of controlling refractory ventricular tachyarrhythmias on an urgent or emergency basis, as has already been noted. Ventricular tachyarrhythmias probably have their origin in the marginal zone of the aneurysm separating the aneurysmal scar from the surrounding viable myocardium. The area is subject to continuous mechanical stress. The presence of uncontrolled supraventricular tachycardias in those instances is more difficult to explain, but it may be related to the increased pressure and volume load in the atrium, or it may be a consequence of the generalized ischemic process. The incidence of symptomatic and potentially lethal ventricular tachyarrhythmias is markedly reduced or abolished following aneurysmectomy, but a few patients continue to have symptomatic tachyarrhythmias that may be difficult to treat following operation. There have been occasional reports of refractory ventricular tachyarrhythmias whose cause was not clear. A variety of therapeutic operations have been performed, but a high failure rate has been reported with most. The operations include sympathectomy, resection of tissue, revascularization, simple ventriculotomy, encircling endocardial ventriculotomy, and section of the His bundle or of the bundle branches.[71,81,82]

CONGENITAL HEART DISEASE IN INFANTS (See also Chapter 17)

The mortality from congenital heart disease is higher in the first six months of life, accounting for approximately 80 to 85% of all deaths in that period. Refinements in pediatric cardiology and cardiac catheterization, along with refinements in the performance of operations, have provided the cardiac surgeon with an increased number of candidates in the first few months of life for emergency, palliative, and, in some instances, corrective procedures.

Patent Ductus Arteriosus

In a few instances, infants under four weeks of age and even premature infants may have severe congestive heart failure secondary to large patent ductus arteriosus. In some instances, the respiratory distress syndrome may be associated with a large patent ductus arteriosus and severe congestive heart failure. Emergency closure of the patent ductus arteriosus via a thoracotomy in the usual manner has been performed in those instances with a mortality of approximately 15 to 20%.

Coarctation of the Aorta

Coarctation of the aorta producing severe congestive heart failure in the first year of life is an emergency. Over two-thirds of infants with coarctation of the aorta have associated lesions, such as patent ductus arteriosus, ventricular septal defect, or an area of tubular hypoplasia (the so-called infantile type of coarctation). The operative mortality in patients of this age is higher than when the operation is performed on an elective basis on patients who are older, largely because of the associated anomalies that may not be amenable to correction at the time of operation. There is usually concomitant pulmonary vascular disease. Nevertheless, emergency operation is required since it is far more successful than conservative medical management alone. The best results are obtained in infants with classic coarctation of the aorta without associated significant cardiac defects and in severe congestive heart failure not responding adequately to medical therapy. In infants operated on during the first year of life, the mortality has been 20 to 55%.

Aortic Stenosis

Congenital valvular aortic stenosis producing intractable congestive heart failure in the first year of life is uncommon, and it may require emergency operation. Associated conditions, such as endocardial fibroelastosis or coarctation of the aorta, should be taken into consideration since they increase the mortality. The infant with critical aortic stenosis should undergo urgent cardiac catheterization and operative correction. Incision of the fused commissures is required to relieve the stenosis. The operative mortality in the first year of life may be as high as 50%, but the emergency surgical management of the critically ill child is imperative since in most patients conservative therapy with medical management will result in death.

Pulmonary Stenosis and Pulmonary Atresia

The prognosis for infants with pulmonary stenosis or pulmonary atresia with an intact septum depends on the severity of the obstruction. In infants with moderate to severe obstruction, the disease is essentially lethal. Sudden death may follow the severe congestive heart failure despite all therapeutic efforts. Most infants with severe obstruction have some degree of cyanosis and usually a patent foramen ovale. Death usually occurs in the first three to six months following the onset of congestive heart failure with attacks of hypoxemia. Emergency operation is indicated when congestive heart failure with dyspnea and fatigue are present along with hypoxic attacks. In infants who have cyanosis due to reversed shunts through a patent foramen ovale, emergency operation is indicated. In infants with pulmonary valve stenosis, the basic principles of operation are incision of the fused commissures of the stenotic pulmonary valve. In infants with pulmonary atresia and an intact septum, a patent ductus arteriosus and atrial septal defect are usually present and required for survival. Emergency operative creation of an aorticopulmonary shunt of the Waterston or Blalock type is performed. In some instances, pulmonary valvulotomy may also be helpful.

Tricuspid Atresia

Congenital tricuspid atresia is an uncommon complex anomaly found in approximately 5% of patients with cyanotic congenital heart disease. Two-thirds of those patients die in the first year of life. Death follows congestive heart failure along with anoxic attacks. The presence of cardiac failure and hypoxic attacks is an indication for emergency operation. When pulmonary flow is adequate, a palliative systemic pulmonary artery shunt should be created by the Waterston or Blalock method. In all instances, the operation should be preceded by cardiac catheterization with balloon atrioseptostomy to insure adequate emptying of the right atrium.[72] Since there may be large blood flows into the lungs when there is an associated transposition of the great vessels, balloon atrioseptostomy should be followed by emergency operative banding of the pulmonary artery. The operative risk is high, and congestive heart failure often develops in the postoperative period.

Transposition of the Great Vessels

In desperately ill infants with transposition of the great vessels, emergency cardiac catheterization with balloon atrioseptostomy is always performed. If after that procedure, the arterial oxygen saturation is found to be over 60%, corrective operation may be deferred to the second or even the third year of life. In infants who are incapacitated by associated pulmonary stenosis and inadequate blood flows, palliation can be achieved by emergency systemic pulmonary artery shunt of the Blalock or Waterston type. Corrective operation may then be deferred until the child is two to three years old. Over 50% of infants with transposition of the great vessels die during the first month of life because of mixing between the two circuits. In many instances, there are few if any associated cardiac lesions, and so those patients are candidates for total correction by the Mustard procedure, even at such an early age. Rather than subject the patient to repeated balloon septostomy or rather than accept the mortality of operative septectomy, early corrective operation is performed when the initial balloon atrioseptostomy yields unsatisfactory palliation. In one series of 15 operative corrections (10 in patients under 21 months of age and four in patients under six months of age), there were only two operative deaths.[73] Those data indicate that total correction by the Mustard procedure can be performed successfully in children under six months of age. Increasing numbers of successful total correction of transposition of the great vessels in infants under one year of age are being reported.

Total Anomalous Venous Return

Approximately 75% of patients with total anomalous venous return die within the first year of life. Early diagnosis and operation are required if death is to be prevented. The natural history and survival of patients with total anomalous venous return are determined by the degree of pulmonary hypertension and obstruction of the pulmonary venous return by constriction of the anomalous venous trunk. When severe pulmonary hypertension associated with pulmonary vascular disease is present, the prognosis is poor and patients usually die in six to 12 months. When there is a good shunt at the atrial level without pulmonary hypertension, cyanosis, or cardiac failure, and when symptoms are not severe, the patient will attain adulthood, and total operative correction at a later date is possible. The mortality following emergency correction of total anomalous venous return is related to the person's age, the pulmonary vascular resistance, and the severity of the cyanosis. The mortality in patients under one year of age as reported in the literature ranges from 47 to 70%. Operative management requires early diagnosis with cardiac catheterization followed by operation. Corrective operation includes connection of pulmonary venous return to the left atrium, closure of the atrial septal defect, and closure of the abnormal venous return to the right atrium. Little or no attempt is made to manage the patient medically. Ventilatory support is maintained postoperatively and the acid-base balance is carefully maintained. Other workers have used extracorporeal circulation with or without surface hypothermia. It is difficult to be certain that the differences in technique are important since satisfactory results have been obtained both with extracorporeal circulation alone and with surface cooling in addition to extracorporeal circulation.

Tetralogy of Fallot

Infants with tetralogy of Fallot may require urgent or emergency operation because of severe cyanosis or apnea. Usually anastomosis of the ascending aorta to the right pulmonary artery as described by Waterston is performed in infants under six months of age although the Blalock shunt is being used more frequently in that age group.

Ventricular and Atrial Septal Defects

Emergency operation in infants with ventricular septal defects and with atrial septal defects and refractory congestive heart failure may rarely be required.

Emergency treatment of infants with congenital cardiac anomalies is a great challenge that must be met with operative intervention as well as with medical care. Most infants with congenital cardiac defects become symptomatic during the first month of life and may not survive without operative intervention. Despite the high risk involved, curative or palliative operations are available and must be performed. Results obtained with those operations continue to be encouraging, and the list of long-term survivors continues to grow rapidly.

COMPLICATIONS OF ARTIFICIAL CARDIAC PACEMAKERS

When a person with a permanently implanted artificial pacemaker develops serious complications (e.g., runaway pacemaker, fracture of pacemaker electrodes, refractory infections), emergency or semi-emergency surgical treatment is necessary. (Artificial pacemakers are discussed in detail in Chapter 11.)

SUMMARY

1. The heart is amenable to urgent or emergency operative repair provided that the facilities are adequate and a knowledgeable team is available.

2. The emergencies that confront the cardiac surgeon include cardiac trauma and a wide variety of acquired and congenital cardiac lesions.

3. The surgeons must be thoroughly familiar with all the basic aspects of traumatic surgery, as well as with the highly specialized techniques of extracorporeal circulation and the circulatory assist devices.

4. In selected patients with refractory tachyarrhythmias, various operative measures may be lifesaving (Chapter 7).

5. Emergency or semi-emergency operative care is necessary for the patient with a permanently implanted artificial pacemaker who develops serious malfunctions or other major complications (Chapter 11).

6. The proper use of the appropriate techniques in emergencies yields excellent overall results.

REFERENCES

1. Rehn, L.: Uber penetrirende herzwanden und herznaht. Arch. Klin. Chir. 55:315, 1897.
2. Hill, L.L.: Report of a case of successful suturing of heart, and table of 37 other cases of suturing by different operators with various terminations and conclusions drawn. Med. Rec. November 29:846, 1902.
3. Tuffier, T.: La chirurgie du coeur. Cinquième Congrès de la Société Internationale de Chirurgie, Paris (July 19–23), 1920. Extrait, Brussels, Hayez, 1920.
4. Blalock, A., and Ravitch, M.M.: Consideration of nonoperative treatment of cardiac tamponade resulting from wounds of heart. Surgery 11:157, 1943.
5. Maynard, A.D.L., Brooks, H.A., and Froix, C.J.L.: Penetrating wound of the heart. Report on a new series. Arch. Surg. 90:680, 1965.
6. Naclerio, E. A.: Penetrating wounds of the heart: Experience with 249 patients. Dis. Chest 46:1, 1964.
7. Borja, A.R., Lansing, A.M., and Ransdell, H.T., Jr.: Immediate operative treatment of stab wounds of the heart. J. Thorac. Cardiovasc. Surg. 59:662, 1970.
8. Sugg, W.L., Rea, W.J., Ecker, R.R., Webb, W.R., Rose, E.F., and Shaw, R.R.: Penetrating wounds of the heart: An analysis of 459 cases. J. Thorac. Cardiovasc. Surg. 56:4, 1968.
9. Beall, A.C., Jr., Ochsner, J.L., Morris, G.C., Cooley, D.A., and DeBakey, M.E.: Penetrating wounds of the heart. J. Trauma 1:195, 1961.
10. Gonzalez, T.A., Vance, M., Helpern, M., and Umberger, C.J.: Legal Medicine Pathology, and Toxicology, 2nd ed. New York, Appleton-Century-Crofts, 1954.
11. Farringer, J.L., Jr., and Carr, D.: Cardiac tamponade. Ann. Surg. 141:437, 1955.
12. Cooley, D.A., Dunn, J.R., Brockman, H.L., and DeBakey, M.E.: Treatment of penetrating wounds of the heart: Experimental and clinical observations. Surgery 37:882, 1955.
13. Reul, G.J., Maddox, K.L., Beall, A.C., and Jordan, J.L., Jr.: Recent advances in the operative management of massive chest trauma. Ann. Thorac. Surg. 16:52, 1973.
14. Elkin, D.C.: Wounds of the heart. Ann Surg. 120:817, 1944.
15. Griswold, R.A., and Drye, J.C.: Cardiac wounds. Ann. Surg. 138:783, 1954.
16. Bolanowski, P.J.P., Suaminathan, A.P., and Neville, W.E.: Aggressive surgical management of penetrating cardiac injuries. J. Thorac. Cardiovasc. Surg. 66:52, 1973.
17. Hutchinson, J.E., Schmidt, D.M., Cameron, A., and McCord, C.W.: The surgical management of intracardiac defects due to penetrating trauma. J. Thorac. Cardiovasc. Surg. 65:103, 1973.
18. Pate, J.W., and Richardson, R.L., Jr.: Penetrating wounds of cardiac valves. J.A.M.A., 207:309, 1969.
19. Hutchinson, J.E., Beach, P.M., Jr., Kaplan, S., and Garvey, J.W.: Management of penetrating cardiac trauma. N.Y. State J. Med. 71:1932, 1971.
20. Ricks, R.K., Powell, J.F., Beall, A.C., and DeBakey, M.E.: Gunshot wounds of the heart: A review of 31 cases. Surgery 57:787, 1965.
21. Carrasquilla, C., Wilson, R.F., Walt, A.J., and Arbulu, A.: Gunshot wounds of the heart. Ann. Thorac, Surg. 13:208, 1972.
22. Parmley, L.F., Manion, W.C., and Mattingly, T.W.: Nonpenetrating traumatic injury to the heart. Circulation, 18:371, 1958.
23. Bright, E.F., and Beck, C.S.: Nonpenetrating wounds of the heart. A clinical experimental study. Am. Heart. J. 10:293, 1935.
24. Kohn, R.M., Harris, R., and Gorham, L.W.: Atrial rupture of the heart: Report of case following atrial infarction and summary of 79 cases collected from the literature. Circulation 10:221, 1954.
25. Ludington, L.G., Boskind, A.S., and Miquel, A.: Rupture of left ventricle from blunt trauma. Review of literature. Ann. Thorac. Surg. 18:195, 1974.
26. Howard, C.P.: Aortic insufficiency due to rupture by strain of a normal aortic valve. Can. Med. Assoc. J. 19:12, 1928.
27. Leonard, J.J., Harvey, W.P., and Hufnagle, C.A.: Rupture of the aortic valve; therapeutic approach. N. Engl. J. Med. 252:208, 1955.

28. Beall, A.C., and Shirkey. A.L.: Successful surgical correction of traumatic aortic valve regurgitation. J.A.M.A. 187:507, 1964.
29. Loop, F.D., Hofmeir, G., and Groves, L.K.: Traumatic disruption of aortic valve. Cleve. Clin. Q. 38:187, 1971.
30. Tchovsky, T.J., Giuliani, E.R., and Ellis, F.H.,: Jr.: Prosthetic valve replacement for traumatic tricuspid insufficiency. Am. J. Cardiol. 26:196, 1970.
31. Liu, S.M., Sako, Y., and Alexander, C.S.: Traumatic tricuspid insufficiency. Am. J. Cardiol. 26:200, 1970.
32. DeBakey, M.E., Henly, W.S., Cooley, D.A., Morris, G.C., Jr., Crawford, E.S., and Beall, A.C.: Surgical management of dissecting aneurysms of the aorta. J. Thorac. Cardiovasc. Surg. 49:130, 1965.
33. Wheat, M.W., Jr., and Palmer, R.L.: Dissecting Aneurysms of the Aorta. Current Problems in Surgery. Chicago, Yearbook, 1971.
34. Wheat, M.W., Jr., Harris, P.D., Malm, J.R., Kaiser, G., Bowman, F.O., and Palmer, R.F.: Acute dissecting aneurysm of the aorta. Treatment and results in 64 patients. J. Thorac. Cardiovasc. Surg. 58:344, 1969.
35. Daily, P.O., Trueblood, W.H., Stinson, E.B., Wuerflein, R.D., and Shumway, N.E.: Management of acute aortic dissections. Ann. Thorac. Surg. 10:237, 1970.
36. Liotta, D., Hallman, G.L., Milam, J.D., and Cooley, D.A.: Surgical treatment of acute dissecting aneurysm of the ascending aorta. Ann. Thorac. Surg. 12:582, 1971.
37. McFarland, J., Willerson, J.T., Dinsmore, R.E., Austen, W.G., Buckley, M.J., Sanders, C.A., and DeSanctis, R.W.: The medical treatment of dissecting aortic aneurysms. N. Engl. J. Med. 286:115, 1972.
38. DeBakey, M.A., Henly, W.S., Cooley, D.A., Crawford, E.S., and Morris, G.C., Jr.: Surgical treatment of dissecting aneurysm of the aorta. Circulation 24:290, 1961.
39. Gerbode, F., Kerth, W.J., and Hill, J.D.: Surgical management of tumors of the heart. Surgery 61:94, 1967.
40. Bahl, O.P., Oliver, G.C., Ferguson, T.B., Schad, N., Parker, B.M.: Recurrent left atrial myxoma: Report of a case. Circulation 40:673, 1969.
41. Vakil, R.J.: Preinfarction syndrome—management and follow-up. Am. J. Cardiol. 14:55, 1964.
42. Krauss, K.R., Hutter, A.M., Jr., and DeSanctis, R.W.: Acute coronary insufficiency. Circulation 45–46(Suppl. I):66, 1972.
43. Levy, H.: The natural history of changing patterns of angina pectoris. Arch. Intern. Med. 44:1123, 1956.
44. Thomas, C.S., Jr., Alford, W.C., Jr., Burrus, G.R., and Stoney, W.S.: Aorta-to-coronary artery bypass grafting. Ann. Thorac. Surg. 16:201, 1973.
45. Wilson, W.S.: Aortocoronary bypass—State of the art 1974. Cardiovasc. Dis. Bull. Texas Heart Inst. 1:270, 1974.
46. Bender, H., Jr., Fisher, D., Faulknes, S., et al.: Unstable coronary disease. Comparison of medical and surgical therapy. Ann. Thorac. Surg. 19:521, 1975.
47. Selden, R., Weill, W.A., Ritzmann, et al.: Medical versus surgical therapy for acute coronary insufficiency. A randomized study. N. Engl. J. Med. 293:1329, 1975.
48. Pifarre, R., Spinazzola, A., Nemickas, R., Scanlon, P.J., and Tobin, J.R.: Emergency aortocoronary bypass for acute myocardial infarction. Arch. Surg. 103:525, 1971.
49. Smullens, S.N., Wiener, L., Kasparian, H., et al.: Evaluation and surgical management of acute evolving myocardial infarction. J. Thorac. Cardiovasc. Surg. 64:495, 1972.
50. Fischl, S.J., Herman, M.V., and Gorlin, R.: The intermediate coronary syndrome— clinical, angiographic, and therapeutic aspects. N. Engl. J. Med. 288:1193, 1973.
51. Cheavechai, C., Effler, D.B., Loop, F.D., et al.: Emergency myocardial revascularization. Am. J. Cardiol. 32:907, 1973.
52. Cohn, L.H., Gorlin, R., Herman, M.V., et al.: Aortocoronary bypass for acute coronary occlusion. J. Thorac. Cardiovasc. Surg. 64:503, 1972.
53. Dawson, J.T., Hall, R.J., Hallman, G.L., et al.: Mortality of coronary artery bypass after previous myocardial infarction. Am. J. Cardiol. 31:128, 1973.
54. Kaiser, G.C., Barner, H.B., Williams, V.L., et al.: Aortocoronary bypass grafting. Arch. Surg. 105:319, 1972.

55. Reul, G.J., Morris, G.C., Howell, J.F., et al.: Current concepts in coronary artery surgery. Ann. Thorac. Surg. 14:243, 1972.
56. Wiener, L., Kasparian, H., Brest, A., and Templeton, J.: Surgical management of acute evolving myocardial infarction. A metabolic and angiographic profile. Am. J. Cardiol. 29:296, 1973 (Abstr.)
57. Cohen, M.V., Cohn, P.D., Herman, M.C., and Gorlin, R.: Diagnosis and prognosis of main left coronary artery obstruction. Circulation 45–46(Suppl. I):57, 1972.
58. Oldham, H.N., Jr., Kong, Y., Bartell, A.G., Morris, J.J., Jr., Behar, V.S., Peter, R.H., Young, G., Jr., and Sabiston, D.C., Jr.: Risk factors in coronary artery bypass surgery. Arch. Surg. 105:918, 1972.
59. Zeft, H.J., Manley, J.C., Huston, J.H., Tector, A.C., and Johnson, W.D.: Direct coronary surgery in patients with left main coronary artery stenosis. Circulation 45–46(Suppl. II):50, 1972 (Abstr.).
60. Pell, S., and Alonzo, C.A.: Immediate mortality and five year survival of employed men with a first myocardial infarction. N. Engl. J. Med. 270:915, 1964.
61. Schlicter, J., Hellerstein, H.K., and Katz, L.N.: Aneurysm of the heart. Correlative study of 102 proved cases. Medicine 33:43, 1954.
62. Najafi, H., Hunter, J.H., Dye, W.S., Javid, H., Ardakani, R.C., and Julian, O.C.: Emergency left ventricular aneurysmectomy for dying patients. J. Thorac. Cardiovasc. Surg. 10:419, 1969.
63. Ritter, E.R.: Intractable ventricular tachycardia due to ventricular aneurysm with surgical cure. Ann. Intern. Med. 71:1155, 1969.
64. Maloy, W.C., Arrants, J.E., Sowell, B.F., and Hendrix, G.H.: Left ventricular aneurysm of uncertain etiology with recurrent ventricular arrhythmias. N. Engl. J. Med. 255:262, 1971.
65. Meister, S.G., and Helfant, R.H.: Rapid bedside differentiation of ruptured interventricular septum from acute mitral insufficiency. N. Engl. J. Med. 287:1024, 1972.
66. Giuliani, E.R., Danielson, G.K., Pluth, J.R., Odyneic, N.A., and Wallace, R.B.: Postinfarction ventricular septal rupture. Surgical considerations and results. Circulation 49:455, 1974.
67. Austen, W.G., Sanders, C.A., Aberill, J.H., and Friedlich, A.L.: Ruptured papillary muscle: Report of a case with successful mitral valve replacement. Circulation 32:597, 1965.
68. Mundth, E.D., Buckley, M.J., Leinbach, R.C., Gold, H.K., Daggett, W.M., and Austen, W.G.: Surgical intervention for the complications of acute myocardial ischemia. Ann. Surg. 178:379, 1973.
69. Sealy, W.C., Wallace, A.J., Ramming, K.R., Gallagher, J.J., and Swenson, R.H.: An improved operation for the definitive treatment of the Wolff-Parkinson-White syndrome. Ann. Thorac. Surg. 17:107, 1974.
70. Sealy, W.C., and Wallace, A.G.: The surgical treatment of the Wolff-Parkinson-White syndrome. J. Thorac. Cardiovasc. Surg. 68:757, 1974.
71. Lloyd, R., Okada, R., Stagg, J., Anderson, R., Brock, H., and Marcus, F.: The treatment of recurrent ventricular tachycardia with bilateral cervicothoracic sympathetic-ganglionectomy: Report of two cases. Circulation 50:382, 1974.
72. Rashkind, W., Waldhausen, J., Miller, W., and Friedman, S.: Palliative treatment in tricuspid atresia. Combined balloon atrioseptostomy and surgical alteration of pulmonary blood flow. J. Thorac. Cardiovasc. Surg. 57:812, 1969.
73. Boncheck, L.I., and Starr, A.: Total correction of transposition of the great arteries in infancy as initial surgical management. Ann. Thorac. Surg. 14:376, 1972.
74. Szentpetery, S., and Lower, R.R.: Changing concepts in the treatment of penetrating cardiac injuries. J. Trauma 17:457, 1977.
75. Ablaza, S.G.G., Ghosh, S.C., and Grana, V.P.: Use of a ringed intraluminal graft in the surgical treatment of dissecting aneurysm of the thoracic aorta. J. Thorac. Cardiovasc. Surg. 76:390, 1978.
76. Hultgren, H.N.: Medical versus surgical treatment of unstable angina. Am. J. Cardiol. 38:479, 1976.

77. Langou, R.A., Geha, A.S., Hammond, G.L., et al.: Surgical approach for patients with unstable angina pectoris: Role of the response to initial medical therapy and intra-aortic balloon pumping in perioperative complications after aortocoronary bypass grafting. Am. J. Cardiol. 42:629, 1978.
78. Hurst, J.W., King, S.B., III, Logue, R.B., et al.: Value of coronary bypass. Part I. Am. J. Cardiol. 42:308, 1978.
79. Takaro, T., Hultgren, H.N., Lipton, M.J., et al.: The V.A. cooperative randomized study of surgery for coronary arterial occlusive disease. II. Subgroup with Significant Left Main Lesions. Circulation 54(Suppl. III): 107–111, 1976.
80. Sealy, W.C., Gallagher, J.J., and Wallace, H.G.: The surgical treatment of Wolff-Parkinson-White syndrome: Evolution of improved methods for identification and interruption of the Kent bundle. Ann. Thorac. Surg. 22:443, 1976.
81. Guirandon, G., Fontaine, G., Frank, R., et al.: Encircling endocardial ventriculotomy: A new surgical treatment for life-threatening ventricular tachycardias resistant to medical treatment following myocardial infarction. Ann. Thorac. Surg. 26:438, 1978.
82. Gallagher, J.J.: Surgical treatment of arrhythmias: Current status and future directions. Am. J. Cardiol: 41, 1035, 1978.

Chapter **19**

RADIOLOGIC DIAGNOSIS IN CARDIOPULMONARY EMERGENCIES

ROBERT M. STEINER

GENERAL CONSIDERATIONS

The interpretation of the chest roentgenogram by the radiologist will yield important information about the status of the patient undergoing a cardiac or pulmonary emergency. The radiologic examination provides important information about the severity of the disease process. Imaging techniques, including plain film radiography, fluoroscopy, and angiographic studies, are important in detecting the complications of various cardiac emergencies. In this chapter, the various roentgenographic findings of the common cardiovascular emergencies are discussed, with particular emphasis on the radiologic differential diagnosis. The cardiac emergencies discussed include pulmonary edema due to the failing ischemic myocardium or to the myocardium compromised by infection or other inflammatory changes. In particular, pulmonary edema following myocardial infarction, as well as the complications of rupture of the interventricular septum and papillary muscle dysfunction secondary to coronary occlusion, are discussed in detail. Other common cardiac emergencies in which the radiologist may play an important role are hemopericardium and pericardial effusion, ventricular aneurysm second-

395

ary to cardiac trauma, infective endocarditis, and acute thoracic aortic dissection. Roentgenographic changes related to surgery, particularly those of the prosthetic valves, and artificial cardiac pacemakers, are also discussed, as are the common pulmonary emergencies associated with the adult respiratory distress syndrome and pulmonary thromboembolism.

The various causes of pulmonary edema are listed in Table 19–1, and the radiographic signs of congestive heart failure are listed in Table 19–2.

Table 19–1. *Various Causes of Pulmonary Edema*

Increased pulmonary capillary pressure
  Cardiac causes
  Fluid overload
  Pulmonary venous pressure
Increased alveolocapillary permeability
Adult respiratory distress syndrome
  Hypoxia
  Oxygen intoxication
  Central nervous system pulmonary edema
Aspiration pneumonia
Infection
Diffuse capillary leak syndrome
Inhaled toxic agents
Radiation pneumonitis
Disseminated intravascular coagulation
  Septicemia
  Immune complex disease post-infectious state
Immunologic reactions
Lymphatic insufficiency
Hypoalbuminemia
Heroin and other drug reactions
Pulmonary embolism
Contusion, hemorrhage
Reexpansion pulmonary edema
High-altitude pulmonary edema

* Source: Adapted from D. Mason: *Cardiac Emergencies.* Baltimore, Williams & Wilkins Co., 1978 (with permission).

Table 19–2. *Radiographic Signs of Congestive Heart Failure*

Cardiac enlargement
Venous and arterial cephalization or upper lobe redistribution
Peribronchial cuffing
Perihilar haziness
Pulmonary interstitial edema characterized by interlobal effusions and fine reticular densities
Thickening of interlobular fissures
Subpleural stripes
Pulmonary alveolar edema
Pleural effusions

ACUTE PULMONARY EDEMA

Probably the most common and the most important cardiopulmonary emergency that all primary physicians encounter is acute pulmonary edema. Accumulation of fluid in the air spaces of the lungs and in the interstitial spaces may be life threatening because it interferes with the carbon dioxide–oxygen exchange. Acute pulmonary edema may be due to an increase in the pulmonary venous pressure, an increased permeability of the alveolocapillary membrane, a decreased pulmonary oncotic pressure due to a reduced serum protein level or to an increased negative interstitial pressure. Reduced lymphatic reserve capacity or lymphatic obstruction may also produce the radiographic appearance of pulmonary edema.

Regardless of the cause of increased fluid density in the air spaces and the interstitial spaces, the basic radiologic pattern is the same. That is,

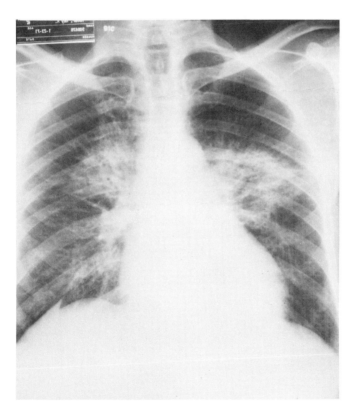

Figure 19–1.   Parahilar air-space infiltrates due to pulmonary edema in a patient with chronic renal failure.

diffuse soft tissue densities in both lung fields with irregular indistinct fluffy and often confluent margins are the usual findings. Those densities may be uniform, or they may be localized to portions of one or both lungs (Fig. 19–1). The patient's position often affects the location of the fluid. If the patient with cardiogenic pulmonary edema is placed in the decubitus position, the fluid may drift to the more dependent part. In pneumonia, however, little or no redistribution of the fluid occurs (Fig. 19–2). On air bronchogram, air-filled alveoli surrounded by fluid-filled acini may be present in an area of air space consolidation unless the bronchi are filled with fluid material, such as mucous plugs, blood, exudate, or other soft tissue densities. Other findings in pulmonary edema are interlobular effusions, or Kerley-B lines. The Kerley-B lines are short, fine densities best seen in the posteroanterior or oblique view along the peripheral lung

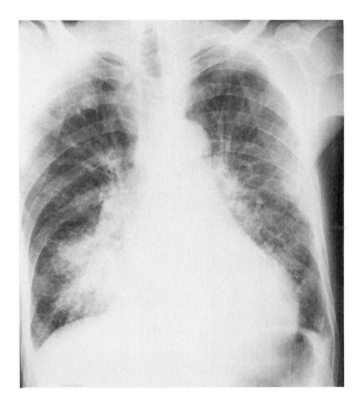

Figure 19–2.   Right middle lobe pneumonia in a patient with congestive heart failure. Note the vascular redistribution of the upper lobes, hazy bronchopulmonary markings, and cardiac enlargement. Right middle lobe pneumonia cannot be differentiated radiologically from an area of pulmonary edema.

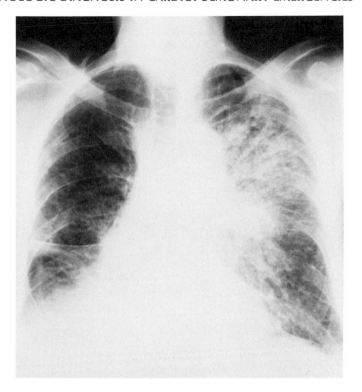

Figure 19–3.   Asymmetrical pulmonary edema due to congestive heart failure in a patient who received radiation therapy of the right lung for carcinoma. The lack of findings of failure in the irradiated area is due to poor pulmonary perfusion.

borders perpendicular to the lateral pleural surfaces. Pleural effusion may or may not be present. There may be alterations in the pulmonary vascular redistribution (Fig. 19–3).

Cardiogenic Pulmonary Edema

The cardiac causes of pulmonary edema are summarized in Table 19–3.

With pulmonary venous hypertension, there is redistribution of both venous and arterial blood flow to the upper lung fields, which reduces the ratio of the lower lobe pulmonary vascular diameters to the upper lobe pulmonary vascular diameters from 2:1 or more to 1:1. That redistribution is an early finding in increased pulmonary venous pressure, and it may be seen even before the auscultatory findings in acute pulmonary edema are noted.[1] Its appearance alerts the clinician to the presence of

Table 19–3.   *Cardiac Causes of Pulmonary Edema*

Systemic hypertension
Acute myocardial infarction
    Left ventricular failure
    Mitral regurgitation
    Left ventricular aneurysm
    Ruptured ventricular aneurysm
Left ventricular outflow obstruction
    Aortic stenosis
    Aortic insufficiency
    Prosthetic malformation
Cardiomyopathy
    Hypertrophic
    Restrictive
    Constrictive
Constrictive pericarditis
Cardiac tamponade
Mitral stenosis
Cardiac tumors (e.g., myxoma)

Source: D. Mason: Cardiac Emergencies. Baltimore, Williams & Wilkins Co., 1978 (with permission).

acute congestive heart failure. Peribronchial thickening or cuffing, perihilar "haziness," and subpleural stripes are often radiographic signs that support the diagnosis of interstitial pulmonary edema (Fig. 19–4).

With higher degrees of pulmonary venous hypertension, bilateral diffuse alveolar infiltrates, often described as having a butterfly or bat-wing pattern, are present in some patients. More commonly, however, a patchy inhomogeneous distribution of alveolar fluid appears, especially early in the development of heart failure. An atypical pattern of pulmonary edema often appears in the presence of underlying pulmonary disease, however. Emphysematous bullae, areas of lung treated with ionizing radiation, or other poorly perfused areas will be clear when fluid is seen in the remainder of the lung field.[2] The use of positive pressure breathing techniques (e.g., positive end-expiratory pressure) reduces the apparent amount of pulmonary fluid by spreading it out over a larger pulmonary surface. This will produce the appearance of improvement, although the pulmonary venous pressure may remain elevated.

Pulmonary edema due to congestive heart failure is usually accompanied by enlargement of the cardiac silhouette, but overt pulmonary edema may occasionally occur following acute myocardial infarction or in advanced chronic pulmonary disease without cardiac enlargement.[3]

As pulmonary venous hypertension and heart failure progresses, pul-

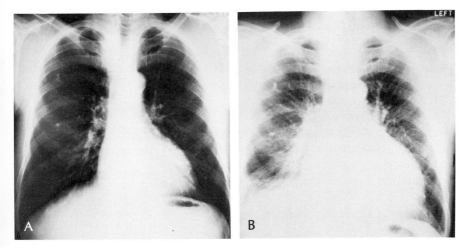

Figure 19–4. Pulmonary edema. A. Roentgenograms made prior to coronary occlusion showed that the lungs were clear. B. Pulmonary edema is present 10 days after myocardial infarction. Note the vascular redistribution, right-sided pleural effusion, and cardiac enlargement.

monary arterial dilatation occurs due to increased pressure. Increased pulmonary resistance places a greater work load on the right ventricle, which eventually fails, and right ventricular dilatation occurs. That phenomenon can be seen on the lateral chest film with filling in the retrosternal space. The right ventricular dilatation is often associated with enlargement of the superior vena cava and the azygos vein.[4]

Pleural effusion is a late manifestation of congestive heart failure, and it is often present together with elevated right ventricular pressures. The coexistence is thought to be related to the anatomy of the pathways of the parietal pleural lymphatics, which fail to drain adequately into the systemic venous system if there is a rise in the central venous pressure.[5]

Pulmonary Edema following Myocardial Infarction

The chest films of patients with acute myocardial infarction may be entirely normal. But if the loss of functioning myocardium is sufficient to cause a rise in left ventricular end diastolic pressure, pulmonary edema develops. Pulmonary edema may occur during an early phase of myocardial infarction, and it is observed in approximately 25% of patients.[6] Often it resolves within a few days. Otherwise it may lead to cardiogenic shock and death when 40 to 50% of the left ventricular myocardium is infarcted.[7]

OTHER COMPLICATIONS OF ACUTE MYOCARDIAL INFARCTION

The radiologist is most helpful to the clinician in diagnosing and evaluating the severity of the other complications of acute myocardial infarction. Those complications include:

1. Interventricular septal defect
2. Papillary muscle dysfunction due to necrosis or ruptured chordae tendineae, with mitral regurgitation
3. Left ventricular myocardial rupture
4. Hemopericardium and pericardial effusion
5. Ventricular aneurysm

Rupture of the Interventricular Septum

Cardiac rupture is the cause of 7 to 9% of deaths following acute myocardial infarction; it usually involves the anterolateral left ventricular wall near the interventricular septum.[8,9] In 1% of fatal myocardial infarctions there is rupture of the septum itself. The defect is usually in the inferior portion of the muscular septum. It may be single, or several communications may be present. Infarction usually involves the anterior septum as well as the left ventricular free wall. The left-to-right shunt may be large, with a systemic-to-pulmonary flow ratio of 2:1 or greater. The shunt, together with the extensive infarction, produces biventricular failure and pulmonary edema.

Clinically, a post-infarction septal communication may be difficult to distinguish from the mitral insufficiency of papillary muscle dysfunction or rupture. A holosystolic murmur and rapid deterioration may be found in both conditions.

Radiologically, overcirculation and dilatation of the main pulmonary artery are demonstrated although the presence of pulmonary edema usually obscures the vascular detail. For that reason, the increased pulmonary arterial vasculature may not be discernible. A specific diagnosis may be made by left ventricular angiography performed in the left anterior oblique projection, which will demonstrate the septum to best advantage. Two-dimensional real-time ultrasonography helps to exclude the mitral valve prolapse syndrome, and it may demonstrate the septal discontinuity.

Papillary Muscle Dysfunction

Acute papillary muscle rupture is a rare and catastrophic event that produces severe mitral regurgitation. The mortality is high; 80% of patients die within two weeks of the rupture.[10] The rupture may involve complete amputation of the papillary muscle, with the rapid onset of pulmonary

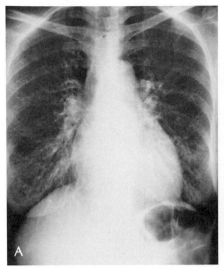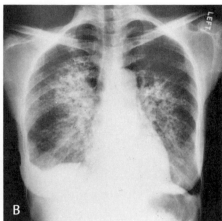

Figure 19–5.   Papillary muscle dysfunction. A. A posteroanterior chest roentgenogram was unremarkable following myocardial infarction. B. Severe pulmonary edema developed 7 days later, following papillary muscle rupture and marked mitral insufficiency. (Courtesy of A. Kurtz, M.D.)

edema or rupture of the chordae tendineae or one or more muscle bundles. Varying hemodynamic derangements under those circumstances are often incompatible with life. The posterior papillary muscle ruptures more frequently because its vascular supply is sparser than that of the anterior papillary muscle.

Radiographically, there is sudden development of pulmonary edema due to the mitral regurgitation and elevated left-sided pressures that usually occur during the first 10 days after acute myocardial infarction. Initially, there is no left atrial enlargement, but if the infarction progresses to scar and if mitral valve prolapse persists, there is gradual enlargement of the left atrium and ventricle (Fig. 19–5).

The presence of papillary muscle dysfunction is suspected following the sudden development of the typical holosystolic murmur and pulmonary edema. As in interventricular septal rupture, ultrasonography and angiography vividly demonstrate the abnormality and confirm the clinical diagnosis.

Hemopericardium and Pericardial Effusion

When hemopericardium or pericardial effusion occurs, the cardiac silhouette enlarges and assumes a globular appearance The normal indentations of the cardiac silhouette are effaced (Fig. 19–6A). The fluid

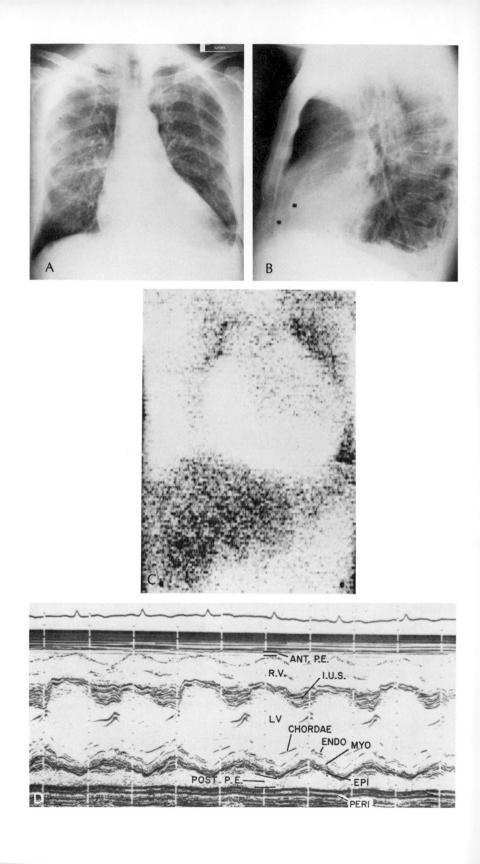

tends to be localized in the caudal portion of the pericardial sac, where the fewest great vessel intrusions are present. As the volume of the fluid increases, the pericardial outline becomes less pulsatile, and the phenomenon is best observed on fluoroscopy. The radiologic diagnosis depends on the separation of the pericardium from the underlying cardiac contour. The most reliable plain film sign of the phenomenon is the displaced epicardial fat sign[11] (Fig. 19–6B). The pericardial space filled with fluid may be seen as a soft tissue band bordered by the radiolucent epicardial fat and the retrosternal fat. That sign may be observed in 40% or less of patients with pericardial effusion.[12] The differential diagnosis includes enlargement of the cardiac shadow due to aneurysm and generalized dilatation due to ischemic or metabolic cardiomyopathy.

Other radiologic modalities of diagnosis are:
1. Radionucleotide imaging (Fig. 19–6C)
2. Carbon dioxide contrast imaging (Fig. 19–7)

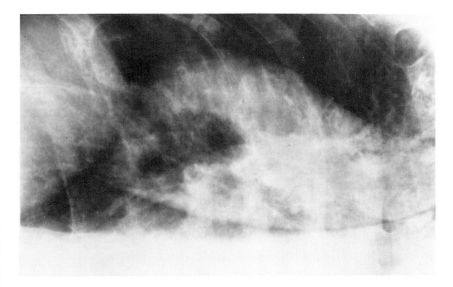

Figure 19–7. Right lateral decubitus roentgenogram following the intravenous injection of carbon dioxide shows air in the right atrium widely separated from air filled lung, a phenomenon that is diagnostic of pericardial effusion. (Courtesy of R. Soulen, M.D.)

Figure 19–6. Pericardial effusion. A. Posteroanterior roentgenogram demonstrates mild cardiac enlargement. B. Lateral examination shows the epicardial and retrosternal fat lines to be 1 cm apart, indicating the presence of pericardial fluid. C. Blood pool isotopic examination shows a wide swath of count-free pericardial fluid about the cardiac chambers in a patient with tuberculous pericarditis. D. Ultrasonographic examination demonstrates a transonic zone of pericardial effusion (Reprinted with permission from R. T. Sandra Hagen-Ansert, *Textbook of Diagnostic Ultrasound.*, St. Louis, C.V. Mosby Co., 1978.) (I.U.S. = interventricular septum)

3. Right atrial angiocardiography

4. Ultrasonography

Today ultrasonography has largely supplanted invasive and isotopic studies in the diagnosis of pericardial effusion. It is the most sensitive study, and it has no known risk. Collections of fluid as small as 16 cc have been detected in that manner[12] (Fig. 19–6D).

Ventricular Aneurysm

Although the formation of a ventricular aneurysm is not an emergency, it is convenient to discuss it here, along with other complications of myocardial infarction. The ventricular aneurysm occurs in an area of dyskinesis or akinesis, and it is a discrete fibrotic area lacking in musculature. A paradoxical motion is seen on fluoroscopy, with an increase in the volume of the aneurysm during ventricular systole.

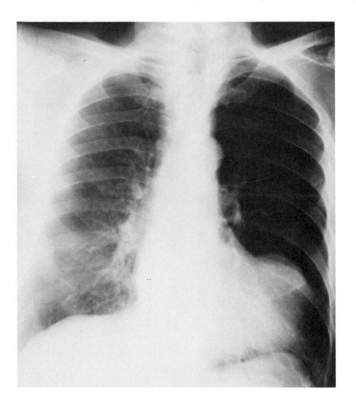

Figure 19–8.   Ventricular aneurysm. A discrete bulge in the area of the left ventricular apex is due to aneurysm, a complication of myocardial infarction. Note the rimlike calcification within the left ventricular wall.

Although the ventricular aneurysm rarely ruptures, it may be the source of emboli and thus lead to cerebrovascular accidents or renal infarctions, and so on. Left ventricular aneurysms often calcify (Fig. 19–8), a phenomenon that can be detected by conventional radiography.

THE ADULT RESPIRATORY DISTRESS SYNDROME (ARDS)

The adult respiratory distress syndrome (ARDS), or noncardiogenic pulmonary edema, is a result of a direct physical or chemical damage to the alveolar lining cells and/or the pulmonary capillary endothelial lining. The damage alters the permeability of the capillary membrane and results in alveolar edema. Hypoxia follows, with right-to-left shunting within the lung and reduced lung compliance. Unlike pulmonary edema of cardiac origin, the pulmonary wedge pressure remains within the normal range, and the roentgenographic signs of increased pulmonary venous pressure are absent (Fig. 19–9).

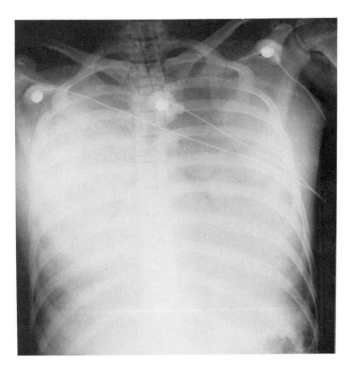

Figure 19–9.   Adult respiratory distress syndrome due to oxygen intoxication. Diffuse air-space consolidation in a patient with viral pneumonia who received 100% oxygen for 24 hours.

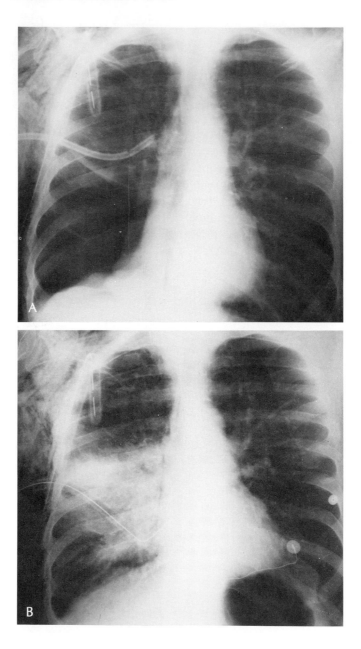

Figure 19–10.   Reexpansion pulmonary edema. A. Right-sided pneumothorax. B. Pulmonary edema following rapid reexpansion.

The adult respiratory distress syndrome is associated with:
1. Shock lung
2. Post-perfusion syndrome
3. Fat embolism
4. Acid aspiration pulmonary edema
5. Chemical inhalation diseases
6. Diffuse viral pneumonia
7. Disseminated intravascular coagulation
8. An immunologic reaction: (a) to drugs, (b) connective tissue disease, or (c) hereditary angioneurotic edema

Other causes of noncardiac pulmonary edema are:
1. Re-expansion pulmonary edema due to a sudden increase in the negative interstitial pressure (Figs. 19–10A and 19–10B).
2. Pulmonary lymphatic block
3. Narcotic overdose
4. High-altitude state
5. Central nervous system pulmonary edema[7]

The chest film is one of the most useful studies in detecting pulmonary edema of cardiac or noncardiac origin but several major limitations in the chest roentgenographic examination should be considered in the emergency patient: (1) the nonspecificity of the roentgenographic pattern and (2) the lag time of both the development and the resolution of pulmonary edema. Up to 72 hours may elapse between the clinical onset of the pulmonary edema and its appearance on the chest film. Many hours may also pass between the correction of pulmonary edema and its disappearance from the film.[16,17]

TRAUMA TO THE HEART AND GREAT VESSELS

Cardiac trauma may be caused by a penetrating object, such as a knife or a bullet. The damage can result in hemopericardium or pseudoaneurysm, and the foreign body may be retained in the heart or pericardium. Atrial or ventricular septal defects or aorticocardiac communications may develop. The right ventricle is most commonly involved because of its anterior location. Fluoroscopy is helpful in localization of the retained foreign body, as are overhead chest roentgenograms with multiple views. Fluoroscopy also demonstrates reduced cardiac motion due to pericardial fluid. Paradoxical motion is demonstrated as a result of aneurysm formation. Angiography and ultrasonography are valuable in excluding injury to valve leaflets and to the valvular supporting structures.

Iatrogenic penetrating trauma may occur during cardiac catheterization. Such trauma is most common during transseptal catheterization, when the right atrial wall (not the interatrial septum) is punctured during the placement of a transvenous pacemaker (Fig. 19–11) or in association with catheter recoil after a high-pressure injection.[13] Although pericardial tamponade may occur following perforation, the patient usually remains asymptomatic and free of significant pericardial fluid.[14]

Nonpenetrating cardiac injury is usually due to contusions secondary to automobile steering-wheel injuries or to cardiac resuscitation. Contusion may result in only transient cardiac arrhythmias, or the damaged myocardium or aorta may rupture, leading to sudden death.

The radiologic signs in trauma to the heart and great vessels include:

1. Sternal fracture or swelling of the soft tissue of the anterior chest wall

2. Enlargement of the cardiac silhouette due to hemopericardium

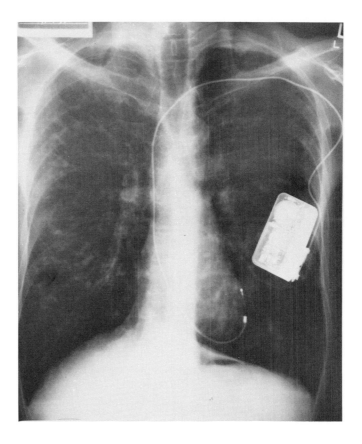

Figure 19–11. Pacemaker electrode perforation. Note the pacemaker leads outside the confines of the cardiac silhouette. (Courtesy of Irving Ehrlich, M.D.)

3. Pulmonary edema due to traumatic valvular insufficiency

4. Signs of infarction, including aneurysm due to thrombosis of the coronary arteries

5. Calcified pericardium, a late finding in pericardial bleeding and trauma.

Of the many techniques for identifying hemopericardium, the most sensitive one is ultrasonography. Ultrasonography can be used to identify even small collections of fluid, either free or loculated within the pericardium. The technique is based on the presence of two separate echos, a pulsatile ventricular myocardial echo synchronous with a peripheral pulse and a nonpulsatile echo of greater amplitude[14] (Fig. 19–6D).

PROSTHETIC VALVE DYSFUNCTION

Dehiscence of the sutures of the prosthetic valve base, or the "sewing ring," is a not infrequent cause of valvular insufficiency. When at least 40% of the circumference of the sewing ring no longer adheres to the valve orifice, the prosthetic valve rocks abnormally. The phenomenon can be seen with fluoroscopy or with cineradiography as an increased arc of excursion. However, since the degree of normal excursion varies greatly from person to person, it is difficult to diagnose an abnormal excursion pattern with certainty, especially when baseline data are not available. But angiography confirms the regurgitation, even when the sewing ring seems to move normally. Regurgitation is the most sensitive indicator of prosthetic valve seat insufficiency. Both fluoroscopy and ultrasonography also demonstrate the abnormalities in ball or disc motion. Ball variance, which was a problem in the early use of prostheses, is rarely encountered today, but disc degeneration resulting in distal embolism of disc material or reduced motion of the disc within the cage struts remains a problem, and it may be a cause of massive valvular insufficiency[13] (Fig. 19–12).

ACUTE VALVULAR INSUFFICIENCY DUE TO INFECTIVE ENDOCARDITIS

Valvular insufficiency may be due to:

1. Perforation of the valve leaflets

2. Rupture of the chordae tendineae

3. Papillary muscle dysfunction or rupture

The radiologic modalities used in the diagnosis of valvular insufficiency due to infective endocarditis are:

1. Plain film radiography

2. Ultrasonography

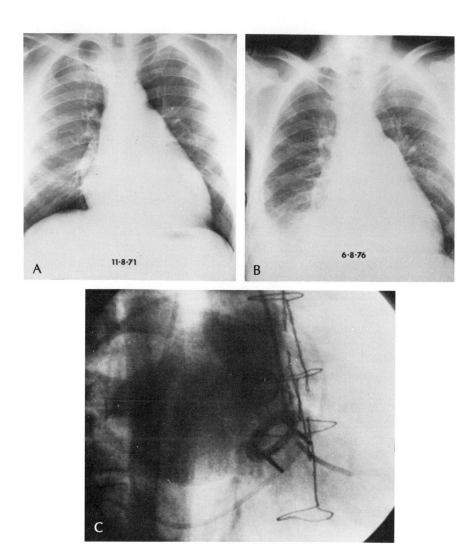

Figure 19–12.   Prosthetic valve malfunction. A. Posterior anterior radiograph of a patient who had undergone mitral valve replacement five months previously. The lungs are clear. B. The patient developed sudden cardiac decompensation 55 months later. Prosthetic valve malfunction was suspected. C. Right anterior oblique left ventricular angiographic study showed +4 mitral regurgitation due to the disc regeneration.

3. Isotopic angiocardiography

4. Positive contrast angiography

Echocardiography, both two-dimensional, real-time and M-mode examinations, can demonstrate evidence of prolapse of the mitral valve apparatus into the left atrium during ventricular systole. If the vegetation is large enough, the vegetation itself may be seen as an area of thickening of the aortic or mitral valve leaflets, or it may be seen as additional structure along the left ventricular wall or at the entrance or exit of a septal defect.

Plain chest roentgenography demonstrates the findings of pulmonary edema. If the infective endocarditis is right sided, septic emboli are seen in the lung fields as rounded, frequently cavitating infiltrates (Fig. 19–13). Multiple septic emboli may also be associated with pelvic and abdominal thrombophlebitis, infected intravenous catheters or needles, infected

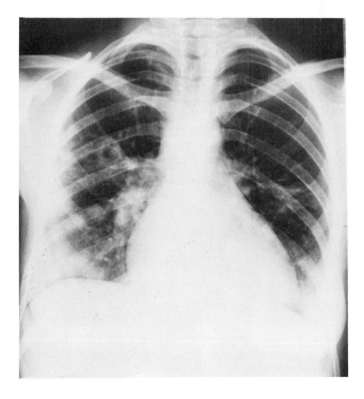

Figure 19–13. A 20-year-old heroin addict developed infective endocarditis with involvement of the tricuspid valve. Multiple cavitating septic emboli are present in both lung fields. Blood cultures grew *Staphylococcus aureus*.

arteriovenous or ventriculoatrial shunts, infected pulmonary emboli, as well as with the infective endocarditis of drug addiction and of other causes.[15]

PULMONARY EMBOLISM AND INFARCTION

In consideration of the radiologic findings in pulmonary embolism and infarction, it is important to note that most thromboembolic episodes are not associated with any detectable radiologic changes. Even in those cases proved by angiography or by isotopic examination, the plain film findings are either entirely negative or negligible.[18] Indeed, the finding most suggestive of pulmonary embolism and infarction is the paucity or absence of radiologic findings in a symptomatic patient.[19]

When embolic disease without hemorrhage or infarct occurs, the most common findings may be described as follows:

1. Oligemia is localized when it is due to lobar or segmental vascular occlusion and generalized when it is due to multiple small emboli.

2. Enlargement of the pulmonary artery is best seen on serial examinations. It is due to thrombosis in the vessel itself or to pulmonary arterial hypertension when 70% or more of the vascular bed is compromised. The size of the pulmonary artery usually decreases rapidly with the lysis and break-up of the thrombus.[19]

3. There is abrupt tapering of the involved vessel—the "knuckle sign."[18]

4. Acute cor pulmonale is most commonly seen with widespread multiple peripheral emboli. Radiologic changes in acute right ventricular insufficiency include cardiac enlargement, increased size of the main pulmonary artery, and a "pruned-tree" appearance of the pulmonary vasculature due to pulmonary arterial hypertension. Dilatation of the azygos vein and the superior vena cava is also found in conjunction with acute cor pulmonale.

5. Elevated diaphragm

6. Areas of discord atelectasis

When infarction or hemorrhage accompanies thromboembolism, the following radiologic findings may be observed:

1. Parenchymal consolidation is found most often at the lung bases, particularly in an area of one or more pleural interfaces. Those changes are usually recognized as ill-defined homogeneous, wedge-shaped infiltrates at the costophrenic or cardiophrenic angles. The infiltrates may develop as early as 10 to 12 hours or as late as seven days after the embolic episode (Fig. 19–14). The size of the infiltrate may vary from 3 to 10 cm, and occasionally central cavitation occurs as a result of necrosis of the infarcted tissue. Resolution may occur as early as seven to 10 days

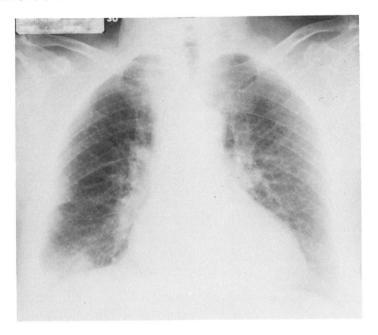

Figure 19–14.   A pleural-based infiltrate in the right costophrenic angle is due to hemorrhage following pulmonary infarction.

when hemorrhage is present without infarction. Following pulmonary infarction, the perfusion deficit may persist for three to five weeks (Fig. 19–15).

   2. Linear shadows (Fig. 19–16)

     a. Linear shadows on the chest film represent platelike atelectasis seen mainly at the lung bases in patients with (1) pulmonary emboli usually due to mucous plugging of the bronchus or (2) adherence of lung tissue due to the loss of surfactant secondary to reduced surface tension.

     b. Parenchymal scarring may appear as long irregular linear densities often terminating at a pleural surface. Those densities may be identified by tenting of the nearby pleura.

   3. Pleural effusion is a more common finding than parenchymal infiltration, and it usually implies infarction rather than embolism alone. The fluid collection is usually unilateral, and the fluid is absorbed when the infarction resolves[18] (Table 19–4).

Pulmonary angiography is the most sensitive radiologic study for the diagnosis of pulmonary embolism and infarction. It should be performed before surgery or on an emergency basis when a massive pulmonary

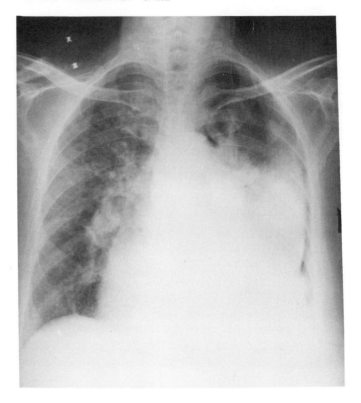

Figure 19–15.   A dense infiltrate involving the left lower lobe and lingular segment of the left upper lobe is due to necrotizing pulmonary infarction in a patient with mitral stenosis.

embolism is suspected. Angiography is of greatest value in the diagnosis of lesions of 2 mm or more that involve the segmental or lobar branches. A positive angiogram exhibits at least one of the following changes:

1. Filling defects within a vessel
2. Cut-off or abrupt termination of the contrast column
3. Reduced venous and arterial flow
4. Reduced segmental perfusion

The perfusion lung scintiscan is a sensitive but nonspecific study that shows the pattern of distribution of the pulmonary vascular flow. However, false-positive results due to perfusion deficits from causes other than pulmonary thromboembolic disease may be obtained. Perfusion abnormalities are seen in chronic obstructive pulmonary disease, pneumonia, pleural effusion, and congestive heart failure. Ventilation scan results are normal in pulmonary embolism, but they show retained

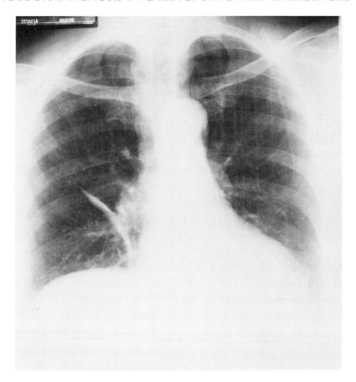

Figure 19–16.   The thin linear density representing atelectasis in the right lower lobe is related to pulmonary embolism in a 75-year-old woman.

Table 19–4.   *Radiologic Findings in Pulmonary Embolism and Infarction*

	University of Michigan	Urokinase Cooperative Study
Normal	18%	15%
Signs of embolism		
Dilated main pulmonary artery	—	23%
Reduced vascularity	3%	15%
Increased right ventricular size	—	5%
Signs of infarction		
Infiltrate	65%	41%
Atelectasis	15%	20%
Elevated diaphragm	—	41%
Pleural effusion	50%	28%
Cavitation	3%	—

Source. D. Mason: *Cardiac Emergencies* Baltimore, Williams & Wilkins Co., 1978 (with permission).

isotope with air trapping in chronic obstructive disease. The lung scan should be performed in conjunction with plain film studies, with the film exposed at the time the isotope examination is performed.

ARTIFICIAL CARDIAC PACEMAKERS (see also Chapter 11)

Although implantation of an artificial cardiac pacemaker is a well-established procedure, pacemaker malfunction is not rare and it may be life threatening. Radiographs can be valuable in detecting the abnormalities associated with pacemaker malfunction, which include:

1. Lead fracture (Fig. 19–17)
2. Electrode dislodgement
3. Electrode malposition (Fig. 19–11)
4. Battery failure

Although the electrodes currently available have improved flex resistance and although the battery life span has increased with the introduction of the lithium-powered batteries, lead fracture is still an important cause of artificial pacemaker failure. Approximately 2.7% of electrodes

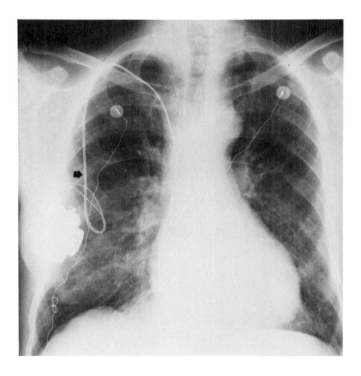

Figure 19–17.   Undisplaced fracture of a transvenous pacemaker lead.

develop fractures, usually at the point of connection with the generator or at the site of venous entry.[20] High-density over-penetrated films demonstrate a break in electrode continuity. If a fracture is not detected by the posteroanterior and lateral projections alone, oblique films, fluoroscopy or cineradiography may be used to identify the break. A fracture may be difficult to recognize, especially when the insulating sheath of the electrode is intact or when the wire is superimposed over the battery pack.[21] Fractures may also occur during trauma to the thorax (Fig.

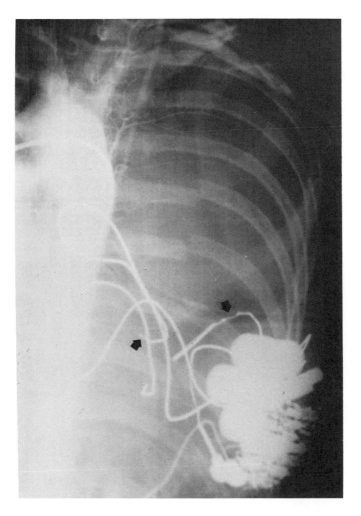

Figure 19–18.   Fractured epicardial pacemaker leads in a young woman who had been injured in an automobile accident. In addition to heart block, she had a ruptured aorta, a left hemothorax, and a ruptured spleen. (Courtesy of Mark Whuley, M.D.)

19–18), and serial films may be needed to show a perforation. Perforation should be suspected when the pacemaker fails to sense either continuously or intermittently. Stimulation, with twitching of the abdominal, diaphragmatic, or intercostal muscles may occur. Although uncommon, cardiac tamponade has been reported after removal of the perforating catheter.

Some other complications are venous thrombosis (Fig. 19–19), pulmonary embolism, and infection.

Thrombosis of the subclavian and axillary venous systems is unusual. When the superior vena caval syndrome is clinically suspected, bilateral upper extremity venography is valuable in demonstrating the negative filing defects of the thrombus. Rerouting of the returning venous flow through the azygous system bypasses the obstructed superior vena cava. The radiologic differential diagnosis includes other conditions causing superior vena caval obstruction, such as:

1. Mediastinal hematoma
2. Carcinoma
3. Lymphoma (Fig. 19–20)
4. Fibrosing mediastinitis

Pain and soft tissue swelling at the generator site may indicate abscess formation. Extrusion of the generator may occur, and infection may travel along the wires to involve the myocardium, causing endocarditis, pulmonary embolism, and bronchocutaneous fistula.[25]

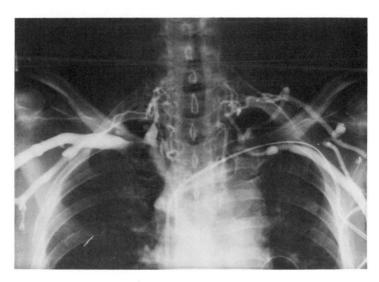

Figure 19–19. Thrombosis of the innominate and jugular venous system related to the presence of a pacemaker electrode. (Courtesy of Bud Bacharach, M.D.)

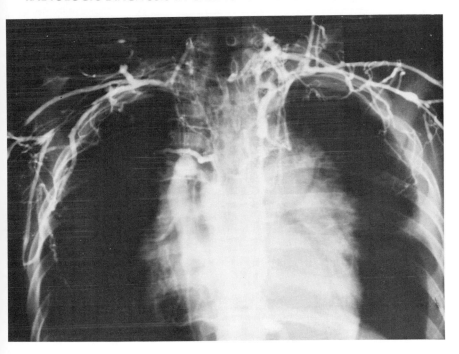

Figure 19–20. Superior vena caval occlusion demonstrated by bilateral upper extremity venography in a young woman with nodular sclerosing Hodgkin's disease. Note the opacification of the accessory hemiazygos veins.

The various complications of artificial pacemaker implantation are described in detail in Chapter 27.

ACUTE THORACIC AORTIC DISSECTION

Acute dissection, or rupture, of the thoracic aorta is one of the most severe medical or surgical emergencies. Although not common, early recognition may permit survival in a majority of cases.[7] Dissection occurs when the intima is perforated and blood enters the wall of the aorta. The systolic pressure of the entering blood allows the dissection to extend both distally and proximally from the point of entry. The new, and false, lumen impinges on the true lumen, reducing its diameter (Fig. 19–21A). There may or may not be an "exit" communication distally.

The causes of acute dissection are:
1. Idiopathic cystic median necrosis
2. Median degenerative disease related to:
   a. Coarctation of the aorta

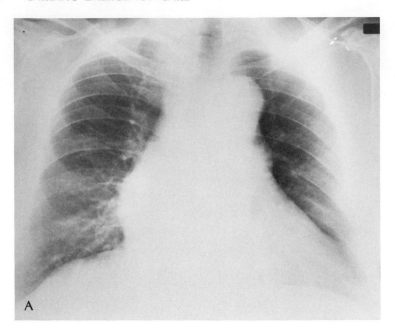

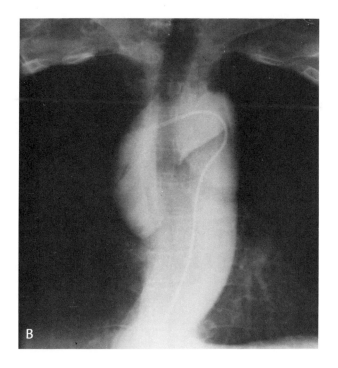

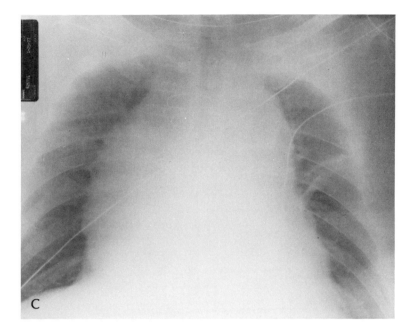

Figure 19–21.   Dissecting aortic aneurysm. A. Cardiomegaly and ectatic aorta in a 50-year-old man with hypertension. B. Aortography demonstrates the radiolucent intimal flap of a dissected ascending aorta. C. Postoperative portable chest roentgenogram shows a wide mediastinum due to bleeding. Signs and symptoms of the superior vena caval syndrome were present.

      b. Marfan's syndrome
      c. Ehlers-Danlos syndrome
      d. Lues
      e. Ankylosing spondylitis
      f. Homocysteinuria
      g. Pregnancy
   3. Hypertension (Figs. 19–21B and 19–21C).

The dissection may begin in the ascending aorta several cm distal to either the sinus of Valsalva or the left subclavian artery. Dissection in the ascending aorta may mimic acute myocardial infarction, but more than 50% of the patients present with aortic insufficiency and a normal ECG or a nonspecific ECG abnormality. When the findings just listed are encountered, the possibility of dissection should be seriously considered. Pulses in the arms and carotid pulses may be unequal due to the involvement of the head and neck vessels in the dissection. The presence of a pericardial rub may suggest rupture into the pericardium. Positive radiologic findings are usually present, but they are often subtle and may be missed or

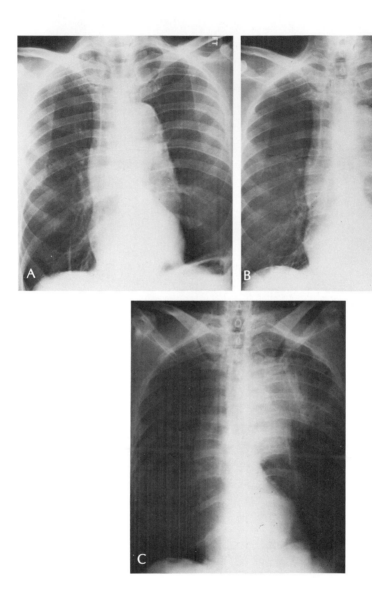

Figure 19–22.   Dissecting aortic aneurysm. A. Posteroanterior chest roentgenogram shows an ectatic aorta with a calcified aortic knob. B. A later film shows a change in the position of the calcified rim with widening of the aortic arch that suggests the presence of a false channel of an aortic dissection. C. A loss of sharpness of the aortic knob and the development of a contiguous infiltrate is due to aortic rupture and pulmonary hemorrhage.

misinterpreted unless one is thinking in terms of a dissecting aortic aneurysm.

The roentgenographic changes suggestive of acute dissection of the thoracic aorta include:

1. Enlargement of the cardiac silhouette due to hemopericardium
2. Mediastinal widening (Fig. 19–21C)
3. Enlargement of the ascending aorta, the knob, or the descending aorta
4. Haziness of the aortic knuckle
5. Change in the position of calcification in the knob as shown in comparison with old films
6. Left pleural effusion
7. Alveolar infiltrates, suggesting bleeding into the lung

If plain film findings and the clinical picture suggest dissection, aortography should be performed (Fig. 19–22). The catheter is passed from the femoral route unless no pulses are present in either femoral artery due to occlusion. The catheter often enters a false lumen through the exit perforation and returns into the true lumen in the ascending aorta. A radiolucent intimal flap localizes the position of the dissection. Multiple views may be needed to demonstrate to best advantage the position of the flap. Other findings include loss of the true lumen and amputation of intercostal and other branch vessels. Injection of contrast material into the root of the aorta is performed in order to estimate the degree of aortic insufficiency.[4] Recently, computed tomography (CT) has been shown to be helpful in evaluating the nature and extent of dissecting thoracic aneurysms.

SUMMARY

1. In this chapter various radiologic approaches to the diagnosis of many of the more important cardiac and pulmonary emergencies have been discussed.

2. The role of the radiologist in cardiac emergencies is a vital one. The radiologist helps the clinician identify the cause or determine the status of many of those emergency conditions.

3. To perform those services, the radiologist must develop his radiologic skills carefully, use the best available equipment, and make sure that both his skills and the equipment are kept up to date.

4. The radiologist's skill and care are especially important in the management of the various cardiopulmonary emergencies, because often the patient is unable to cooperate (owing to his illness) and because often portable filming techniques must be used.

5. The fastest, most responsive equipment and personnel should be

available for cardiac emergencies. High-penetrant, rapid-filming techniques that require modern, sophisticated equipment are most useful in such emergencies.

6. A radiologist and technicians must be available around the clock.

7. Many of the cardiopulmonary emergency conditions discussed in this chapter initially have similar or even identical roentgenographic patterns.

8. An appropriate and complete history of each patient is needed to help the radiologist and the clinician make an accurate diagnosis and decide on the proper management.

9. The radiologist, the cardiologist, the cardiovascular surgeon, and the primary physician must work as a team if they are to provide the best cardiac emergency care.

REFERENCES

1. Milne, E.: Correlation of physiologic findings with chest roentgenology. Radiol. Clin. North Am. 9:17, 1973.
2. Hublitz, U.F., and Shapiro, J.: Atypical pulmonary patterns of congestive failure in chronic lung disease. Radiology 93:995, 1969.
3. Ravin, C., Kelley, M., and Greenspan, R.: Chest pain in the non-traumatized patient. Radiol. Clin. North Am. 16:3, 1978.
4. Phalen, J.J., Dobry, C.A., and Baltaxe, H.A.: The use of chest roentgenograms in cardiac emergencies. In R.S. Eliot, Cardiac Emergencies. Mt. Kisco, N.Y., Futura, 1977, Pp. 119–138.
5. Mellins, R.B., Levine, O.R., Fishman, A.P., et al.: Effect of systemic and pulmonary venous hypertension on pleural and pericardial fluid accumulation. J. Appl. Physiol. 25:564, 1970.
6. Soulen, R.L., and Freeman, E.: Radiologic evaluation of myocardial infarction. Radiol. Clin. North Am. 9:567, 1971.
7. DeMotes, H., Rahimtoola, S.H., McAnulty, J.H., Mason, D.T., and Murphy, E.S.: Acute pulmonary edema. In D.T. Mason, Cardiac Emergencies. Baltimore, Williams & Wilkins Co., 1978. P. 175.
8. Heikkila, J., Karesoja, M., and Luomanmaki, K.: Ruptured interventricular septum complicating myocardial infarction. Chest 66:675, 1974.
9. Oblath, R.W., Levinson, D.C., and Griffith, G.C.: Factors influencing rupture of the heart after myocardial infarction, J.A.M.A. 149:1276, 1952.
10. Debusk, R.F., and Harrison, D.C.: The clinical spectrum of papillary muscle disease. N. Engl. J. Med. 286:1458, 1969.
11. Lane, E.J., and Carsky, E.W.: Epicardial fat: Plain film analysis in normals and pericardial effusion. Radiology 91:1, 1968.
12. Boal, D., and Soulen, R.L.: The diagnosis of pericardial effusion. Weekly Radiol. Science Update. IV. 50:2, 1977.
13. Morse, D., and Steiner, R.: Pacemaker and Valve Identification Guide. Garden City, N.Y., Medical Examinations, Inc., 1978.
14. Soulen, R.L., and Freeman, E.: Radiologic evaluation of traumatic heart disease. Radiol. Clin. North Am. 9:285, 1971.
15. Tuddenham, W.J., Barden, R.P., Campbell, R.E., et al.: Chest Disease Syllabus. Chicago, American College of Radiology, 1978.
16. McHugh, T., Forrester, J., and Adler, L.: Pulmonary vascular congestion in acute myocardial infarction: hemodynamic and radiologic correlations. Ann. Intern. Med. 76:29, 1972.

17. Kostuk, W., Ran, J., Simon, A., et al.: Correlations between the chest film and hemodynamics in acute myocardial infarction. Circulation 48:624, 1973.
18. Fraser, R., and Pare, J.: Diagnosis of Diseases of the Chest. Philadelphia, W.B. Saunders Co., 1970.
19. Figley, M., Gurdes, A., and Ricketts, H.: Radiographic aspects of pulmonary embolism. Semin. Roentgenol. 2:398, 1967.
20. Green, G.: The Assessment and Performance of Implanted Cardiac Pacemakers. London, Butterworths, 1976.
21. Tegtmeyer, C.J.: Roentgenographic assessment of causes of cardiac pacemaker failure and complications. CRC Crit. Rev. Diagnostic Imaging 9:1, 1977.
22. Krozon, I., and Mehta, S.S.: Broken pacemaker wire in multiple trauma. J. Trauma 14:82, 1974.
23. Bayliss, C., Beanlands, D., and Baird, R.: The pacemaker twiddler's syndrome: A new complication of the implantable transvenous pacemakers. Can. Med. Assoc. J. 99:371, 1968.
24. Tegtmeyer, C.: The radiographic diagnosis of pacemaker failure and complications. In D. Morse and R. Steiner, Pacemaker and Valve Identification Guide. Garden City, N.Y., Medical Examinations, Inc., 1978.
25. Tegtmeyer, D., Hunter, J., and Keats, T.: Bronchocutaneous fistula as a late complication of permanent epicardial pacing. Am. J. Radiol. 121:614, 1974.

Chapter *20*

THE NURSING ASPECTS OF CARDIAC EMERGENCY CARE*

MARTHA I. SPENCE
LOUIS LEMBERG

GENERAL CONSIDERATIONS

The nurse is frequently the first line of defense in the management of cardiac emergencies. Her ability to make critical judgments—by correlating pathophysiology with presenting signs and symptoms—may significantly affect the course of an illness. Knowledge of the mechanism of action and toxic effects of cardiovascular drugs, skill in handling emergency equipment, and skill in performing cardiopulmonary resuscitation are prerequisites to the pursuit of logical and appropriate lines of action.

Cardiac emergencies can generally be categorized as those resulting from electrical dysfunction and those resulting from mechanical dysfunction although both types are closely interrelated. For example, congestive heart failure and cardiogenic shock are often preceded by serious cardiac arrhythmias, and vice versa. Cardiac tamponade is discussed in the section on mechanical dysfunction because it results in mechanical failure. Two vascular emergencies that may compromise cardiac

*Supported in part by a grant from Morris D. Logan

function—pulmonary embolism and hypertensive crisis—are discussed briefly.

The preventive aspects of nursing management, as well as the principles and rationale for crisis intervention, are discussed in each section. The rationale for drug therapy is emphasized.

The Basis for Nursing Action

Cardiac emergencies exist when failure to deliver adequate amounts of oxygen to the tissues is traceable to a variable in cardiac function. A cardiac problem becomes an emergency when the patient experiences a symptomatic fall in cardiac output as manifested by:

1. Changes in sensorium—restlessness, confusion, and agitation that may progress to loss of consciousness
2. Cool or clammy skin that may be dusky
3. Decreased urinary output
4. Tachycardia (usually sinus tachycardia).

The sensorium changes are a manifestation of hypoperfusion of the brain, with resultant tissue hypoxia. The changes in skin color and temperature occur as the body attempts to compensate for the falling cardiac output by shunting blood to more critical areas, and the arterial oxygen tension falls. The urinary output decreases as the renal blood flow is reduced. Tachycardia (usually sinus tachycardia) often occurs as in compensation for the reduced cardiac output.

A cardiac emergency may be averted if the nurse is skilled in assessing the early signs and symptoms of compromised cardiac function. The variables that maintain the integrity of the cardiovascular system are the four determinants of cardiac output:

1. The heart rate and rhythm
2. The venous blood volume (the preload)
3. The arterial vascular tone (peripheral vascular resistance—the afterload)
4. The inotropic (contractile) state of the myocardium.

Assessment of those four determinants in the light of their effects on the myocardial oxygen demand often enables the nurse to avert a crisis or to determine the most appropriate line of action when a crisis occurs.

Emergencies related to disturbances in each of the four determinants of cardiac output are discussed in the following paragraphs. Dysfunctions in heart rate and rhythm are discussed first because they occur so frequently. The pathophysiologic aspects, preventive aspects, the nursing management with regard to drug therapy, and the specific features of each problem are covered.

CARDIAC EMERGENCIES DUE TO ELECTRICAL DYSFUNCTION
(See also Chapters 7 and 8)

Generally, cardiac arrhythmias occur as a result of disturbances in automaticity or in conduction or in both. Automaticity is the ability of the heart to initiate or generate electrical activity. Enhanced automaticity can result in tachyarrhythmias originating from any area of the heart: the sinus node, the atria, the AV junctional tissue, and the His-Purkinje system. Tachyarrhythmias also occur as a result of altered or non-uniform conduction. Frequently those tachyarrhythmias are the result of a uni-directional block occurring in a Purkinje fiber due to ischemia. On finding a single pathway refractory, a normal impulse proceeds to depolarize normal tissue and then reenters the previously refractory tissue, producing an ectopic beat. Once established, such a circuit can result in the generation of a reciprocating tachyarrhythmia.

Tachyarrhythmias are clinically significant because:

1. They may result in a symptomatic fall in cardiac output.
2. They decrease the time needed for coronary artery filling.
3. They increase the myocardial oxygen consumption (MVO_2).

Depressed automaticity and/or conduction results in bradyarrhythmias. When automaticity is depressed, the rate of discharge from automatic centers decreases and slow heart rates occur. When conduction is slowed in any part of the conduction system, the transmission of a cardiac impulse may be delayed or blocked. Bradyarrhythmias are clinically significant when:

1. They are slower than 45 beats per minute
2. They result in a symptomatic fall in cardiac output
3. They allow a breakthrough of serious tachyarrhythmias resulting in brady-tachyarrhythmias.

When a patient presents with various cardiac arrhythmias, the nurse should mentally review a list of possible causative factors. The review will help her to decide on a line of action. The following is a list of possible causative factors:

1. Myocardial ischemia or acute myocardial infarction
2. Electrolyte imbalance
3. Drugs
4. Alterations of parasympathetic or sympathetic tone
5. Surgical trauma
6. Acid-base disturbances
7. Stress—an excess of catecholamines (catecholamine-induced stress)
8. Heart failure and/or cardiogenic shock
9. Pericarditis, myocarditis, or bacterial endocarditis

10. The Wolff-Parkinson-White (WPW) syndrome
11. Hypoxia.

Supraventricular Tachyarrhythmias

Supraventricular arrhythmias are arrhythmias that arise above the ventricles; that is, in the sinus, atrial, or AV junctional tissue. Supraventricular ectopic tachyarrhythmias are clinically significant when they:

1. Produce significant symptoms and/or a very rapid rate (more than 180 beats per minute)
2. Result in a symptomatic fall in cardiac output
3. Cause heart failure or aggravate preexisting heart failure
4. Precipitate angina pectoris.

The most serious of those effects is the symptomatic fall in cardiac output. The persistent supraventricular tachyarrhythmias should alert the nurse or physician to look for evidence of heart failure (i.e., pathologic gallops, rales, a rising central venous pressure, and a positive fluid balance). Digitalis intoxication (Chapter 16) should be ruled out when certain supraventricular tachycardias occur; that is, nonparoxysmal AV junctional tachycardia, atrial tachycardia with varying degrees of AV block (so-called PAT with block). Drugs that have a positive chronotropic effect (beta-adrenergic) should also be considered as possible causative agents.

The initial therapy for supraventricular tachyarrhythmias is directed toward decreasing the ventricular rate. The subsequent therapy is directed toward depressing atrial or AV junctional automaticity, with possible conversion to sinus rhythm and correcting the underlying cause, such as heart failure or digitalis intoxication.

Pharmacologic Management of Supraventicular Tachyarrhythmias. The drugs capable of slowing the ventricular rate are the beta-adrenergic blocking drugs, such as propranolol and the parasympathomimetics (the digitalis glycosides). Propranolol and digoxin are synergistic in their effects on delaying AV conduction time. The synergism results in a slower ventricular rate.

Propranolol (Inderal). Propranolol is the only beta-blocker available for clinical use in the United States. Propranolol decreases the heart rate (in a negative chronotropic effect), depresses AV conduction (in a negative dromotropic effect), depresses contractility (in a negative inotropic effect), and depresses atrial and ventricular automaticity.

● *What Nurses Should Know/Do About Propranolol Therapy*

1. Atropine sulfate and isoproterenol should be available for intravenous use to counteract a serious bradycardia.

2. The drugs should be given slowly intravenously, 0.5 mg at 3-minute intervals.

3. Watch the monitor for signs of a therapeutic effect (slowing of the heart rate).

4. Observe the patient for rales, wheezing, and hypotension during administration (because of negative inotropic effects and bronchoconstriction).

5. Propranolol may potentiate the effects of oral hypoglycemic drugs.

6. Special care about the dosage of propranolol should be taken in the presence of renal insufficiency because propranolol is excreted primarily through the kidneys.

Digitalis. The digitalis glycosides slow the ventricular rate in supraventricular tachyarrhythmias by depressing AV conduction. Digoxin, a rapidly acting glycoside, is usually the glycoside of choice because of its rapid onset of action.

The undesirable effects of an excess of digitalis are shown by enhanced automaticity in the atria, AV junctional tissue, and ventricles. As a result, arrhythmias, such as paroxysmal atrial tachycardia with varying AV block, nonparoxysmal AV junctional tachycardias, and ventricular arrhythmias, may occur (Chapter 16). A rule to remember is, almost every type of arrhythmia can be induced by an excess of digitalis.

One's potential for digitalis intoxication is enhanced in the presence of hypokalemia. Since digoxin is primarily excreted through the kidneys, special care in dosage is required in the presence of renal impairment. Anorexia, nausea, and vomiting may be the initial symptoms of digitalis intoxication.

- *What Nurses Should Know/Do About Digitalis Therapy*

1. Observe the patient for the effects of digoxin:
   a. Slowing of the ventricular rate
   b. Development of new tachyarrhythmias
   c. Improvement in heart failure.

2. Determine the serum potassium and BUN levels.

3. Monitor the patient carefully for ectopic arrhythmias (especially in acute myocardial infarction, where the potential for intoxication is enhanced).

4. Observe the patient for symptoms of intoxication—anorexia, nausea, and vomiting.

5. Diphenylhydantoin or lidocaine may be used to manage digitalis-induced tachyarrhythmias.

6. Propranolol is also useful in the digitalis-induced tachyarrhythmias.

7. Digoxin causes vasoconstriction when it is given intravenously as a bolus.

8. Except as a last resort, direct current shock is contraindicated when digitalis intoxication is suspected or diagnosed.

Electrical Management—Cardioversion (See also Chapter 10). Cardioversion, the electrical management of tachyarrhythmias, is often effective in terminating atrial tachycardia, atrial flutter, atrial fibrillation, and ventricular tachycardia.

Cardioversion is the delivery of a synchronized charge to the myocardium. The cardioverter releases a charge synchronous to the QRS deflection. Therefore, a QRS must be present for that type of countershock to work. The equipment needed for cardioversion are a power generator, paddles, and a monitor with an ECG print-out. A good quality ECG should be obtained before cardioversion is attempted, and the machine should be checked for synchronization. The patient should be in the supine position for delivery of the direct current shock.

There is usually a brief period of electrical instability following cardioversion. The following factors enhance electrical instability, and they should be taken into consideration prior to cardioversion:

1. Hypokalemia
2. Hypoxia
3. Digitalization
4. Acid-base imbalance.

Problems in premedication may occur with cardioversion. Commonly, drugs such as diazepam and sodium methohexital are used intravenously. On some occasions, those drugs may cause hypoventilation and respiratory depression.

The nursing measures to prevent postcardioversion respiratory complications include:

1. Watching for hypoventilation
2. Having an airway, oxygen, and ambu at the bedside
3. Removing the patient's dentures, to prevent airway obstruction
4. Encouraging coughing and deep breathing.

Transient arrhythmias may occur immediately after the elective charge is delivered. Cardioversion should be documented by ECG monitoring. Antiarrhythmic drugs should be available. Failure to convert the arrhythmia may be related to hypoxia, acidosis or alkalosis, or drug intoxication. Embolism is a rare complication of cardioversion, especially in patients with chronic atrial fibrillation.

- *What Nurses Should Know/Do About Cardioversion*

1. Explain the procedure to the patient.
2. Connect the patient to a monitor and, with the patient supine, obtain a good quality ECG tracing.
3. Secure a patent intravenous line.

4. Check the cardioverter and the ECG machine for proper grounding and synchronization.

5. Remove the patient's dentures.

6. Have resuscitation equipment (airway, oxygen, ambu, and crashcart) at the patient's bedside.

7. Have available all the commonly used cardiac emergency drugs (e.g., lidocaine, atropine sulfate, epinephrine, and isoproterenol).

8. Check the patient's serum potassium and blood gases levels; find out whether the patient has been taking digitalis.

9. Have premedications available.

10. Charge the machine, apply the conductive paste, and deliver the charge as ordered.

11. Make sure that no one is in contact with the bed or the patient.

12. Monitor the ECG for postcardioversion rhythm.

13. Observe the patient for hypoventilation and initiate respiratory supportive measures as indicated.

14. Observe the patient for any new cardiac arrhythmias, especially during the first hour.

15. Observe the patient for clinical manifestations of thromboembolic phenomena, especially postcardioversion atrial fibrillation.

● *What Nurses Should Know/Do About Supraventricular Tachyarrhythmias*

1. Anticipate the need for digoxin or propranolol.

2. Observe the patient for evidence of heart failure (e.g., gallops, rales, dyspnea, and distended neck veins).

3. Rule out drugs that could cause arrhythmias.

4. If medication is indicated, observe the patient for therapeutic effects (especially with intravenous administration).

5. Reduce the peripheral demands for oxygen by maintaining a calm environment for the patient.

6. Remember that oxygen is often indicated.

Ventricular Arrhythmias

Ventricular arrhythmias may occur as a manifestation of increased automaticity or altered conduction in the ventricles. The ventricular premature contraction (VPC) is the earliest sign of electrical instability in the ventricles. VPCs are easily recognizable, and they are harbingers of the most serious ventricular arrhythmias—ventricular tachycardia and ventricular fibrillation or flutter—and of sudden death.

Ventricular arrhythmias are clinically significant because:

1. They often result in a symptomatic fall in cardiac output.

2. They may result in ventricular fibrillation and even death.

Since only one VPC in the presence of acute myocardial infarction may result in ventricular fibrillation, the treatment of even a few VPCs in acute myocardial infarction is mandatory. VPCs in other clinical conditions may be tolerated without serious consequences.

Ventricular Tachycardia. The term ventricular tachycardia is used when six or more VPCs occur consecutively. The term ventricular group beats is used when three or more VPCs occur consecutively. The rate of ventricular tachycardia is 100 to 180 beats per minute, but it is usually faster than 160 beats per minute. Accelerated idioventricular rhythm (slow ventricular tachycardia or nonparoxysmal ventricular tachycardia) occurs when the sinus rate slows; it is usually initiated by a "late" VPC. The ventricular rate is 60 to 130 beats per minute. The term late VPC refers to the appearance of the contraction late in diastole. Accelerated idioventricular rhythm is usually benign and transient, lasting less than a few minutes, and it is not treated. In general, nonparoxysmal ventricular tachycardia occurs most commonly during the first 24 to 72 hours of acute myocardial infarction. The condition is self limited. Paroxysmal (ordinary) ventricular tachycardia, on the other hand, is a more malignant arrhythmia. It is often initiated by an early VPC (the R–on–T phenomenon). Therapy is directed toward depressing the ectopic ventricular focus through pharmacologic intervention or electrical countershock.

Ventricular Fibrillation. Ventricular fibrillation represents chaotic electrical activity in the ventricles with characteristic ECG features. Mechanical action is likewise disorganized and wholly inadequate, resulting in clinical death. Ventricular fibrillation may appear as rapid, high-amplitude waves or slow, low-amplitude waves. Primary ventricular fibrillation occurs in acute cardiac disease, and it shows rapid high-amplitude waves. That form of ventricular fibrillation is easily terminated. Secondary ventricular fibrillation represents a more chaotic waveform that is slow and low in amplitude and is seen in prolonged anoxic and depressive states of cardiac muscle (prolonged shock and congestive heart failure). In those instances, drugs and cardiopulmonary resuscitation are prerequisites to defibrillation. The prognosis is extremely poor in secondary ventricular fibrillation.

Pharmacologic Management of Ventricular Tachyarrhythmias. The antiarrhythmic drugs are classified as group I or group II drugs, based on their mechanisms of action.

Group I drugs generally have three effects:

1. They depress automaticity (both atrial and ventricular).
2. They depress AV conduction.
3. They depress intraventricular conduction.

Their primary route of excretion is the kidneys. Included in group I drugs are procainamide, quinidine sulfate, propranolol, and disopyramide phosphate.

Group II drugs have two effects:

1. They depress automaticity.

2. They may enhance AV conduction.

Their primary route of excretion is through the liver. Included in group II drugs are lidocaine and diphenylhydantoin. Lidocaine, procainamide, and propranolol are the three most commonly used drugs, and they are easily administered intravenously.

● *What Nurses Should Know/Do About Lidocaine (Xylocaine) Therapy*

1. Anticipate the need for lidocaine in acute ventricular arrhythmias.

2. Lidocaine is usually given intravenously in a bolus of 50 to 100 mg.

3. Observe the patient for hypotension when lidocaine is given intravenously.

4. Signs of central nervous system depression or stimulation can occur with lidocaine intoxication—excitement, twitching, irritability, nervousness, tremor, convulsions, or lethargy.

5. A continuous intravenous infusion of lidocaine is titrated to achieve the therapeutic response. It is best administered with an infusion pump to avoid accidental administration of toxic doses. The usual infusion dosage is 2 to 4 mg/min.

6. Patients with hepatic dysfunction and congestive heart failure may show signs of intoxication at dosages in lower ranges because of decreased metabolism.

● *What Nurses Should Know/Do About Procainamide (Pronestyl) Therapy*

1. Anticipate the need for procainamide when the patient fails to respond to lidocaine.

2. Give the drug slowly intravenously and watch for hypotension (it is a peripheral vasodilator); the usual dosage is a 100-mg bolus every 2 minutes.

3. Watch for QRS widening with intravenous administration (the drug slows intraventricular conduction).

4. *Note:* The cardiac output may decrease because of the drug's depressant effects on contractility.

5. Procainamide may cause gastrointestinal disturbances when it is given orally; it should be given with food or milk.

6. Patient with renal insufficiency should be observed for signs of intoxication because the kidneys are the major route of excretion.

7. A reversible lupus erythematosus–like syndrome manifested by joint pain, pleural effusion, pericardial friction rub, and fever may occur with long-term use (six months or more).

8. Although procainamide is the most commonly used drug (oral) for chronic ventricular arrhythmias or the preventive measure, its major disadvantage is that because of its short half-life, it has to be given every three hours in order to maintain the therapeutic blood level.

Propranolol was discussed on pages 432–433.

Electrical Management—Cardioversion and Defibrillation. Cardioversion is indicated in ventricular tachycardia if the patient loses consciousness or is unresponsive to drugs. Cardioversion is discussed in the section on supraventricular tachyarrhythmias (pp. 432 to 435).

Defibrillation is the delivery of a nonsynchronized high-intensity electrical charge to the myocardium. The charge completely depolarizes the myocardium and thus interrupts ventricular fibrillation.

- *What Nurses Should Know/Do About Ventricular Arrhythmias*
  1. Evaluate the possible causes of the ventricular arrhythmias:
     a. Myocardial ischemia, injury, or infarction
     b. Electrolyte imbalance
     c. Drugs
     d. Increased circulatory catecholamines
     e. Stress
     f. Hypoxia
     g. Acid-base imbalance
     h. Heart failure
     i. Preexisting or underlying bradycardia.
  2. Have a cardioverter (defibrillator), ambu bag, and oxygen available:
     a. Initiate countershock as indicated
     b. Institute measures as indicated to prevent the recurrence of the arrhythmia.
  3. Have an intravenous infusion of lidocaine secured and started.

Bradyarrhythmias

Bradyarrhythmias generally require less oxygen consumption by the myocardium and they are less hazardous than the tachyarrhythmias. However, marked bradyarrhythmias (less than 45 beats per minute) may result in a reduced minute volume and symptoms of poor peripheral perfusion. Bradyarrhythmias may also enhance automaticity, resulting in brady-tachyarrhythmias.

The initial therapy in the management of symptomatic bradycardia is directed toward increasing the ventricular rate. The increase may be accomplished by:

1. Increasing the sinus rate when AV transmission is intact
2. Accelerating AV conduction when AV transmission is impaired

3. Stimulating AV junctional automaticity

4. Stimulating ventricular automaticity.

Pharmacologic Management of the Bradyarrhythmias. Drugs capable of increasing the ventricular rate by one or more of those mechanisms are (1) the parasympathetic (vagal) blocking drugs (e.g., atropine sulfate) and (2) the beta-adrenergic stimulators (e.g., isoproterenol).

Atropine Sulfate. Atropine sulfate, a vagolytic drug, allows sympathetic effects on the heart to dominate. Atropine sulfate thus increases the sinus rate and accelerates AV conduction. It is a rapidly acting drug, easily administered intravenously as a bolus, and is thus frequently the drug of choice in treating a symptomatic bradycardia. Small intravenous increments of atropine sulfate (0.4 to 0.6 mg) allow for more judicious management of the heart rate and less occasion for excessive rate response.

Other undesirable effects of atropine that relate to its parasympathetic-blocking effect are urinary retention, dryness of the mouth, flushing of the face, and dilatation of the pupils. Atropine is contraindicated in the presence of glaucoma because it increases intraocular pressure. However, even in the presence of glaucoma it may be used in emergencies, provided that pilocarpine-type eye drops are promptly used to counteract the effects of atropine. Mental confusion, which has been labeled atropine madness and atropine psychosis, has been attributed to prolonged therapy with atropine. Atropine is primarily excreted through the kidney and thus its effects may be accentuated in the presence of renal insufficiency.

● *What Nurses Should Know/Do About Atropine Sulfate Therapy*

1. Continuous ECG monitoring for rate and rhythm is needed to prevent excessive acceleration of the heart rate.

2. Observe the patient for urinary retention due to atropine.

3. *Note*: Atropine is contraindicated in glaucoma (but in an emergency, the effects of atropine may be counteracted by pilocarpine–type eye drops).

4. With prolonged atropine therapy, observe the patient for changes in sensorium. (A mnemonic for the side effects of atropine: Red as a beet, dry as a bone, and mad as a hare.)

5. *Note:* Children are more susceptible to the effects of atropine than are adults.

6. *Note:* Atropine is most effective in those settings in which the bradycardia (particularly sinus bradycardia) is due to enhanced vagal tone (i.e., vasovagal reactions, acute diaphragmatic myocardial infarction, and digitalis intoxication).

Isoproterenol (Isuprel). Isoproterenol is a beta-adrenergic stimulator, and thus it selectively affects the beta-receptors of the sympathetic nervous system. Beta-receptors are found primarily in the heart and lungs. Isoproterenol increases the heart rate by:

1. Increasing automaticity in the sinus node
2. Accelerating AV conduction
3. Enhancing AV junctional pacemakers
4. Enhancing ventricular pacemakers.

Isoproterenol also stimulates myocardial contractility (in a positive inotropic effect) and causes bronchodilatation and peripheral vascular dilatation. Isoproterenol is administered as an intravenous drip and, ideally, with an infusion pump so that dosages can be carefully regulated. The patient must be carefully observed for therapeutic effects and for signs of overdose, such as atrial or ventricular premature beats and atrial or ventricular tachyarrhythmias. Isoproterenol is indicated as an emergency measure to temporarily increase the heart rate when atropine is ineffective; that is, in block below the AV junctional tissue (Mobitz type II AV block). It may also be used in symptomatic AV nodal block during an acute diaphragmatic myocardial infarction when atropine is ineffective and provided that AV transmission and the heart rate improves. Isoproterenol increases oxygen consumption. But when the drug improves AV conduction and the heart rate, the increase in oxygen consumption is usually more than balanced by the benefits of the improved heart rate and rhythm.

Artificial Pacemaker Therapy for Bradyarrhythmias. Anticipating the need for an artificial pacemaker before an emergency occurs may be lifesaving. The capable nurse is skilled in diagnosing hemiblocks and bundle branch blocks from the ECG and knows the morbidity and mortality in bradyarrhythmias (Chapter 8). The nurse must be familiar with the operation of locally used pacing units so that they can be made to function smoothly in an emergency. (Artificial pacing is described in detail in Chapter 11.)

● *What Nurses Should Know/Do About Bradyarrhythmias*

1. Evaluate the patient's tolerance to the slow heart rate by observing the patient for:
   a. Signs of a critical decrease in cardiac output
   b. Changes in sensorium
   c. Cool or clammy skin
   d. Hypotension
   e. Heart failure
   f. Bradycardia-related ventricular arrhythmias (brady-tachy-arrhythmias).

Note: Raising the patient's legs to augment the venous return and stroke volume may eliminate symptoms during a transient bradycardia. It may be used while the patient is awaiting drug or electrical management.

2. Have atropine, isoproterenol, and an external pacemaker available.
3. Consider the possible causes of bradyarrhythmias:
   a. Drugs or electrolyte imbalance
   b. Enhanced vagal tone due to acute diaphragmatic myocardial infarction, drugs, or vagal stimulating maneuvers
   c. Anterior wall myocardial infarction
   d. Mobitz type II AV block
   e. Bradyarrhythmia due to the sick sinus syndrome (Chapter 9).

CARDIAC EMERGENCIES DUE TO MECHANICAL DYSFUNCTION

Four main factors affect the pumping function of the heart:
1. The peripheral vascular resistance, or the afterload
2. The venous return, or the preload
3. The inotropic or contractile state of the myocardium
4. The cardiac rhythm.

Disturbances in any one of those four factors can result in heart failure.

Congestive heart failure causes symptoms related to:
1. Failure to deliver sufficient blood to the tissue
2. Congestion—the damming of blood in the vessels leading to the heart.

Pulmonary Edema (See also Chapter 1)

The clinical manifestation of acute left ventricular failure is pulmonary edema. When the left ventricle fails, there is an increase in left ventricular filling pressure and volume because of damming of the blood in the ventricles. The rise in pressure and volume is transmitted retrogradely to the left atrium and then back to the pulmonary veins and capillaries.

A rise in pulmonary capillary pressure in excess of 18 mm Hg results in pulmonary edema. Contributory factors may be alterations in the permeability of the pulmonary capillary membrane (acute respiratory distress syndrome), a fall in plasma oncotic pressure, or alteration in interstitial lymphatic flow.

Pulmonary congestion may be manifested by the following symptoms: (1) dyspnea, (2) cough, (3) orthopnea, (4) rales and/or wheezing, and (5) frothy sputum (often it is blood tinged).

The heart rate increases in compensation for the falling stroke volume. Other compensatory symptoms of a falling cardiac output are cool or clammy skin, changes in sensorium, and decreased urinary output.

Therapy for pulmonary edema is directed at decreasing congestion and improving cardiac output.

Pharmacologic Management of Pulmonary Edema. Three drugs are generally used in the management of acute pulmonary edema: (1) morphine, (2) diuretics, and (3) aminophylline. The digitalis glycosides may be used subsequently.

Morphine Sulfate. The drug used initially in the management of pulmonary edema is morphine sulfate. Morphine has four important effects in pulmonary edema: (1) venodilatation, resulting in a reduction of the preload, (2) a decrease in anxiety, (3) a decrease in the rate of respiration, alleviating the severe dyspnea, and (4) a decrease in pulmonary venous pressure.

Diuretics. Rapidly acting diuretics, such as furosemide (Lasix) and ethacrynic acid (Edecrin), are given intravenously. An immediate response to intravenous furosemide is peripheral venous dilatation, resulting in a decrease in the preload.

Aminophylline. Aminophylline is a pulmonary vasodilator and bronchodilator. It also stimulates myocardial contractility and has a mild diuretic effect.

Digitalis. Digitalis is *not* a primary drug for the treatment of acute pulmonary edema, but many patients require digitalization (Chapters 1 and 7).

Additional Measures Used in Managing Acute Left Ventricular Failure. *Rotating Tourniquets.* Decreasing venous return in pulmonary edema may also be effected by the application of tourniquets. The principles of tourniquet application are: (1) apply the tourniquet high in the groin and axilla and reduce only the venous flow, (2) occlude only three limbs at a time, (3) rotate the tourniquets every 10 to 15 minutes, (4) discontinue using the tourniquets one at a time to prevent sudden increases in the venous return, and (5) do not apply the tourniquets if the patient is hypotensive, and discontinue the use of the tourniquets if hypotension occurs during their use.

Oxygen. Oxygen is administered to the patient in pulmonary edema to increase arterial oxygen saturation and to reduce cardiac workload. Intermittent positive pressure breathing (IPPB) may be used to decrease venous return and to enhance ventilation. Alcohol may be used as a defoaming agent to assist in the removal of fluid. A mask may be used in mouth breathers.

Parameters to Be Evaluated Frequently. Evaluation of the lungs and respiratory status is continuously made by (1) observation of the rate and character of respiration, (2) auscultation of the lungs, and (3) analysis of blood gases.

Avoid Suction. Suctioning should be avoided in pulmonary edema, because it may produce bronchospasm and further decrease oxygen transport.

Evaluation of the Efficacy of Treatment. The efficacy of the treatment should be evaluated constantly, and the results should be documented.

● *What Nurses Should Know/Do About Pulmonary Edema*

1. Place the patient in the high Fowler's position (chair rest is ideal).
2. Administer oxygen.
3. Start an intravenous infusion to keep a vein open.
4. Have tourniquets at bedside. Apply them as indicated, but do not apply them if the patient is hypotensive.
5. Anticipate the need for morphine, diuretics, aminophylline, and, possibly, digitalis
   a. With the intravenous administration of morphine, watch for hypotension and respiratory depression.
   b. With the administration of diuretic drugs, record the diuretic response; watch for electrolyte depletion.
   c. With the administration of aminophylline, watch for nausea and vomiting, tachycardia, and ventricular premature contractions.
   d. Have rapidly acting digitalis preparations ready (e.g., digoxin, deslanoside, and ouabain).
6. Have resuscitation equipment at the patient's bedside.
7. Explain any procedures that might frighten the patient (e.g., tourniquets, IPPB, and phlebotomy) and stay with him to decrease his anxiety.
8. Examine the patient's lungs and heart every two to five minutes until his condition stabilizes.
9. Monitor the patient's blood pressure, level of consciousness, skin color, and temperature for signs of decreased cardiac output.
10. If central venous pressure lines or a Swan-Ganz catheter is in place, monitor pressure changes to determine the effectiveness of drug therapy.
11. Avoid tracheal suctioning; it may induce bronchospasm.

Shock (See also Chapter 3)

Shock is a hypotensive state accompanied by clinical signs of poor peripheral perfusion; that is, cold or clammy skin, poor mentation, and reduced urinary output.

Hypovolemia, the most frequent cause of shock, is due to a reduction in circulatory volume per se or to a decrease in the effective circulating volume. A decrease in the effective circulating volume can result from (1) sequestration of fluid in one or more of the vascular compartments in which there has been an alteration in venous, capillary, or arterial tone or (2) shifting of fluid into interstitial tissues.

Marked tachyarrhythmias or bradyarrhythmias that result in a significant reduction in cardiac output will produce shock. The hypotension is a direct consequence of a critically reduced minute volume (the quantity of blood ejected by the heart each minute).

Cardiogenic shock has all the clinical manifestations of shock, but it is due to extensive myocardial damage with a serious impairment in contractility that causes a low cardiac output. During shock, the reduced peripheral perfusion creates tissue hypoxia and forces anaerobic metabolism and lactic acidosis.

Constant monitoring of circulatory volume and fluid balance is of paramount importance in all forms of shock so that an adequate fluid volume is maintained in the vascular space. Shifts of volume occur within the vascular space as a result of the compensatory responses to hypoxia and hypotension. Depending on the integrity of the vascular bed, there are various degrees of vascular constriction and dilatation in the organ systems. Blood flow is distributed in such a way that nonvital areas receive less blood than do the vital organs—the heart, brain, and kidneys.

Management. Therapy is primarily directed to the cause of shock:

1. In hypovolemic shock, replace the circulatory volume.

2. In arrhythmic shock, change the rate or rhythm to improve cardiac output and to provide an adequate minute volume.

3. In cardiogenic shock, improve the relationship between oxygen supply and demand to ischemic and injured myocardium by (1) reducing cardiac work, and (2) improving coronary perfusion by augmenting diastolic volume and pressure (the time when the coronaries are perfused), using vasoactive drugs or mechanical cardiac support.

The selection of the appropriate intravenous fluid for volume challenge is based on the hemoglobin and hematocrit values, the oncotic pressure, the state of the myocardium, and the pulmonary artery wedge pressures. The nurse's job in fluid challenge management is the careful hemodynamic monitoring of the patient with regard to those parameters. Before manipulating fluid administration, it is important to find out from the attending physician what the target pressure is.

The initial goal in managing cardiogenic shock is lessening the discrepancy between myocardial oxygen supply and demand. Therapy is directed toward (1) minimizing the demands for myocardial oxygen consumption and (2) improving coronary blood supply.

The demands for myocardial oxygen consumption are minimized by:

1. Controlling the heart rate and rhythm
2. Decreasing the preload (ventricular filling pressure)
3. Decreasing the afterload by the use of vasodilators
4. Taking general ambient measures to lower tissue demands and thus

reduce cardiac work; that is, making the patient comfortable and creating a calm, reassuring surrounding.

Myocardial oxygen demands may be decreased by vasodilator therapy, which decreases the preload and afterload. Coronary blood supply may be improved by vasoconstrictor drugs and by surgical revascularization. The intra-aortic balloon pump will decrease demands, increase cardiac output, and improve coronary blood supply.

Sodium Nitroprusside (Nipride). Sodium nitroprusside is commonly used to reduce myocardial oxygen demands. The drug acts directly on the blood vessels to produce vasodilatation. It affects both arteries and veins and thus is able to reduce both the preload and afterload. It is a better vasodilator than the other antihypertensive drugs because it does not significantly affect the heart rate and because it does not alter the sensorium. Patients receiving sodium nitroprusside should have an arterial line and a Swan-Ganz catheter in place. The drug should be administered by an infusion pump, with meticulous monitoring of the left atrial and systemic arterial pressures. Before starting the drug, the nurse must find out from the physician what the target pulmonary artery wedge pressure and the systemic arterial pressure are. Because sodium nitroprusside deteriorates rapidly when it is exposed to light, the intravenous bottle and the tubing should be wrapped in foil. And because of the rapid deterioration, sodium nitroprusside that is four or more hours old must be discarded.

In the body, sodium nitroprusside is converted to thiocyanide. Thiocyanate levels should be determined if the patient has taken sodium nitroprusside for more than 24 hours. Cyanide poisoning causes depression of cellular respiration and results in confusion and psychosis. Cyanide poisoning antidote kits should be at hand when sodium nitroprusside is used.

● *What Nurses Should Know/Do About Sodium Nitroprusside Therapy*

1. For initiating therapy with sodium nitroprusside, an arterial line and a Swan-Ganz catheter should be in place.

2. Wrap the bottle and tubing to protect the drug from light, and indicate the time the solution was prepared; the unused portion must be discarded in four hours. Administer the drug with an infusion pump; do not add other medications to the intravenous solution containing sodium nitroprusside.

3. Before starting therapy, find out from the physician what the target wedge, systolic, and diastolic pressures are.

4. Titrate the intravenous infusion to achieve a therapeutic response. A nurse should be in constant attendance to maintain the target pressures.

5. If the wedge or arterial pressure falls below the determined critical levels, immediately slow down or discontinue the sodium nitroprusside infusion.

6. Thiocyanate levels should be determined if the patient has been taking sodium nitroprusside for more than 24 hours. If the serum levels exceed 12 mg/100 ml, sodium nitroprusside should be discontinued to avoid intoxication, which is manifested by deterioration of the patient's condition (a decreased pH and oxygen tension), psychosis, and confusion.

Dopamine (Intropin). Dopamine is a sympathomimetic drug that has alpha-, beta-, and gamma-adrenergic properties. Dopamine can selectively increase myocardial contractility without increasing the heart rate or inducing any ectopic arrhythmia. Thus the effects of dopamine on myocardial oxygen consumption are much less than those of isoproterenol. At low to moderate doses, dopamine is uniquely able to selectively produce vasoconstriction in some vessels and vasodilatation in others. At low dosage, dopamine produces vasodilatation in the renal, mesenteric, coronary, and cerebral beds.

● *What Nurses Should Know/Do About Dopamine Therapy*

1. Find out from the physician the target blood and wedge pressures.

2. Find out from the physician the dosage in mcg/min. Therapeutic effects are most evident at low to moderate dosages.

3. Administer dopamine via an infusion pump; do not mix it with other medications.

4. Monitor the patient's blood pressure and urinary output during infusion.

Norepinephrine (Levophed). Norepinephrine may be used to support arterial pressure and thus improve coronary blood flow. Norepinephrine causes vasoconstriction of the blood vessels (in an alpha-adrenergic effect) and produces a slight positive inotropic effect (in a beta-adrenergic effect). By enhancing afterload and stimulating contractility, norepinephrine may increase oxygen consumption. However, if therapeutic blood pressure levels are attained, the benefits derived from improved coronary perfusion outweigh the slight increase in oxygen consumption.

● *What Nurses Should Know/Do About Norepinephrine Therapy*

1. Find out from the physician the end point of therapy.

2. Administer epinephrine with an infusion pump, via an Intracath.

3. Monitor the patient's blood pressure and cardiac status.

4. Avoid infiltration into subcutaneous tissue; norepinephrine can cause severe tissue sloughing.

Note: The antidote for norepinephrine that infiltrates the tissue is phentolamine (Regitine) injected into the tissues involved.

5. Patients receiving norepinephrine often have cold or clammy skin because of the drug's vasoconstriction effects.

- *What Nurses Should Know/Do About Shock*

1. Place the patient flat (to maximize the blood flow to the cerebrum).
2. Maintain oxygen therapy.
3. Have resuscitation equipment at the bedside.
4. Swan-Ganz catheters and arterial lines are needed for sodium nitroprusside and dopamine therapy.
5. Evaluate and treat the underlying causes:
   a. Correct cardiac arrhythmias
   b. Fluid discharge for hypovolemia
   c. Elevate the patient's legs to increase venous return, and observe the patient's response.
   d. Check the central venous, pulmonary artery, and wedge pressures to determine whether they are low or low normal.
   e. Rule out vasoactive mechanisms as the cause of shock; determine whether the shock is drug related (morphine, nitroglycerin, meperidine hydrochloride), is a vasovagal reaction or is caused by infection (sepsis).
6. Evaluate the patient's lung status:
   a. Examine the patient for rales
   b. Investigate whether shock is due to depressed oxygen and carbon dioxide transport at lung level.
7. Evaluate the patient's tissue metabolism:
   a. Analyze the blood gases. Is metabolic acidosis present, or is there a respiratory component?
   b. Evaluate the rate and character of respirations. Are Kussmaul's respirations present?
   c. Watch for signs of deterioration in tissue perfusion.
   d. Evaluate the effectiveness of drugs.
8. Evaluate the patient's renal perfusion status:
   a. Is the patient uremic and/or oliguric?
   b. Is the urine concentrated in appearance (is there volume depletion)?
   c. Observe the urine output closely (every hour) and correlate it with the intravenous therapy and oral intakes.
9. If shock is determined to be cardiogenic:
   a. Reduce the myocardial oxygen demand
   b. Treat fever if present
   c. Maintain the patient's heart in optimal contractile state by correcting acid-base electrolyte imbalances and by checking the

central venous, pulmonary artery, and wedge pressures and the cardiac output.
d. Support the patient with drugs as ordered.
10. Monitor the cardiac and vascular effects of drug therapy (e.g., sodium nitroprusside, dopamine, norepinephrine, and furosemide). Observe the patient closely and correlate his signs and symptoms with his:
a. Arterial pressure
b. Wedge pressure
c. Central venous pressure
d. Cardiac rhythm
e. Fluid intake and urinary output.

CARDIAC TAMPONADE (See also Chapter 14)

Cardiac tamponade results when an increase in intrapericardial pressure due to fluid accumulation results in an impairment of the diastolic filling of the heart. The ability of the pericardium to accommodate or comply with the increase in fluid volume depends on the length of time over which the fluid accumulates. The pericardium, if stretched over a period of days or weeks, may accommodate a liter or more. However, if an increase in contents occurs suddenly, as little as 100 to 200 cc may cause mechanical embarrassment and produce severe symptoms.

Tamponade can be readily recognized and even prevented if the possibility of its occurrence is considered in certain clinical states. Infection, inflammation, trauma, acute myocardial infarction, or neoplasm of the heart may cause tamponade. A complete list of causative factors is given in Chapter 14.

Signs and Symptoms

Cardiac tamponade is characterized by the following signs and symptoms: (1) a rising venous pressure, (2) a falling blood pressure and cardiac output—narrowing pulse pressure, (3) pulsus paradoxus, (4) distant heart sounds, (5) dyspnea, (6) electrical alternans and/or diminished voltage of the QRS complexes on the ECG, and (7) tachycardia. Those manifestations correlate with the pathophysiologic aspects of tamponade.

Elevation of the venous pressure and distention of the neck veins result from impedance to right ventricular diastolic filling. A greater increase in neck vein distention occurs on inspiration. The fall in arterial pressure and cardiac output is a manifestation of decreasing left ventricular stroke volume. Pulsus paradoxus is defined as a greater than normal inspiratory decline in systolic arterial pressure (8 to 10 mm Hg is considered the upper limits of normal). That definition was first used by Kussmaul (in 1873) to describe the marked diminution of the peripheral pulse volume on inspiration in patients with tamponade.

The exaggerated fall in arterial pressure on inspiration can be measured by an arterial pressure monitor; or it can be detected by palpating the peripheral pulse; or it can be heard with the use of a brachial sphygmomanometer.

The low voltage of the QRS complexes due to cardiac tamponade represents decreased transmission of electrical activity through the pericardial effusion.

Management

Therapy for cardiac tamponade is directed toward decreasing the intrapericardial pressure. Pericardiocentesis and surgical drainage are the usual modes of therapy. The technique used in pericardiocentesis is described in Chapter 14. A large-bore needle and/or catheter is used so that pus or blood can be readily evacuated. Preparation by skin anesthesia is desirable if time permits. The needle should be connected by an alligator clamp to the chest lead of an ECG apparatus to permit monitoring of the course of the needle. The S–T segment elevation (seen in subepicardial injury) appears if the needle comes in contact with the ventricle. Emergency equipment should be at the patient's bedside during the procedure, and an intravenous line should be kept running. If no fluid is aspirated during attempted pericardiocentesis and if the diagnosis of effusion is reasonably certain, a pericardiotomy is indicated.

● *What Nurses Should Know/Do About Cardiac Tamponade*

1. Be aware of the settings in which tamponade could occur; that is, chest trauma, pericarditis, postcardiac surgery, and acute myocardial infarction.

2. Monitor the venous pressure of the patient suspected of having tamponade:
   a. Check the central venous pressure
   b. Check for neck vein distention and rate increases on inspiration
   c. Watch for narrowing pulse pressure
   d. Rule out other causes of an increasing venous pressure.

3. Examine the patient for pulsus paradoxus:
   a. Palpate the peripheral pulse and note if there is a diminution on inspiration.
   b. Obtain the systolic brachial blood pressure reading with a sphygmomanometer. Deflate the cuff on expiration; after noting the peak systolic pressure, slowly deflate the cuff until inspiration and note the difference in systolic peak pressure between

expiration and inspiration. A fall greater than 15 mm Hg is a sign of possible tamponade.

   c. Watch for narrowing of the pulse pressure.

   d. If the patient has an arterial line in place, note from the pulse wave patterns whether there is marked fall on inspiration.

4. Auscultate the chest frequently for heart sounds:

   a. Establish a baseline for the patient's normal heart sounds.

   b. Note if the heart sounds become distant.

   c. Listen for pericardial friction rubs; alert the physician if you hear any. (*Note:* If friction rubs are present, anticoagulation therapy should be discontinued.)

5. Examine the patient for increased cardiac dullness by percussing his chest wall.

6. Look for electrical alternans.

7. Note the heart rate and rhythm change.

8. Look for signs of decreased cardiac output:

   a. Cool or clammy skin

   b. Sensorium changes

   c. Decreased urinary output

   d. Acceleration of the heart rate.

9. Note the character of respiration—look for dyspnea, orthopnea, and a changing respiratory rate.

10. Make sure an intravenous route is available.

11. Have emergency equipment available.

● *What Nurses Should Know/Do About Pericardiocentesis*

1. Explain the procedure to the patient and stay with the patient during the procedure.

2. Have a crashcart and defibrillator at the patient's bedside.

3. Start a slow intravenous infusion.

4. Connect the patient to a monitor (a dual-channel monitor or a monitor and an ECG machine should be used).

5. Have a pericardiocentesis tray available (if one is not available, a large-bore needle or an Intracath may be used). Lidocaine and a syringe for local skin infiltration should also be available.

6. Connect the alligator clamp to the chest lead of the electrode cable and to the needle.

7. Monitor simultaneously for cardiac rhythm and needle position.

8. Have culture bottles available.

HYPERTENSIVE CRISIS (See also Chapter 15)

Acute hypertensive crisis is a life-threatening emergency characterized by a marked elevation in arterial pressure with diastolic levels above 140 mm Hg. It is manifested by acute encephalopathy and acute left ventricular failure.

Most hypertensive crises develop in patients who are known to be hypertensive. The usual history is of a patient who has neglected or discontinued treatment for hypertension. The hypertensive crisis can usually be avoided by educating the patient about the need to adhere to his diet and to long-term drug management.

Acute hypertensive encephalopathy is accompanied by a severe headache, a decreasing level of consciousness, blurred vision, or other visual disturbances. Nausea, vomiting, or focal neurologic sensory or motor disturbances may be the presenting signs. Funduscopic examinations frequently reveal exudates, papilledema, and hemorrhage. Those findings are manifestations of cerebral edema and increased intracranial pressure. The treatment of pulmonary edema in such a setting is similar to the usual drug regimen for pulmonary edema plus antihypertensive drugs.

The primary therapy for an acute hypertensive crisis is directed toward decreasing the arterial pressure with acute antihypertensive drugs and decreasing the cerebral edema with diuretics. Care must be taken to avoid precipitous drops in blood pressure, which may compromise the cerebral, coronary, and renal blood flows.

Pharmacologic Management

The primary nursing responsibility is the monitoring of the patient's response to therapy. The monitoring is done by:

1. Checking the blood pressure every 5 to 15 minutes (as drug therapy indicates)

2. Monitoring the heart rate and rhythm

3. Monitoring the neurologic states—level of consciousness, pupil responsiveness, general movement, and focal neurologic signs

4. Monitoring the renal status, measuring the intake and output and the BUN and creatinine levels.

Direct Vasodilators. *Diazoxide (Hyperstat).* Sodium nitroprusside and hydralazine are rapid vasodilators. Diazoxide, a potent antihypertensive drug, is given as a rapidly acting intravenous bolus to dilate the arterioles. It is given in that way because it binds with serum proteins, which inactivate the drug. Renal blood flow remains stable, and the heart rate and cardiac output increase reflexly. Sodium retention may occur with continued therapy with diazoxide and necessitates the use of diuretics. Hyperglycemia may also occur with diazoxide, just as it does with other thiazide drugs.

Sodium Nitroprusside. Sodium nitroprusside causes direct vasodilatation. It is administered in an intravenous infusion and titrated to achieve the decreased pressure. The drug may be especially helpful in acute left ventricular failure because of its effects on reducing the preload.

Hydralazine (Apresoline). Hydralazine is a direct vasodilator, and, like diazoxide, it increases the heart rate and cardiac output. Hydralazine is usually given intravenously slowly over a five-minute period. A continuous intravenous infusion may be given subsequently. The drug usually begins to act in 15 to 20 minutes. Hydralazine has been reported to have unpredictable effects on encephalopathy in some patients.

The Ganglionic Blockers (Sympathetic Blockers). The ganglionic blocking drugs produce their effects by blocking the transmission of impulses at autonomic ganglia. By that mechanism, they block the effects of both sympathetic and parasympathetic nerves. The inhibition of sympathetic signals produces vasodilatation and thereby decreases blood pressure.

Antihypertensive drugs classified as ganglionic blockers or sympathetic blockers include: trimethaphan (Arfonad) and pentolinium (Ansolysen). To enhance the effects of those drugs, it is recommended that the head of the patient's bed be elevated on shock blocks 10 to 12 inches—so that.the patient will maintain a more upright posture.

Because the ganglionic blockers produce parasympathetic as well as sympathetic blockage, complications, such as urinary retention, paralytic ileus, and dilatation of the pupil, occur if therapy is continued. Inactivation of pupillary reflexes interferes with the evaluation of the patient's neurologic status. Reduction in the glomerular filtration rate may also be seen with the ganglionic blockers.

Catecholamine Depleters. For practical purposes, drugs that deplete the stores of norepinephrine and epinephrine (catecholamines) at the nerve terminals or that deplete the level of circulating catecholamines may be considered as sympathetic blockers. That is so because the catecholamines are the chemical transmitters of the sympathetic nervous system.

The drugs classified as catecholamine depleters are reserpine and methyldopa.

Reserpine (Serpasil). Reserpine acts by depleting the stores of norepinephrine and epinephrine at the nerve terminals in the central nervous system. It begins to act 1 to 2 hours after administration.

Methyldopa (Aldomet). Methyldopa depletes the stores of catecholamines by replacing them with a false transmitter in both the peripheral and central nervous systems. Like reserpine, methyldopa has a gradual onset of action (4 to 6 hours), and it may cause somnolence secondary to central nervous system depression. Therefore, it is generally not used in crisis therapy as the initial drug.

Alpha-Adrenergic Blockers. *Phentolamine (Regitine).* Another drug used specifically to manage hypertensive crisis associated with increased levels of catecholamines is phentolamine. Phentolamine blocks the alpha receptors of the sympathetic nervous system, which are found primarily in the blood vessels, and thus produces vasodilatation. Phentolamine is used in patients with pheochromocytoma and crisis associated with monoamine oxidase (MAO) inhibition. For more information regarding those two disorders, see Chapter 15.

Diuretics. Furosemide and ethacrynic acid, rapidly acting diuretics, are administered intravenously in a hypertensive crisis. They are used to enhance the antihypertensive action of the drugs already discussed. Furosemide can produce transient peripheral venous dilatation when infused rapidly as a bolus.

● *What Nurses Should Know/Do About Hypertensive Crisis*

1. Administer oxygen.

2. Place the patient in the reverse Trendelenburg's position, if possible, to minimize cerebral pressure and to maximize the effects of drugs, especially the ganglionic blockers.

3. Intravenous infusion and infusion pump—have an arterial line available.

4. Have the crashcart and other emergency equipment at the patient's bedside.

5. Anticipate the need for rapidly acting antihypertensive drugs:
   a. Diazoxide and hydralazine—for patients without primary cardiac involvement
   b. Sodium nitroprusside and trimethaphan—for patients with left ventricular failure or other types of comprised cardiac function
   c. Phentolamine and sodium nitroprusside—for patients with pheochromocytoma or crisis associated with MAO inhibition.

6. Know the physician's criteria for a therapeutic response:
   a. The target systolic and diastolic pressures
   b. The amount of time allotted to reach the goal (*Note:* Precipitous drops in blood pressure may compromise the coronary, cerebral, and renal blood flows.)
   c. The maximum infusion rate to titrate.

7. Establish and document baseline data about the patient's:
   a. Neurologic status
   b. Blood pressure
   c. Wedge pressure
   d. Renal status
   e. Urinary output
   f. BUN and creatinine levels.

8. Anticipate the need for rapidly acting diuretics—furosemide and ethacrynic acid:
   a. Monitor the fluid intake and urine output
   b. Monitor the serum electrolytes

9. Keep the peripheral vascular demands for oxygen down by:
   a. Sedating the patient
   b. Maintaining a calm environment to decrease the patient's anxiety
   c. Explaining all frightening procedures
   d. Controlling the traffic into the room.

10. With diazoxide therapy, watch especially for tachycardia, fluid retention, and hyperglycemia.

11. With sodium nitroprusside, protect the drug from light, change the bottle every four hours, and monitor the thiocyanide levels after 24 hours of therapy.

12. With the ganglionic blockers, trimethaphan and pentolinium, watch for urinary retention, paralytic ileus, and inactivation of pupillary reflexes.

13. With reserpine and methyldopa, watch for increasing somnolence.

14. During intravenous therapy with antihypertensive drugs, be in constant attendance and have levarterenol and metaraminol available in case of hypotension.

PULMONARY EMBOLISM AND INFARCTION (See also Chapter 2)

Pulmonary embolism and infarction are apt to occur in people who are bedfast. In most cases, the source of pulmonary embolism is the deep veins of the legs, but there may be no clinical evidence of deep vein thrombosis.

Pulmonary embolism may be manifested clinically by the signs and symptoms of pulmonary infarction or of acute hemodynamic disturbance or both.

The clinical manifestations of pulmonary embolism depend on the size of the artery occluded, the percentage of pulmonary circulation involved, and the previous state of the cardiovascular system.

The symptoms of pulmonary embolism and/or infarction include:
1. Dyspnea and tachypnea when the person is apprehensive
2. Precordial and/or retrosternal chest pain
3. Pleuritic chest pain (with infarction)
4. Cough and hemoptysis (with infarction)
5. Diaphoresis
6. Distended neck veins
7. Fever and leukocytosis (with infarction)
8. S_3 and S_4 gallop
9. ECG manifestations of cor pulmonale (e.g., right axis deviation, P pulmonale, S_1, Q_3 pattern, inverted T waves in leads II, III, and aVF, and/or inverted T waves in leads V_{1-3}, acute right bundle branch block, and acute atrial tachyarrhythmias)

10. Increased cardiac dullness
11. Signs of decreased cardiac output:
    a. Cool or clammy skin
    b. Fall in blood pressure
    c. Tachycardia (most commonly marked sinus tachycardia).
12. Wide and fixed splitting of the second heart sounds with a loud pulmonic component
13. Pulmonary rales.

When pulmonary embolism occurs, blood flow to the area distal to the occlusion is obstructed. If a large area of tissue is not being perfused, the oxygen tension in the arterial blood falls significantly. The patient develops dyspnea and then tachypnea in an effort to compensate for the underperfusion. Left ventricular output falls concomitantly, contributing to the increased respiratory drive. Chest pain occurs as a result of ischemia to the lung tissue and as a result of pulmonary infarction with pleural rub. Hemoptysis results from hemorrhagic necrosis of the lung tissue distal to the obstruction. Distention of the neck veins is due to increased pressure in the right heart, which represents a retrograde build-up of the elevated pulmonary artery pressure. A symptomatic fall in cardiac output may result in syncope. Syncope occurs when the embolic obstruction is significant enough to reduce left atrial and left ventricular filling and the reflex tachycardia and peripheral vascular constriction cannot support cardiac output. The pulmonary component of the second heart sounds is loud, and there is wide and fixed splitting of the second heart sounds because right ventricular ejection time is prolonged against a high pulmonary artery pressure.

Therapy for pulmonary embolism is primarily medical. The main therapeutic intervention is the administration of anticoagulants (heparin and warfarin). Thrombolytic drugs, such as urokinase and streptokinase, may also be used.

● *What Nurses Should Know/Do About Pulmonary Embolism and Infarction*

1. Anticipate and look for the signs and symptoms of pulmonary emboli in patients who may be at risk:
    a. Patients after surgery
    b. Patients with leg injuries
    c. Patients who are postpartum
    d. Patients taking contraceptive drugs
    e. Patients with chronic peripheral vascular disease
    f. Patients with chronic congestive heart failure
    g. Patients with cardiovascular disease
    h. Patients with a history of thromboembolic phenomena
    i. Patients who are obese.

(*Note:* The only presenting symptoms may be dyspnea, pain, tachycardia, and loud pulmonic component of the second heart sounds with wide splitting.)

2. Use anti-embolic stockings and foot and leg exercise for patients at risk.

3. Administer oxygen when pulmonary embolism and/or infarction are suspected.

4. Place the patient in Fowler's position when embolization is suspected.

5. Anticipate the use of heparin. Investigate the patient's clotting times (the prothrombin time and the Lee-White clotting time), explain the need for the tests to the patient.

6. Perform serial blood gases analyses to monitor the effectiveness of therapy.

7. Monitor the patient's vital signs closely.

8. Ease the patient's anxiety.

9. Explain the diagnostic procedures to patient (e.g., lung scan, and angiography)

CARDIOPULMONARY RESUSCITATION (See also Chapter 12)

● *What Nurses Should Know/Do About Cardiopulmonary Resuscitation (CPR)*

The nurse has a primary role in CPR. Her ability to perform CPR according to the established guidelines give the patient the best chances for survival. The American Heart Association has established CPR certification programs at both the basic and the instructor levels. It is recommended that all nurses be certified at one of those levels to establish the highest standard of care.

Other nursing responsibilities in cardiac arrest are related to the preparation and administration of drugs. The nurse who understands the mechanism of action and potential hazards of drugs commonly used in cardiac arrest can act appropriately when a crisis occurs.

Drug Therapy

The five most commonly used drugs in a cardiac arrest are (1) epinephrine, (2) sodium bicarbonate, (3) calcium, (4) atropine, and (5) lidocaine. The nursing aspects of atropine and lidocaine were discussed in the section on arrhythmias (pp. 437–440). Sodium bicarbonate, epinephrine, and calcium are discussed in the following paragraphs.

Sodium Bicarbonate. Sodium bicarbonate, a naturally occurring buffer in the body, is used to correct metabolic acidosis in cardiac emergencies.

A normal pH improves the response of the myocardium to resuscitative measures. Analyses of arterial blood gases should be made after every two ampules of sodium bicarbonate are given in order to prevent an overdose. It is worth noting that sodium bicarbonate may increase the osmolarity of the serum and result in cellular dehydration.

Epinephrine. Epinephrine is one of the chemical mediators of the sympathetic nervous system. It has both alpha- and beta-adrenergic effects. Epinephrine stimulates the heart; it causes pulmonary vasodilatation and peripheral vasoconstriction. Its use during cardiac arrest can help change the slow and low-amplitude fibrillatory waves to more rapid and higher-amplitude deflections, which are generally more responsive to electrical defibrillation.

The usual dose of epinephrine is 0.5 cc of a 1:1000 solution or 5 cc of a 1:10,000 solution by the intravenous route. It is also given in an intracardiac injection by trained personnel. Since epinephrine can be rapidly absorbed in the lungs, it may be given with an endotracheal tube as an alternative route in an emergency.

Calcium. Calcium is less commonly used in CPR. It stabilizes the permeability of the cell to sodium and potassium and thus affects electrical activity. It is also a direct stimulant to muscle contractility. An excess of calcium results in cardiac standstill in systole (rigor). The mechanism of action of calcium is similar to those of the digitalis glycosides. Calcium is sometimes used in cardiac arrest to enhance the susceptibility of the heart to defibrillation. Calcium preparations are administered intravenously slowly and may produce sloughing of tissues if intravenous fluid infiltrates. Calcium precipitates if it is mixed with sodium bicarbonate. It is important to remember that calcium and digitalis produce a synergistic action.

SUMMARY

1. The role of the nurse in cardiac emergencies has become a vital one with the advent of intensive care units. Since cardiac emergencies may take place anywhere in the hospital, all nursing personnel should be required to have a working knowledge of cardiac emergencies.

2. In this chapter, cardiac emergencies have been discussed with emphasis on pathophysiology and pharmacology in order to provide a better understanding of diagnosis and management.

3. The cardiac emergencies have been divided into two broad categories: those resulting from electrical dysfunction and those resulting from mechanical dysfunction.

4. Tachyarrhythmias and bradyarrhythmias have been discussed with electrical dysfunction, whereas pulmonary edema, shock, cardiac tam-

ponade, hypertensive crisis, and pulmonary emboli have been discussed with mechanical dysfunction.

5. Arrhythmias are considered to result from disturbances in automaticity and/or conduction. The possible causes must be reviewed when a patient presents with an arrhythmia.

6. Ventricular arrhythmias generally have greater clinical significance because of their frequency and the fact that they may precipitate ventricular fibrillation, as well as because a symptomatic fall in cardiac output often accompanies those arrhythmias.

7. The symptoms and the pathophysiologic aspects of pulmonary edema as a manifestation of acute left ventricular failure have been discussed. Therapy is directed toward acutely decreasing the preload and cardiac work and thus indirectly improving the cardiac output. Thus the acute management of pulmonary edema includes the use of morphine, diuretics, sublingual nitroglycerin, and in certain instances aminophylline, whereas digitalis may be used in the later management.

8. Shock is defined as a hypotensive state accompanied by signs of poor peripheral perfusion. Hypovolemic, arrhythmogenic, and cardiogenic shock have been discussed with emphasis on the collaboration of the nurse and physician in monitoring the patient's hemodynamic status and fluid balance, minimizing the myocardial oxygen demands, and carrying out vasoactive drug therapy.

9. The presence of cardiac tamponade has to be considered whenever there is infection, inflammation, trauma, acute myocardial infarction, or neoplasm of the heart. Nursing considerations for the early detection of tamponade have been discussed.

10. Hypertensive crisis is characterized by an acute and marked elevation in the arterial pressure with manifestation of acute encephalopathy or acute left ventricular failure. The primary therapy is directed toward decreasing the arterial pressure with antihypertensive drugs and decreasing the cerebral edema with diuretics. Care must be taken to avoid precipitous drops in blood pressure, which may compromise cerebral, coronary, and renal blood flow.

SUGGESTED READINGS

1. AMA Committee on Hypertension. The treatment of malignant hypertension and hypertensive emergencies. J.A.M.A. 228:1673, 1974.
2. Bell, W.R.: Reaching the correct diagnosis of pulmonary thromboembolism. Geriatrics 30:49, 1975.
3. Burrel, Z.L., and Burrell, L.O.: Critical Care. St. Louis, Mosby, 1977.
4. Cosio, F.G., Martinez, J.P., Concepcion, M., Carlos, S., et al.: Abnormal septal motion in cardiac tamponade with pulsus paradoxus. Chest 71:787, 1977.
5. Conn, H.F.: Current Therapy. Philadelphia, Saunders, 1977.
6. Dhar, S.K., and Freeman, P.: Clinical management of hypertensive emergencies. Heart Lung 5:571, 1976.

7. Frater, R.W.: Postoperative care in the pediatric cardiac patient. Heart Lung 3:903, 1974.
8. Gifford, R.W.: Managing hypertension. Postgrad. Med. 61:153, 1977.
9. Gulhoed, G.W.: Blunt and penetrating chest trauma. Fam. Physician 17:100, 1978.
10. Goodman, L.S., and Gilman, A.: The Pharmacologic Basis of Therapeutics. New York, Macmillan, 1975.
11. Harken, D.W.: Postoperative care following heart-valve surgery. Heart Lung 3:893, 1974.
12. Holt, J.P.: The normal pericardium. Am. J. Cardiol. 26:455, 1970.
13. Hurst, J.W., Logue, B., and Wenger, N.K.: The Heart. New York, McGraw-Hill, 1974.
14. Sawaya, M.P.: Hemorrhagic cardiac tamponade complicating the post-myocardial infarction syndrome in the absence of anti-coagulation. Heart Lung 4:770, 1975.
15. Scroder, J., and Daily, E.: Techniques in Bedside Hemodynamic Monitoring. St. Louis, Mosby, 1976.
16. Shabetai, R., Fowler, N.O., and Guntheroth, W.G.: The hemodynamics of cardiac tamponade and constrictive pericarditis. Am. J. Cardiol. 26:480, 1970.
17. Sharma, G.V.R.K., Sashara, A.A., and McKintyre, K.M.: Pulmonary Embolism: The Great Imitator. Disease-a-Month, 22:4, 1976.
18. Skillman, J.J.: Intensive Care. Boston, Little, Brown, 1975.
19. Sodeman, W.A., Jr., and Sodeman, W.A.: Pathologic Physiology: Mechanisms of Disease. Philadelphia, Saunders, 1974.
20. Spodick, D.H.: Medical history of the pericardium. The hairy heart of hoary heroes. Am. J. Cardiol. 26:447, 1970.
21. Vinsant, M., Spence, M., and Hagen, D.: A Commonsense Approach to Coronary Care, ed. 2. St. Louis, Mosby, 1975.
22. Wagner, H.R.: Paradoxical pulse: 100 years later. Am. J. Cardiol. 32:91, 1973.

INDEX

Page numbers in *italics* refer to illustrations.
Page numbers followed by t refer to tables.

461